2nd edition

genetics

National Medical Series

In the basic sciences

anatomy, 2nd editon
the behavioral sciences in
   psychiatry, 3rd edition
biochemistry, 3rd edition
clinical edpidemiology and
   biostatistics
genetics, 2nd edition
hematology
histology and cell biology,
   2nd edition

human developmental anatomy
immunology, 3rd edition
introduction to clinical medicine
microbiology, 2nd edition
neuroanatomy
pathology, 3rd edition
pharmacology, 4th edition
physiology, 3rd edition
radiographic anatomy

In the clinical sciences

medicine, 2nd edition
obstetrics and gynecology,
   3rd edition
pediatrics, 3rd edition
preventive medicine and
   public health, 2nd edition
psychiatry, 3rd editon
surgery, 3rd edition

In the exam series

review for USMLE Step 1,
   3rd edition
review for USMLE Step 2
geriatrics

The National Medical Series for Independent Study

2nd edition
genetics

J. M. Friedman, M.D., Ph.D.

Professor and Head, Department of Medical Genetics
University of British Columbia
Vancouver, Canada

Fred J. Dill, Ph.D.
Associate Professor, Department of Medical Genetics
University of British Columbia
Vancouver, Canada

Michael R. Hayden, M.B., Ch.B., Ph.D.
Professor, Department of Medical Genetics
Director, Centre for Molecular Medicine and Therapeutics
University of British Columbia
Vancouver, Canada

Barbara C. McGillivray, M.D.
Professor, Department of Medical Genetics
University of British Columbia
Vancouver, Canada

Williams & Wilkins
A WAVERLY COMPANY

BALTIMORE • PHILADELPHIA • LONDON • PARIS • BANGKOK
BUENOS AIRES • HONG KONG • MUNICH • SYDNEY • TOKYO • WROCLAW

Editor: Elizabeth A. Nieginski
Managing Editor: Amy G. Dinkel
Development Editors: Donna Siegfried, Rebecca Krumm
Production Coordinator: Danielle Santucci
Designer: Karen Klinedinst
Typesetter: Maryland Composition
Printer: Port City Press
Binder: Port City Press

351 West Camden Street
Baltimore, Maryland 21201-2436 USA

Rose Tree Corporate Center
1400 North Providence Road
Building II, Suite 5025
Media, Pennsylvania 19063-2043 USA

Printed in the United States of America

Library of Congress Cataloging in Publication Data

Genetics / Jan M. Friedman . . . [et al.].—2nd ed.
   p. cm.—(National medical series for independent study)
Includes index.
ISBN 0-683-06217-4
1. Medical genetics. I. Friedman, J. M. (Jan Marshall), 1947–
II. Series.
   [DNLM: 1. Genetics, Medical—outlines. 2. Genetics, Medical—
examination questions.   QZ 18.2 G327 1995]
RB155.G3874 1995
616′.042′076—dc20
DNLM/DLC
for Library of Congress   95-33364
                                           CIP

                                         96 97 98 99
                          1 2 3 4 5 6 7 8 9 10

Reprints on chapters may be purchased from Williams & Wilkins in
quantities of 100 or more. Call Isabella Wise in the Special Sales Department, (800) 358-3583.

Dedication

To our spouses and children
Peg, Laura, and David
Barbara
Sandy, Sarah, Anna, Jessica, and Gideon
Bob, Karen, and Andrea

Contents

Preface

NMS Genetics has been written for medical students and house officers by four experienced medical geneticists. As geneticists and physicians, we have grown increasingly excited as modern genetic research has transformed our understanding of human biology and pathophysiology. Our goal in writing this book is to help tomorrow's physicians gain a basic understanding of medical genetics so that as family physicians and specialists of all types they will be able to incorporate genetic medicine into their practices. Moreover, we hope to encourage all aspiring physicians to share in the excitement that comes from "thinking genetically."

J. M. Friedman

Acknowledgments

This book grew out of our combined experience of more than 50 years in teaching genetics to medical students. Our approach has been greatly influenced by our students, by our colleagues in the University of British Columbia Department of Medical Genetics, and by Drs. James Miller and Patricia Baird, who developed and taught the UBC Medical Genetics 440 course before us.

We are grateful to Donna Siegfried for her excellent editorial work. This book never would have been completed had not Deb Furlong-Raher kept kicking us in the seat of the pants to get it done. We are grateful not only for her kindness and good humor, but also for her persistence.

To the Reader

Since 1984, the *National Medical Series for Independent Study (NMS)* has been helping medical students meet the challenge of education and clinical training. In this climate of burgeoning knowledge and complex clinical issues, a medical career is more demanding than ever. Increasingly, medical training must prepare physcians to seek and synthesize necessary information and to apply that information successfully.

The *National Medical Series* is designed to provide a logical framework for organizing, learning, reviewing, and applying the conceptual and factual information covered in basic and clinical studies. Each book includes a concise but comprehensive outline of the essential content of a discipline, with up to 500 study questions. The combination of an outlined text and tools for self-evaluation allows easy retrieval of salient information.

All study questions are accompanied by the correct answer, a paragraph-length explanation, and specific reference to the text where the topic is discussed. Study questions that follow each chapter use current USMLE format to reinforce the chapter content. Study questions appearing at the end of the text in the Comprehensive Exam vary in format depending on the book. Wherever possible, Comprehensive Exam questions are presented as a clinical case or scenario intended to simulate real-life application of medical knowledge. The goal of this exam is to challenge the student to draw from information presented throughout the book.

All of the books in the *National Medical Series* are constantly being updated and revised. The authors and editors devote considerable time and effort to ensure that the information required by all medical school curricula is included. Strict editorial attention is given to accuracy, organization, and consistency. Further shaping of the series occurs in response to biannual discussions held with a panel of medical student advisors drawn from schools throughout the United States. At these meetings, the editorial staff considers the complicated needs of medical students to learn how the *National Medical Series* can better serve them. In this regard, the staff at Williams & Wilkins welcomes all comments and suggestions.

Chapter 1

Nature of the Genetic Material

J. M. Friedman
Fred J. Dill
Michael R. Hayden

I. GENETICS IN MEDICINE

A. Introduction. Because the role that genetic factors play in pathologic processes is now better understood, the importance of genetics in medicine has increased. Scientific advances have made it possible to identify genetic diseases more precisely, to provide better genetic counseling and more accurate prenatal diagnosis for genetic diseases, and to improve the health of many people affected with such conditions. Some areas of genetic medicine are listed below.

1. **Medical genetics** is a branch of medicine that deals with the inheritance, diagnosis, and treatment of diseases caused by single gene mutations, chromosome abnormalities, and multifactorial predispositions. Genetic counseling and screening are also part of medical genetics.

2. **Clinical genetics** is the application of genetics to clinical problems in individual families and patients.

3. **Dysmorphology** is the study of abnormalities of morphologic development.

4. **Molecular medicine** is the clinical application of molecular biology to the diagnosis and treatment of disease.

B. Major types of genetic disease

1. **Single gene (mendelian or monogenic) disorders** (see Chapter 3) are conditions that are produced by the effects of one gene or a gene pair. Such traits are usually transmitted in simple patterns as originally described by Gregor Mendel.
   a. **Autosomal dominant traits** are transmitted on the **autosomes** (i.e., chromosomes other than the X or Y) and are expressed when only a single copy of the mutant gene is present. **Huntington disease** is an example of an autosomal dominant disorder.
   b. **Autosomal recessive traits** are transmitted on the autosomes and are only expressed when both copies of a gene are mutant. **Cystic fibrosis** is an autosomal recessive disorder.
   c. **X-linked traits** are transmitted on the X chromosome. An example of an X-linked disorder is **Duchenne-type muscular dystrophy.**

2. **Chromosome abnormalities** (see Chapter 2) are deviations from the normal chromosome number or structure. Examples include **Down syndrome** and **Turner syndrome.**

3. **Multifactorial traits** (see Chapter 9) result from the combined effects of multiple genetic and nongenetic influences. Examples include common kinds of **cancer** and **atherosclerotic heart disease.**

C. The incidence of genetic disease and other congenital anomalies apparent by 25 years of age is about 79/1000 livebirths. This excludes most of the common diseases of adulthood such as hypertension, noninsulin-dependent diabetes mellitus, coronary artery disease, and cancer, which have a multifactorial etiology but have an age of onset usually older than 25 years.

1. **Single gene (mendelian) disorders** occur with an incidence of 3.6/1000 livebirths.
   a. **Autosomal dominant diseases** have an incidence of 1.4/1000 livebirths.
   b. **Autosomal recessive conditions** have an incidence of 1.7/1000 livebirths.
   c. **X-linked disorders** have an incidence of 0.5/1000 livebirths.

2. **Chromosome abnormalities** occur with an incidence of 1.8/1000 livebirths.

3. **Multifactorial conditions** with onset before 25 years of age have an incidence of 46.4/1000 livebirths.

4. **Conditions that appear to be genetic but for which no precise mechanism has been defined** have an incidence of 1.2/1000 livebirths. Included in this category are conditions such as retinitis pigmentosa, which can be inherited as an autosomal dominant, autosomal recessive, or X-linked trait. The precise etiology may be unknown in an individual case.

5. The incidence of **other congenital anomalies** is about 26/1000 livebirths. Most isolated limb reduction defects would fall into this category, for example.

D. **Effect of genetic disease on society**

1. The **societal burden** of genetic disorders and congenital anomalies is particularly great because they often produce disease that begins in childhood and continues throughout life.

2. **Hospital admissions.** Genetic diseases are responsible for **30%–50% of pediatric hospital admissions** and **10% of adult hospital admissions.**

3. **Infant mortality.** Congenital anomalies, many of which are caused by genetic factors, at least in part, are the leading cause of infant mortality.

E. **Thinking genetically**

1. **The etiologic approach to disease.** In medical genetics, determination of the etiology of a patient's illness is a primary goal. However, consideration of etiology is a principle that is applicable throughout all branches of medicine. Physicians often treat the physical or functional manifestations of disease in a patient symptomatically, but disease prevention or cure requires an understanding of etiology and pathogenesis.

2. **The family as the unit of concern.** All physicians need to be aware that a disease in one person can have important repercussions for the entire family. This is especially true in medical genetics.
   a. There may be a substantial **risk for similar disease in the relatives** of an affected individual.
   b. In addition to this risk for recurrence, diagnosis of a genetic disease or congenital anomaly in one family member often has major **psychological and social implications** for the patient's parents, siblings, and children.

3. **Consideration of the patient as a whole.** In medical genetics, it is essential to view the patient as a whole person in the course of assessment, diagnosis, counseling, and treatment.
   a. Inherited gene or chromosome mutations **affect all cells** of the body and may **manifest in many different organs and systems.** Moreover, genetic diseases may produce **varying symptoms at different ages.**
   b. Because of the personal and social burden associated with many genetic diseases and birth defects, **secondary psychological effects** in both the patient and his or her relatives are common and must be considered in the management of affected patients and their families.
   c. Many genetic diseases are familial, and many patients are concerned about the **reproductive consequences** of a genetic diagnosis.

II. STRUCTURE AND FUNCTION OF GENES

A. **Gene structure.** Genes are composed of deoxyribonucleic acid (DNA), which codes for the production of specific amino acid residues. These amino acids are then joined to form the proteins that comprise living organisms.

1. The **human genome** consists of all DNA and consequently all the genes in one set of human chromosomes. In humans, there are 23 chromosome sets, each of which consists of approximately 3×10^9 base pairs. In contrast, the chromosome of Escherichia coli contains only 4×10^6 DNA base pairs.

2. **DNA molecules** consist of two complementary chains twisted about each other in the form of a double helix—the "twisted ladder" model.

   a. **Composition of DNA** (Figure 1-1). Each chain is composed of four nucleotides, each of which contains a deoxyribose residue, a phosphate, and a pyrimidine or a purine base. The **pyrimidine bases** are thymine (T) and cytosine (C); the **purine bases** are adenine (A) and guanine (G).

      (1) The **"sides" of the ladder** consist of the deoxyribose residues linked by phosphates.

      (2) The **"rungs" of the ladder** are made up of the pyrimidine and purine bases. The two strands of DNA are joined together by hydrogen bonds existing between the pyrimidine and purine bases: Adenine is always paired with thymine (AT), and guanine is always paired with cytosine (GC).

      (3) The **ends of the DNA strands** are designated 5' and 3'. By convention, the 5' end of a sequence is written to the left and indicates the sequence closer to the beginning of the gene; the 3' end is written to the right and indicates the

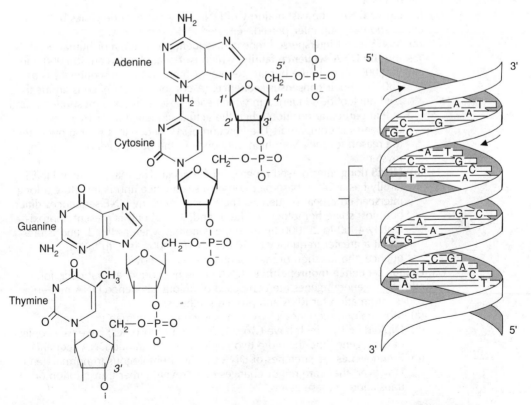

FIGURE 1-1. DNA molecule and nucleotide bases. (Reprinted from Gelehrter TD, Collins FS: *Medical Genetics*. Baltimore, Williams & Wilkins, 1990, p 10.)

sequence closer to the end of the gene. New DNA is synthesized in the 5' to 3' direction (Figure 1-2).

b. Replication, transcription, and translation

(1) Replication. During cell division, the DNA content of the parent cell is replicated by separation of the two strands of the double helix and synthesis of two new complementary strands according to the stated rules of base pairing.

(2) Transcription. The DNA acts as a template for messenger ribonucleic acid (mRNA). The process of creating mRNA complementary to the DNA in a gene is called transcription.

   (a) The mRNA is **transported from the nucleus to the cytoplasm.** Less than 10% of human DNA is transcribed into mRNA.

   (b) Two major **chemical differences** exist between DNA and RNA.

     (i) Ribose is the **sugar** in the structure of RNA; deoxyribose is the sugar in DNA.

     (ii) RNA has the **pyrimidine base** uracil (U) instead of thymine, as in DNA. So, in RNA, the correlating purine and pyrimidine bases are GC and AU.

(3) Translation is a process that occurs on the ribosomes in the cytoplasm, in which the information coded by the mRNA is translated into a chain of specified amino acids, constituting a polypeptide.

   (a) The first and second bases within an mRNA triplet are fixed with regard to the particular amino acid. However, the base in the **third position** often is less crucial. For example, the mRNA triplet that specifies arginine can be CGU, CGC, CGA, or CGG.

   (b) All amino acids are coded for by three base pairs. Therefore, the number of base pairs in the translated portion of a gene is three times the number of amino acids in the corresponding polypeptide chain.

c. Classes of DNA

(1) Repetitive DNA. The vast majority of DNA does not encode genes but is present as short or long interspersed, repeated DNA sequences.

   (a) SINES (short interspersed repeated sequences). The major human SINE is the *Alu* **DNA sequence family,** which is repeated between 300,000 and 900,000 times in the human genome. Common to *Alu* sequences is a 300–base-pair **consensus sequence.** (A consensus sequence is an idealized nucleotide sequence in which each base is the one most often found at that particular position when the actual sequence in many individuals or species is compared.) The function of *Alu* sequences is unknown, and the reason for their very high frequency in the human genome remains a mystery.

   (b) LINES (long interspersed repeated sequences). The major human LINES family has a 6400–base-pair consensus sequence and is therefore a long interspersed repeat sequence. The 5' ends of many LINE sequences differ, but most share homology on the 3' end. The 5' end is present approximately 4000 to 20,000 times in the genome, whereas the 3' end is present at a greater frequency of 50,000 to 100,000. As with the *Alu* sequence, the function of these sequences is unknown.

(2) Unique sequence (nonrepetitive) DNA contains sequences that code for mRNA. In general, genes are composed of unique sequence DNA that encodes information for RNA and protein synthesis.

   (a) Most unique sequence DNA occurs once in the human genome.

   (b) Diploid cells, which have two sets of 23 chromosomes, have two copies of each gene, and therefore two copies of each unique DNA sequence.

   (c) Pseudogenes are stretches of DNA that are homologous to normal genes. However, there are minor changes that prevent either transcription or translation of these genes.

3. Organization of genes (Figure 1-3)

a. Exons are the functional portions of gene sequences that code for proteins.

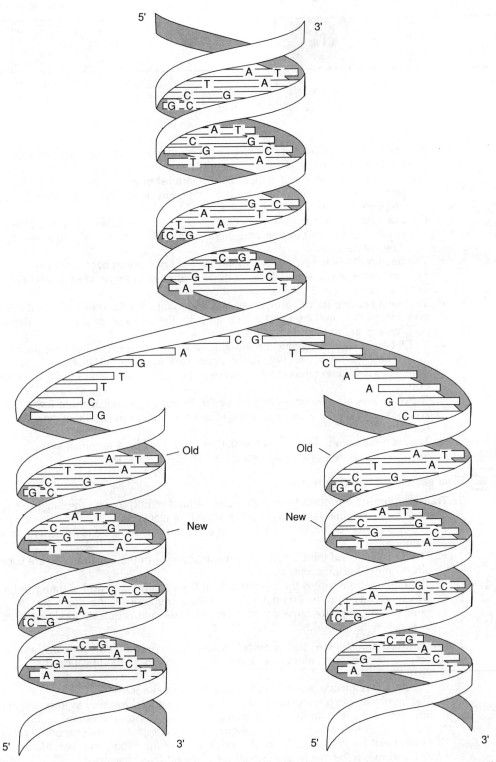

FIGURE 1-2. DNA synthesis. (Reprinted from Gelehrter TD, Collins FS: *Medical Genetics*. Baltimore, Williams & Wilkins, 1990, p 13.)

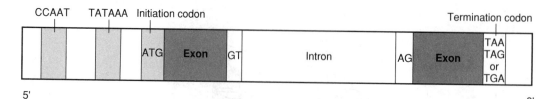

FIGURE 1-3. A human gene.

   b. Introns are the noncoding DNA sequences of unknown function that interrupt most mammalian genes. The number and size of introns vary in different genes.
     (1) In certain instances, the **evolutionary relationship** of specific genes can be discerned by their similar organization with equivalent numbers of introns at appropriate locations within the gene.
     (2) Examples include the apolipoprotein and globin genes, which have a similar number and size of introns and share a common ancestry. All, however, have different functions.
   c. The **boundaries** between exons and introns are not random base sequences. In most instances, the first two bases at the 5′ end of each intron are GT, and the last two bases at the 3′ end of each intron are AG.
   d. The **open reading frame** is the sequence beginning with the triplet **ATG**—the universal translation initiation codon that specifies the initiation of protein synthesis. ATG resides at the 5′ end of genes.
   e. TATA boxes. AT-rich regions are found in most genes. These regions are about 20–30 bases to the 5′ end (left) of the open reading frame (ATG). TATA boxes are thought to help direct important enzymes to the correct initiation site for transcription.
   f. CCAAT boxes are sequences that occur 70–90 base pairs upstream (prior to the ATG starting point) and are also thought to be important in regulating transcription.
   g. Termination codon. The end of translation is signified by a termination triplet at the 3′ end of genes. The triplet could be TAA, TAG, or TGA.

B. **From gene to protein (Figure 1-4)**

   1. Transcription is the process that synthesizes a strand of mRNA with the same sequences as the original strand (the coding strand) of DNA.
     a. The two strands that compose DNA can each serve as separate templates for transcription.
     b. The TATA box and the CCAAT sequence that are 5′ to the initiation site are usually required for transcription.
     c. The primary transcript is the large strand of RNA synthesized during transcription, which extends from the original 5′ to 3′ ends and comprises the exons and introns of the gene. This large strand is very unstable and is quickly modified at its 5′ and 3′ ends into mRNA.

   2. RNA processing. At the 5′ end of mRNA, a **cap** structure is added, while a string of adenylic acid (poly A) residues is added to the 3′ end. These modifications help to stabilize the mRNA.
     a. The **poly A sequence** acts as a stop signal to terminate transcription.
     b. The introns are then removed, and the exons are spliced together to form the mature mRNA, which can then be transported to the cytoplasm for translation.
     c. The precise mechanisms of RNA splicing are not completely understood, but it is evident that the sequences at the 5′ and 3′ ends of the exon/intron boundaries (GT and AG, respectively) are crucial for efficient RNA cleavage.

   3. Translation is the process that converts the mRNA sequences derived from the coding strand of DNA into the sequences that make up polypeptides. This process occurs on the ribosomes in the cytoplasm in a 5′ to 3′ direction.

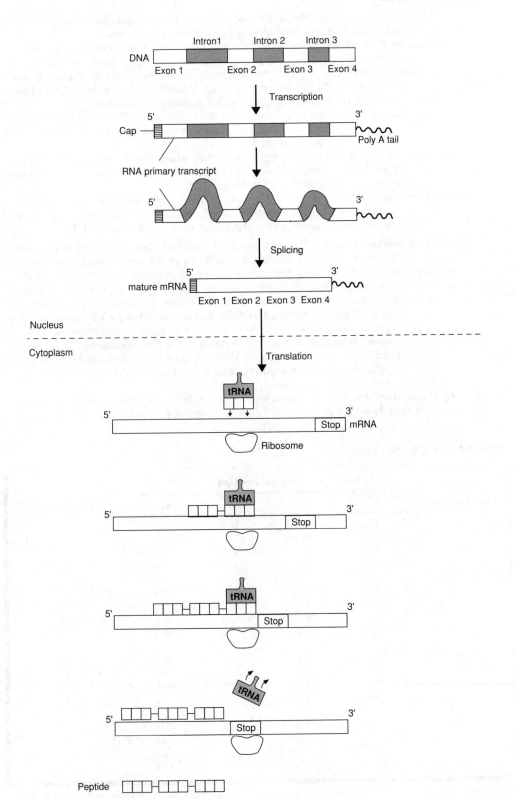

FIGURE 1-4. Transcription, RNA processing, and translation.

a. The mRNA moves over the surface of the ribosome, bringing successive groups of nucleotides that code for an amino acid (codons) into position.

b. Transfer RNA (tRNA) is an RNA molecule that brings the amino acids to the mRNA–ribosome complex. The amino acid–tRNA complex lines up next to the codons of mRNA and is joined to the previously synthesized polypeptide chain by a peptide bond. As this happens, the tRNA is released, and the mRNA moves further over the ribosome, bringing another codon into position.

c. This process is repeated in a 5′ to 3′ direction until a specific **termination codon** (UAA, UAG, or UGA) is reached. The peptide is then released, and the tRNA molecule and ribosomes are separated.

d. There are 20 naturally occurring amino acids, which are the building blocks for proteins. With four different bases, and amino acids specified by groups of three bases, there are 64 possible coding triplets.

e. Degenerate code. Most amino acids are coded for by more than one triplet, which means the code is degenerate. The alternate triplets for a given amino acid often vary only by a change in the third base of the triplet (Table 1-1).

4. Levels of protein structure. Proteins are often modified after translation to become active. For example, insulin is produced initially as an 82–amino acid proinsulin. Subsequently, 31 amino acids are removed before it becomes an active hormone.

a. The **primary structure** of the protein is constituted by the number of polypeptide chains and the sequence of the amino acid residues. In some instances, proteins have nonprotein groups attached to them that are essential for functional activity. For example, the globin polypeptide is attached to heme to form hemoglobin.

b. The **secondary structure** of the protein refers to the configuration of the polypeptides influenced by bonding between different peptides. For example, hydrogen bonding between groups on a polypeptide chain leads to twisting of the polypeptide backbone to form an α-helix.

c. The **tertiary structure** of a protein refers to its three-dimensional form. Many proteins have helical and nonhelical regions. The three-dimensional structure repre-

TABLE 1-1. The Genetic Code

First Position	Second Position				Third Position
	U	**C**	**A**	**G**	
U	Phe	Ser	Tyr	Cys	U
	Phe	Ser	Tyr	Cys	C
	Leu	Ser	STOP	STOP	A
	Leu	Ser	STOP	Trp	G
C	Leu	Pro	His	Arg	U
	Leu	Pro	His	Arg	C
	Leu	Pro	Gln	Arg	A
	Leu	Pro	Gln	Arg	G
A	Ile	Thr	Asn	Ser	U
	Ile	Thr	Asn	Ser	C
	Ile	Thr	Lys	Arg	A
	Met	Thr	Lys	Arg	G
G	Val	Ala	Asp	Gly	U
	Val	Ala	Asp	Gly	C
	Val	Ala	Glu	Gly	A
	Val	Ala	Glu	Gly	G

Amino acid abbreviations: Ala = alanine; Arg = arginine; Asn = asparagine; Asp = aspartic acid; Cys = cysteine; Gln = glutamine; Glu = glutamic acid; Gly = glycine; His = histidine; Ile = isoleucine; Leu = leucine; Lys = lysine; Met = methionine; Phe = phenylalanine; Pro = proline; Ser = serine; Thr = threonine; Trp = tryptophan; Tyr = tyrosine; Val = valine.

sents the most favorable arrangement of the polypeptide chain for efficient and optimal activity.

5. **Control of gene expression.** All cells have the DNA available to code for every cellular function. Yet cells are specialized, with specific functions due to differential expression of different genes.
   a. **DNA sequences** coexist in human and animal genomes in **methylated and non-methylated forms.**
      (1) **Methylation** appears to have a significant repressor effect on gene expression.
      (2) Many genes that are expressed have regions of nonmethylated DNA at their 5′ end.
   b. Sequences on the mammalian X chromosome that are expressed tend to be nonmethylated, whereas sequences that are inactive tend to be methylated.
   c. Numerous **other factors** affect expression. These include:
      (1) Sequences 5′ to the gene, including TATA and CCAAT
      (2) Sequences 3′ to the gene
      (3) Occasionally, intronic sequences within the gene

6. **Mitochondrial genes.** Mitochondria are the only organelles outside the nucleus that contain their own DNA in the form of two to ten copies of double-stranded DNA, measuring about 16 kilobases (kb) in length (Figure 1-5).
   a. **Mitochondrial DNA (mt-DNA)** differs from nuclear DNA in the following ways.
      (1) It is circular, rather than linear.
      (2) It consists mostly of unique-sequence DNA rather than repetitive DNA.
      (3) It is exclusively transmitted to the next generation by mothers.
      (4) It uses the triplet TGA to code for tryptophan rather than as a stop codon.
   b. Mitochondrial DNA **codes for 13 proteins,** which are components of the mitochondrial respiratory chain and oxidative phosphorylation system, as well as **2 rRNAs** and **22 tRNAs.**
      (1) **Mutations** in the mt-DNA coding for these proteins may result in disease.
      (2) In such disorders, the mutation is transmitted through the ovum from an affected mother to all of her children, regardless of gender. Examples include diseases affecting the central nervous system (CNS; e.g., Leber optic atrophy) or diseases affecting muscle (e.g., mitochondrial myopathies).

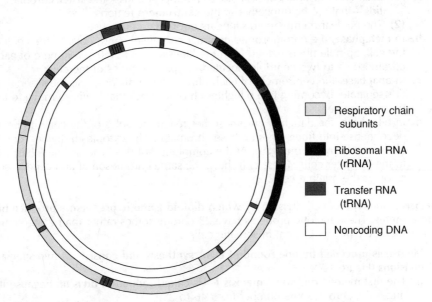

FIGURE 1-5. Ring structure of mitochondrial DNA (mt-DNA).

(3) However, only the daughters would transmit this trait in subsequent generations—an example of nonmendelian inheritance.

III. MITOSIS AND MEIOSIS

A. **Mitosis** is the type of division in which a cell with 46 chromosomes produces two daughter cells, each of which also has 46 chromosomes.

1. **Somatic cells** undergo mitosis to produce genetically identical progeny.

2. **Germ cells** also undergo mitosis to increase their numbers within the gonads before the onset of meiosis.

3. Mitosis is the **shortest portion of the cell cycle,** which can be arbitrarily divided into **four stages.**
    a. Just after mitosis is completed, the cell enters a phase called G_1, during which all of the DNA is present in an unreplicated state. G_1 ends when DNA synthesis begins.
    b. DNA synthesis occurs during the **S** phase of the cell cycle. The DNA is reproduced in units called **replicons,** each of which makes a single copy of itself by **semiconservative replication** of each strand of the DNA double helix.
    c. At the completion of the S phase, each chromosome has doubled and consists of two chromatids. The stage that begins at the completion of DNA synthesis and lasts until the onset of mitosis is called G_2.
    d. The entire **cell cycle** is thus the sequence of phases $G_1 \rightarrow S \rightarrow G_2 \rightarrow$ **mitosis,** which is repeated for each replicating somatic cell.
        (1) Terminally differentiated cells, such as neurons, stop dividing. They are arrested in a prolonged G_1 phase, which is sometimes called G_0.
        (2) The part of the cell cycle between mitoses (i.e., the entire period between the onset of G_1 and the end of G_2) is called **interphase.**

4. Although mitosis is a continuous dynamic process, for purposes of description this segment of the cell cycle is divided into **four stages** (Figure 1-6).
    a. At the conclusion of interphase, mitotic **prophase** begins with the condensation of the chromosomes into filaments that are visible under the light microscope.
        (1) Each chromosome consists of two parallel strands—the **sister chromatids**—that are held together at the **centromere** region.
        (2) The nuclear membrane disappears during late prophase.
    b. In **metaphase,** the chromosomes contract completely and move to the center of the cell. Spindle fibers extend from the **kinetochore** at the centromere of each chromosome to two centrioles located in opposite poles of the cell.
    c. In **anaphase,** the centromere of each chromosome divides, and the sister chromatids separate, becoming two daughter chromosomes that begin to move to the poles of the cell.
    d. In **telophase,** the daughter chromosomes reach the poles of the cell and begin to decondense into fibers of interphase chromatin. The cytoplasm divides, and nuclear membranes form again. At the completion of this process, interphase begins in the daughter cells. These cells have the same chromosomal and genetic composition as the original cells.

B. **Meiosis** is the type of cell division by which **diploid gametic precursors produce haploid gametes.** These meiotic products have 23 chromosomes rather than the 46 chromosomes that are typically present in somatic cells.

1. **Meiosis is preceded by one round of DNA synthesis and consists of two special cell divisions** (Figure 1-7).
    a. The first meiotic division—**meiosis I**—is called **reduction division** because it reduces the chromosome number from 46 to 23.
        (1) At the beginning of **meiosis I prophase (prophase I),** each chromosome has

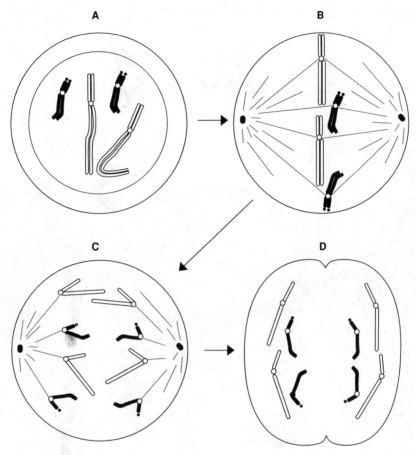

A

B

C

D

FIGURE 1-6. Mitosis: (*A*) Prophase; (*B*) Metaphase; (*C*) Anaphase; (*D*) Telophase.

completed replication and consists of two sister chromatids attached at the centromere. For descriptive purposes, **prophase I** is divided into several sequential stages.

(a) **Leptotene.** The chromosomes first become visible under the light microscope as thin threads. Separate sister chromatids cannot be distinguished.

(b) **Zygotene.** Homologous chromosomes, one of which originates maternally and the other of which originates paternally, pair along their entire lengths.

  (i) The process of pairing, which brings corresponding DNA sequences on the homologous chromosomes into close physical proximity, is called **synapsis.**

  (ii) Synapsis is mediated by the **synaptonemal complex,** which is a specialized structure that can be seen by electron microscopy lying between the chromatin fibers. The synaptonemal complex is thought to be involved in the process of genetic recombination.

(c) **Pachytene.** The chromosomes condense further and appear as **bivalents** because homologous chromosomes are tightly apposed in synapsis. Recombination takes place between individual chromatids of homologous chromosomes through **crossing over.**

(d) **Diplotene.** The pair of homologous chromosomes (i.e., the bivalents) begin to separate but are held together at the sites of crossing over, which appear as cross-shaped structures (**chiasmata**).

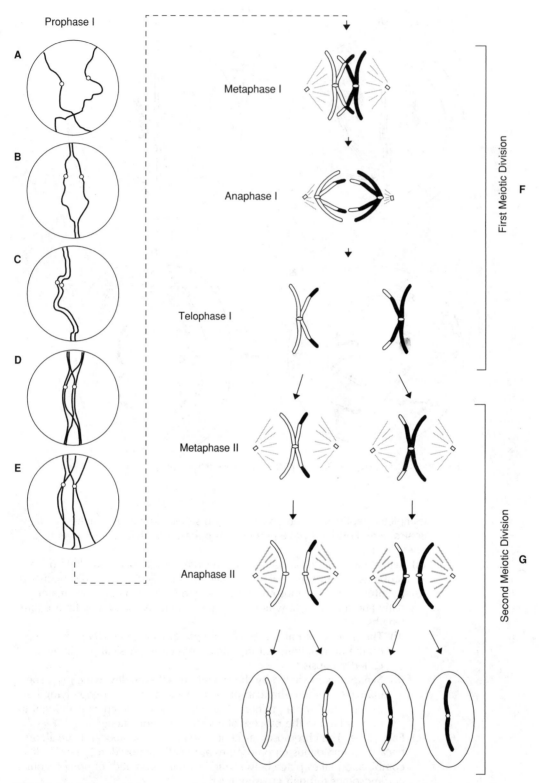

FIGURE 1-7. Meiosis. (*A*) Leptotene of prophase I; (*B*) Zygotene of prophase I; (*C*) Pachytene of prophase I; (*D*) Diplotene of prophase I; (*E*) Diakinesis; (*F*) Remainder of first meiotic division; (*G*) Second meiotic division.

(e) **Diakinesis.** The chromosomes reach maximal condensation.

(2) In **metaphase I,** the nuclear membrane disappears and the bivalents align on a plane in the center of the cell. A spindle connects the centromeres to centrioles in opposite poles of the cell.

(3) In **anaphase I, the homologous chromosomes comprising each bivalent separate** from each other and move to opposite poles of the cell.

   (a) **The sister chromatids of each chromosome remain attached at the centromere, which does not divide in meiosis I.**

   (b) The chromosomes in each homologous pair segregate independently in meiosis I; that is, there is no tendency for the chromosomes orginally obtained from the mother to move to one pole and those obtained from the father to move to the other pole. The movement of the chromosomes from each bivalent is random.

(4) During **telophase I,** the two haploid sets of chromosomes reach opposite poles of the cell and the cytoplasm divides.

b. The second meiotic division, **meiosis II,** is preceded by a brief interphase in which **DNA synthesis does not occur.**

   (1) **Meiosis II is similar to mitosis** in that the chromosomes, each consisting of two sister chromatids attached at the centromere, align on a central plane in the cell, a spindle forms, the centromeres split, and the daughter chromosomes move to opposite poles of the cell.

   (2) The essential difference is that **in meiosis II there are only 23 chromosomes** in the original cell and in each of the daughter cells, whereas in mitosis there are 46.

2. **Meiosis differs from mitosis** in the following ways.

   a. **Meiosis occurs only in germ cells;** mitosis occurs in all somatic cells as well as in germ cells before they enter their final stages of development.

   b. **Meiosis consists of two sequential cell divisions;** mitosis occurs in a single division.

   c. **Pairing of homologous chromosomes occurs in meiosis** but not in mitosis.

   d. **Recombination between homologous chromosomes is a regular feature of meiosis** but not of mitosis.

   e. **Meiosis results in a reduction of the chromosome number from 46 to 23.** Mitosis produces two daughter cells with 46 chromosomes, the same number that was present in the original cell.

3. **The genetic consequences of meiosis** are:

   a. **Reduction of the chromosome number from diploid to haploid**

   b. **Segregation of alleles** so that only one member of the original gene pair is included in each gamete

   c. **Independent assortment of homologous chromosomes** so that a gamete contains some chromosomes that were inherited from the mother and other chromosomes that were inherited from the father

   d. **Crossing over** between homologous chromosomes so that every chromosome in the gamete is likely to contain some genes that were inherited from the mother and other genes that were inherited from the father

C. **Gametogenesis** is the formation of the ova or sperm. In males, the process is called **spermatogenesis;** in females, it is called **oogenesis.**

1. **Spermatogenesis** begins to occur in the seminiferous tubules of the testes at the time of puberty and continues throughout life.

   a. Mitotic germ cell precursors called **spermatogonia** produce **primary spermatocytes,** each of which undergoes meiosis I to produce two **secondary spermatocytes.**

   b. Each secondary spermatocyte undergoes meiosis II to form two **spermatids,** which mature without further division to form sperm.

   c. The production of mature sperm from a spermatogonium takes about **75 days.**

2. **Oogenesis** differs in several important ways from spermatogenesis.

   a. Much of oogenesis occurs during fetal life. Mitotic division of germ cell precursors in females is restricted to the first few months after conception.

   b. Oogonia produce **primary oocytes,** which initiate meiosis I by about the third month of gestation. No primary oocytes are formed after birth.

   c. The primary oocytes become arrested in prophase I in a stage called **dictyotene** before birth and remain so until after the female reaches sexual maturity.

   d. After menarche, individual ovarian follicles mature, releasing their primary oocytes from dictyotene as ovulation occurs.

   e. Meiosis I in females results in unequal division of the cytoplasm, with most going to the **secondary oocyte** and relatively little going to the other meiotic product, **the first polar body.**

   f. Meiosis II is not completed until after fertilization has occurred. Meiosis II also results in an unequal division of the cytoplasm, with most going to the **ovum** and relatively little going to a **second polar body.**

   g. The ovum functions as a gamete, but the polar bodies normally do not. Thus, **each female meiosis produces only one functional gamete,** whereas each male meiosis produces four functional gametes.

   h. The prolonged arrest of female gametes in prophase I, which lasts from fetal life until the ovum is ovulated, may account for the increased risk of nondisjunction associated with advanced maternal age (see Chapter 2 II A 3 b).

IV. CHROMOSOME STRUCTURE

A. **Packaging of DNA into chromatin and chromosomes.** Each chromosome contains a single molecule of DNA organized into several orders of packaging to construct a metaphase chromosome. The length of a metaphase chromosome is about 0.0001 times the length of its DNA.

  1. Levels of packaging and organization of chromatin (Figure 1-8)

    a. DNA in chromosomes is associated with DNA-binding proteins; the DNA–protein complex is called **chromatin.** These proteins may mediate gene transcription or DNA replication or be the structural proteins that organize the DNA.

    b. Histones are the structural proteins of chromatin and are the most abundant proteins in the nucleus. Five histones—H1, H2A, H2B, H3, and H4—provide the framework for the fundamental chromatin packaging unit, the **nucleosome.**

    c. Each **nucleosome** consists of a tightly bound package of eight histones (two each of H2A, H2B, H3, and H4) with a DNA helix wound twice around the surface.

      (1) Each nucleosome core binds 146 base pairs of the DNA helix, and the cores are linked by about 60 bases into a bead-like structure.

      (2) The width of the nucleosome package is 11 nanometers (nm) compared to 2 nm for a DNA double helix.

      (3) Nucleosomes are packed tightly together with the aid of histone H1 to form a 30–nm-wide fiber, which is the basic chromatin unit seen in interphase nuclei when using electron microscopy.

    d. The 30-nm fiber is further packaged into a system of **looped domains.**

      (1) The loops, which contain from 20,000 to 100,000 base pairs of DNA, are **formed by nonhistone proteins binding specific sites along the 30-nm fiber.**

      (2) Evidence suggests that the loops house individual units of DNA transcription and replication. Therefore, they have both a structural and a functional significance.

  2. Higher-order organization

    a. Prophase and metaphase chromosomes. Chromatin in metaphase chromosomes is highly condensed compared with interphase chromatin.

      (1) The process of condensation during prophase of mitosis is thought to proceed by coiling and compaction of the looped domain structure. In the condensed

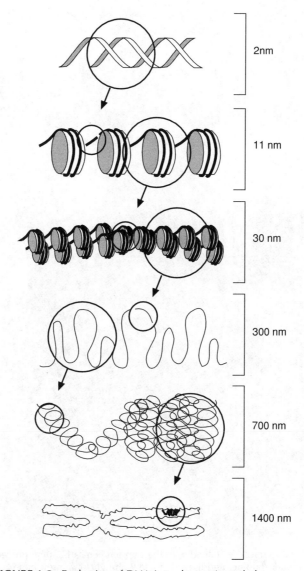

FIGURE 1-8. Packaging of DNA into chromatin and chromosomes.

state, nearby loops are held together by protein interactions that form a network or scaffold.
   (2) The chromatin network is arranged in a helical fashion along the axis of the chromosome.
   (3) The width of an individual chromatid of a metaphase chromosome is about 700 nm, reflecting a high degree of compression of the 30-nm fiber.
   b. Chromosome bands. Prophase and metaphase chromosomes exhibit alternating light and dark bands under appropriate staining conditions (see IV C 1 b; Figure 1-9). These bands reflect the differential folding of clusters of looped domains and also define regions of the genome that have different properties and functions.

B. **Special features of chromosomes**

   1. Euchromatin forms the main body of the chromosome and has a relatively high density of coding regions or genes. The **chromosome bands** define alternating partitions of euchromatin with differing properties.

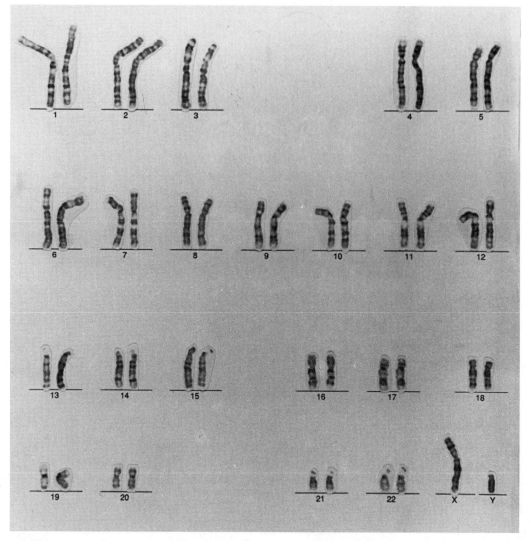

FIGURE 1-9. A normal male karyotype stained with the trypsin/Giemsa banding procedure. With this method, the G bands are dark staining, and they alternate with light-staining R bands.

  a. **R bands** are areas that:
   (1) **Stain light** with G banding procedures [see IV C 1 b (1)]
   (2) Replicate DNA early in the S phase of the cell cycle
   (3) Have a relatively high content of guanine and cytosine
   (4) Have the majority of **SINES** [see II A 2 c (1) (a)]
   (5) Have the highest gene density
  b. **G bands** are areas that:
   (1) **Stain dark** with G banding procedures [see IV C 1 b (1)]
   (2) Replicate late in the S phase
   (3) Have a higher content of adenine and thymine than R bands
   (4) Have the majority of **LINES** [see II A 2 c (1) (b)]
   (5) Have relatively fewer genes than R bands

 2. **Heterochromatin** is chromatin that is either devoid of genes or has inactive genes (i.e., gene transcription has been turned off). Heterochromatic segments of the genome remain more condensed in interphase than euchromatin and replicate very late in the S phase of the cell cycle.

    a. Constitutive heterochromatin is located around the centromeres of all chromosomes, in the long arm of the Y chromosome, and in the satellites of the acrocentric chromosomes [see IV C 2 a (1)].

      (1) These areas contain various families of highly repetitive elements of DNA with no known function.

      (2) Constitutive heterochromatin can be highlighted on metaphase chromosomes using banding procedures such as C banding or Q banding [see IV C 1 b (3), (5)].

    b. Facultative heterochromatin is euchromatin in a transcriptionally inactive state. In humans, the clearest example is lyonization (see V B): One of the two X chromosomes in females is inactivated as a means of compensation for the double dosage of X chromosome genes, compared with the single copy in males (i.e., **dosage compensation**).

      (1) Early in the development of the female embryo, one of the two X chromosomes in each cell is altered so that the majority of the genes become inactive in transcription, and thus cannot be translated into functioning proteins. This inactivation process is permanent for that chromosome, and inactivation is maintained through subsequent cell divisions.

      (2) The mechanism of inactivation is not known, but one of the outcomes of the process is modification of the methylation patterns of cytosine nucleotides in the areas around genes that regulate transcription. X chromosome inactivation is also accompanied by a change in timing of DNA replication to later in the S phase. The inactive X chromosome remains highly condensed and stains darkly during interphase, forming a **Barr body.**

3. The **centromere** appears as a constricted area of the metaphase chromosome. Normally, each chromosome has one centromere. During cell division, the centromere is the last segment of the chromosome to replicate and separate.

    a. Structure. The centromere consists of specific DNA sequences that bind proteins, which can be identified by their antigenic properties.

    b. Function. Centromeric proteins form the **kinetochore,** which participates with spindle-fiber microtubules to facilitate the separation of sister chromatids or chromosomes at anaphase of mitosis or meiosis [see III A 4 c, B 1 a (3)].

4. Telomeres are DNA sequences found at **the ends of chromosomes,** which are required to maintain chromosome stability. Chromosomes without telomeres tend to recombine with other chromatin segments and are generally subject to breakage, fusion, and eventual loss.

    a. Structure. The terminal segments of all chromosomes have a similar DNA sequence (**TTAGGG),** which is tandemly repeated in several thousand copies.

    b. Function. Intact telomere structure facilitates the DNA replication process at the ends of chromosomes.

C. **Chromosome analysis and classification**

1. Cytogenetic studies. Diagnostic cytogenetic analysis can be performed with **metaphase** or **prometaphase chromosomes** obtained from rapidly dividing cells in tissue culture or, in some cases, directly from tissues with high mitotic activity (e.g., tumor cells).

    a. Source of cells

      (1) Chromosomes from cultured lymphocytes provide the shortest and most convenient method for routine cytogenetic analysis. These cultures can be established from peripheral lymphocytes and can be used to prepare metaphase chromosome spreads after 3 days.

      (2) Cell cultures from other cell types (e.g., fibroblasts, amniocytes, chorionic villus cells, tumor cells) require 1 to 2 weeks to accumulate sufficient cells for cytogenetic analysis. Fibroblast and other cell cultures can be subcultured and maintained for weeks or months. They also can be frozen in liquid nitrogen and stored for years for future analysis.

(3) **Direct preparation of cells** for chromosome analysis can be performed on bone marrow cells from leukemia patients or on some solid tumors. This technique takes advantage of the relatively high mitotic rate in these tissues.

b. **Procedures for chromosome analysis**

(1) **G banding,** the most common procedure, uses **Giemsa stain** after enzymatic treatment of metaphase chromosomes to differentiate chromosome bands.

(a) Viewed under the light microscope, metaphase chromosomes have alternating dark-staining and light-staining bands (see Figure 1-9). The dark bands by convention are called **G bands;** the light bands are **R bands.**

(b) In an average conventional metaphase preparation, approximately 400 dark and light bands can be resolved in a haploid set of chromosomes.

(2) **High-resolution banding procedures** capture chromosomes in prophase or prometaphase, when they are markedly less condensed than in metaphase. The procedure involves partial synchronization of mitosis in the culture by arresting DNA synthesis, which allows the cells to accumulate at this point in the cell cycle. Then, the cells are released from arrest so that many cells proceed into mitosis together. In high-resolution preparations, each band seen in metaphase chromosomes can be resolved into sub-bands, which allows for resolution of 800 or more bands. Analysis of prophase chromosomes with higher resolution than 850 to 900 bands, although possible, is not generally technically practical.

(3) **Q banding** uses **quinacrine** to stain chromosomes, which are viewed with fluorescence microscopy. Alternating bands of bright and dull fluorescence correspond to those seen by G banding for most areas of the chromosomes. Bright Q bands are equivalent to dark-staining G bands. Areas lacking this similarity are called variable bands [see IV C 2 a (2) (c)].

(4) **R banding,** or **reverse banding,** uses Giemsa dyes under elevated temperatures to produce the reverse of the pattern seen in G banding or Q banding. Fluorescent dyes with a high-binding affinity to GC-rich DNA (e.g., olivomycin) can also produce R banding.

(5) **C banding** requires heating in an alkali solution and staining with Giemsa. C bands are areas of **constitutive heterochromatin** [see IV B 2 a] located adjacent to the centromeres of all chromosomes and in the long arm of the Y chromosome (Yq).

(6) **Fragile site analysis** can be accomplished by growing the culture under specific conditions for induction of each type of fragile site. For example, to detect the **folate-sensitive X-chromosome fragile site** that is associated with **X-linked mental retardation** (see Chapter 2 IV A 1), cells must be grown in medium with no folic acid or treated with methotrexate or fluorodeoxyuridine (FdUR), which interferes with folate metabolism.

(7) **In situ hybridization of DNA probes to metaphase and interphase cells.** Methods for detecting DNA probes for **single-copy genes, chromosome-specific centromeric heterochromatin,** or **individual whole chromosomes (chromosome painting)** are available to clinical cytogenetic laboratories.

(a) These procedures involve **in situ hybridization** of specially labeled DNA probes to metaphase chromosomes or to interphase chromatin.

(b) The DNA probes are labeled with **reporter molecules,** such as biotin, digoxigenin, and dinitrophenyl, which can be visualized under the microscope by coupling the reporter molecule to a fluorescent signal or other dye. Fluorescent dyes are most widely used, giving rise to the term **fluorescence in situ hybridization (FISH).**

(i) **FISH tools are powerful.** For example, they can be used to determine the origin of small marker chromosomes that cannot be fully characterized by banding (see Chapter 2 IV B 4).

(ii) A more common use of FISH is for the detection of **submicroscopic deletions,** such as those associated with Prader-Willi syndrome (see Chapter 2 III A 3 a; Table 1-2), or for the determination of gain or

TABLE 1-2. Recognizable Microdeletion Syndromes Detectable By Fluorescence In Situ Hybridization (FISH)

Syndrome	Deletion	Clinical Description
Prader-Willi	15q12	Hypotonia, obesity, mental retardation (MR), early feeding problems
Angelman	15q12	Seizures, lack of speech, hand flapping
Velocardiofacial	22q11.2	Narrow face, cleft palate, cardiac anomalies
Miller-Dieker	17p13.3	Lissencephaly, wrinkled brow, early death
Williams	7q11.2	Prominent lips, cardiac defects, friendly behavior, MR
Wolf-Hirschhorn	4p16.3	Severe MR, prominent nose

loss of chromosomes in interphase tumor cells by probing with chromosome-specific centromere probes.

2. **Chromosome classification** is based on the International System for Human Cytogenetic Nomenclature (ISCN).

   a. **The normal human karyotype** (see Figure 1-9) consists of 23 pairs of chromosomes: 22 homologous pairs of **autosomes** and 1 pair of **sex chromosomes (XX or XY).** The autosomes, by convention, are divided into seven groups, arranged by size and position of the centromere. The standard ISCN idiogram of banded human chromosomes is shown in Figure 1-10.

   (1) Chromosome features

      (a) Metaphase chromosomes are divided longitudinally into two sister **chromatids** [see III A 4 a (1)] held together at the **centromere,** which delineates the chromosome into a **short arm (p)** and a **long arm (q).**

      (b) The position of the centromere is used in the morphologic description of a chromosome: **Metacentric** chromosomes have central centromeres, whereas **submetacentric** and **acrocentric** chromosomes have a centromere that is slightly or markedly closer to one end. For example, chromosomes 13 and 21 are described as acrocentric.

      (c) Satellites are small segments of heterochromatin at the tips of the short arms of the acrocentric chromosomes (numbers 13, 14, 15, 21, and 22).

   (2) Bands. Each chromosome has alternating dark and light bands.

      (a) Band numbering. Starting at the centromere, each arm is divided into one or more regions (e.g., 1, 2). The bands are then numbered from the centromere progressing to the telomere (e.g., 11, 12, 21). High-resolution banding resolves bands into sub-bands (Figure 1-11). These are numbered as a subset. For example, band 18q22 (band 22 on the long arm of chromosome 18) may be divided into 18q22.1, 18q22.2, and 18q22.3. Higher-resolution preparations have a higher "band level" and more detail.

      (b) Most bands (depicted by solid black or white areas in Figure 1-10) have constant morphology between members of a homologous pair of chromosomes and between normal individuals. A change in morphology is usually associated with an abnormal clinical presentation (see Chapter 2 III).

      (c) Chromosome **heteromorphic bands,** or **variable regions,** are evident on many chromosomes. These areas of **heterochromatin** (see IV B 2) are depicted as shaded areas in the ideogram in Figure 1-10. Deletions or duplications to these regions have no clinical significance.

   b. **Nomenclature for normal and abnormal karyotypes.** ISCN formulas can be written to describe any chromosome complement. Box 1-1 provides a list of some abbreviations used in human cytogenetic nomenclature.

   (1) Basic formula. In describing the karyotype, the first item is the number of

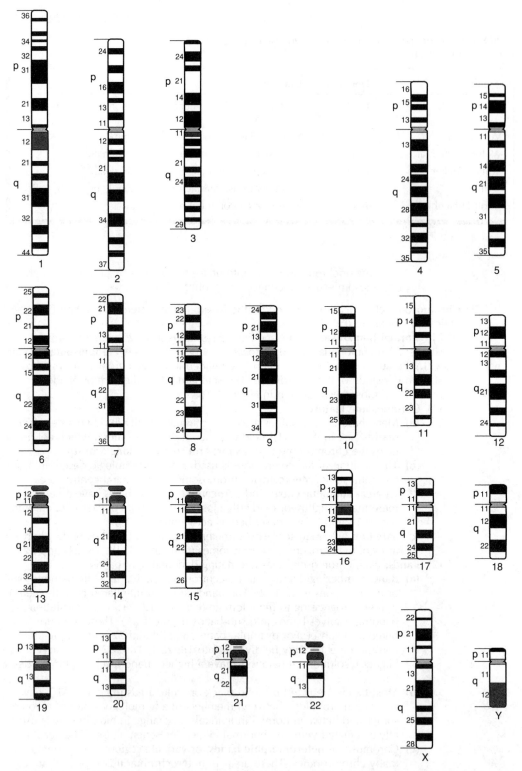

FIGURE 1-10. Diagrammatic representation (ideogram) of human chromosomes showing specific morphologic features and band numbering system. Each chromosome arm is divided into one or more regions, and the regions are divided into bands. Numbering starts at the centromere and proceeds to the telomere (all numbers are not included here). The *light-shaded areas* are the centromeres, the *dark-shaded areas* denote heteromorphic, or variable, regions. Short arms of the chromosomes are indicated by *p*; long arms by *q*. [Based on the International System for Human Cytogenetic Nomenclature (ISCN), 1985.]

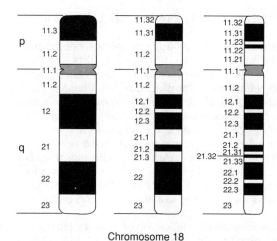

Chromosome 18

FIGURE 1-11. Diagrammatic representation of chromosome 18, showing standard to high resolution of chromosome bands. The level of resolution for the chromosome on the *left* is 400 bands, for the *middle* chromosome is 550 bands, and for the *right* chromosome is 850 bands.

chromosomes; second is the sex chromosome constitution. The normal female karyotype is 46,XX; the normal male karyotype is 46,XY. Autosomes are specified only if there is an abnormality.

(2) **Formulas for karyotypes with abnormal numbers of chromosomes.** A plus or minus sign before a chromosome number indicates that the entire chromosome is extra (trisomy) or missing (monosomy). Triploidy (three copies of each chromosome) or tetraploidy (four copies of each chromosome) is evident from the chromosome number. Mosaicism (i.e., cell populations of differing karyotypes in an individual) is indicated by a diagonal line. Examples include the following.

  (a) **45,X** indicates a total of 45 chromosomes with only one X chromosome.
  (b) **47,XY,+21** indicates 47 chromosomes, XY sex chromosomes, and an extra chromosome 21 (trisomy 21).
  (c) **45,X/46,XX/47,XXX** indicates mosaicism for three cell lines.

(3) **Formulas for karyotypes with structurally altered chromosomes** may or may not use the band-numbering system to define chromosome rearrangements ac-

BOX 1-1.	Sample of Symbols Used in Cytogenetic Nomenclature
del	= deletion
der	= derivative chromosome
dic	= dicentric chromosome
fra	= fragile site
i	= isochromosome
idic	= isodicentric chromosome
inv	= inversion
m	= marker chromosome
mat	= derived from mother
p	= short arm of chromosome
pat	= derived from father
q	= long arm of chromosome
r	= ring chromosome
rec	= recombinant chromosome
t	= translocation
ter	= terminal (end of chromosome)
pter	= terminal end of p arm
qter	= terminal end of q arm
→	= from → to

cording to the points of breakage and reunion (**breakpoints**). Examples include the following.

(a) **46,X,i(Xq)** indicates a female karyotype of 46 chromosomes, one normal X chromosome, and an isochromosome (see Chapter 2 III C) of Xq.

(b) **46,XX,-13,+t(13q21q)** indicates a female karyotype with 46 chromosomes and an **unbalanced robertsonian translocation** (see Chapter 2 III E 3 a) between chromosomes 13 and 21. A normal chromosome 13 is replaced by a translocation chromosome combining the long arms of chromosome 13 and chromosome 21. The long arm of chromosome 21 is present in triplicate because there is one copy on each of the normal chromosomes 21 and a third copy on the translocation chromosome. The breakpoints are not indicated, but the translocation chromosome is a fusion of the long arms of chromosomes 13 and 21 near the centromeres. The short arms of both chromosomes were lost after formation of the translocation.

(c) **45,XX,t(14;21)(p11;q11)** indicates a female karyotype with 45 chromosomes, a **balanced robertsonian translocation** (see Chapter 2 III E 3 b) between chromosomes 14 and 21, and breakpoints at p11 on 14 and q11 on 21. The term **balanced** in human cytogenetics usually refers to karyotypes with structural rearrangements with no gain or loss of essential chromosome material. Although **robertsonian** translocations between any of the acrocentric chromosomes are described as balanced because they present a clinically normal phenotype, material is deleted from the short arms of the chromosomes involved. The short arms of these chromosomes contain multiple copies of rRNA genes as well as heterochromatin. Loss of heterochromatin and some copies of rRNA genes is compatible with a normal phenotype.

(d) **46,XY,r(4)(p16q34)** indicates a male karyotype of 46 chromosomes with one chromosome 4 in the form of a ring. The breakpoints are at p16 and q34.

(e) **46,XY,t(2;12)(p24;q21)** indicates a male karyotype of 46 chromosomes with a **balanced reciprocal translocation** (see Chapter 2 III F) between chromosomes 2 and 12. The breakpoints are at band p24 on chromosome 2 and on band q21 on chromosome 12.

(f) **46,XX,-2,+der(2),t(2;12)(p24;q21)pat** indicates an unbalanced female karyotype of 46 chromosomes with a derivative chromosome 2, from a balanced reciprocal translocation between chromosomes 2 and 12. There is only one normal chromosome 2, but two normal chromosomes 12. The karyotype has trisomy for segment 12q21 to the 12q telomere (12qter) and monosomy for segment 2p24 to the 2p telomere (2pter). The derivative chromosome is from the father (pat = paternal).

V. EPIGENETIC CONTROL OF GENE EXPRESSION

A. **Epigenetic factors affect the expression of genes without altering the genotype.** Many of these factors exist (see II B 5). **X inactivation** and **genomic imprinting** are examples of epigenetic mechanisms that are known to be involved in the pathogenesis of disease in some patients.

B. **X chromosome inactivation.** In normal female somatic cells, there are two X chromosomes, but most of the genes on one of the X chromosomes are inactive. The process by which this occurs is called **X inactivation** or **lyonization.**

1. The X chromosome with most of the genes turned off is called the **inactive X chromosome.** The other one is called the **active X chromosome.**

2. **If a mammalian somatic cell contains more than one X chromosome, all but one are inactivated.** For example:

a. In a **47,XXY** cell, there is one active and one inactive X chromosome (the Y chromosome is irrelevant to the process of X inactivation).

b. In a **49,XXXXX** cell, there is one active X chromosome and four inactive X chromosomes.

3. **X inactivation occurs early in embryogenesis,** in the morula and blastula stages of development. The process is completed at different times in different embryonic tissues.

4. The **process of X inactivation is random** in any single cell. Either the X chromosome inherited from the mother (called X^m) or the X chromosome inherited from the father (called X^p) may be inactivated, with equal likelihood.

5. Once X inactivation occurs in an embryonic cell, the **same X chromosome remains inactivated in all of the progeny** of that cell. Thus, if an embryonic cell happens to inactivate X^m, both of its daughter cells, all four of its granddaughter cells, all eight of its great-granddaughter cells, and so on also have X^m as the inactive X chromosome.

a. Females are **mosaics** with many small patches of cells containing an inactive X^m interspersed with small patches of cells containing an inactive X^p.

b. On the average, **half** of the cells in a female have an inactive X^m and half have an inactive X^p, but some tissues (and some women) may have substantially more cells with one or the other X chromosome active by chance.

6. X inactivation involves **most, but not all, genes** on the X chromosome.

a. A cluster of genes on the tip of the short arm of the X chromosome escapes X inactivation. These genes lie in or adjacent to the region of the X chromosome that pairs with the Y chromosome during meiosis in males.

b. Some genes in the more proximal short arm and in the proximal long arm of the X chromosome also escape X inactivation despite the fact that many surrounding genes are inactivated in the usual fashion.

7. The inactive X chromosome may be visible in an interphase cell as a condensed mass of chromatin, the **Barr body.**

a. The **maximum number of Barr bodies seen in a cell is equal to the number of inactivated X chromosomes** (i.e., one less than the total number of X chromosomes in the cell). For example:

(1) One Barr body may be seen in a 47,XXY cell (the presence of a Y chromosome is irrelevant to the process of X inactivation).

(2) Up to four Barr bodies may be seen in a 49,XXXXX cell.

b. Counting the number of Barr bodies in somatic cells (usually in smears of buccal mucosa) is the basis of the **sex chromatin test** for sex chromosome aneuploidy. This test is no longer used clinically because karyotyping is much more accurate.

8. The **inactive X chromosome replicates later** in the S phase of the cell cycle than the active X chromosome and the autosomes.

9. The **molecular mechanisms** responsible for X inactivation are only partially understood.

a. Separate mechanisms appear to exist for **initiation of inactivation** and for **maintaining it with high fidelity** during cell division.

b. A basic mechanism underlying X inactivation is **inhibition of transcription.** Transcriptional inhibition seems to be maintained on a locus-by-locus basis, although initial events in X inactivation involve the chromosome as a whole.

c. The DNA of inactive X chromosomes is extensively **methylated,** whereas the DNA of the active X chromosome and active genes on the autosomes is largely unmethylated. Methylation appears to be involved in maintaining rather than initiating X inactivation.

d. *XIST* is a gene that seems to be involved in X inactivation.

(1) *XIST* is located in Xq13, a region that is required for rearranged or deleted X chromosomes to be inactivated.

(2) *XIST* is transcribed from the inactive X chromosome but not from the active X.

(3) *XIST* activity is thought to turn off most genes on the chromosome on which it is expressed, thus initiating X inactivation.

10. **Dosage compensation.** Females normally have two X chromosomes, and males normally have one.
    a. Although the X chromosome contains many essential genes, most do not have homologues on the Y chromosome. In fact, most of the Y chromosome appears to be "junk DNA," that is, repetitive sequences that are without function.
    b. Despite the fact that females have **double doses of most X-linked genes** in comparison to males, the **amount of X-linked gene products is usually about the same** in males and females.
    c. X inactivation produces this **dosage compensation.**

11. **Clinical implications of X inactivation**
    a. A female who carries an **X-linked recessive mutation** (see Chapter 3 I D) on one of her two X chromosomes **may express the mutant phenotype if most of her cells happen to have inactivated the X chromosome carrying the normal gene.**
    b. A female **carrier of an X-linked recessive disease** (see Chapter 3 I D) **may not be detectable** by gene product assays (e.g., amount of protein or enzyme activity) if most of her cells happen to have inactivated the X chromosome carrying the mutant gene.
    c. Although **monosomy** (i.e., the presence of only one instead of the normal two copies) **for any autosome is lethal early in embryogenesis,** monosomy for the X chromosome is rather common in liveborn infants and produces a relatively mild phenotype (**Turner syndrome;** see Chapter 2 II C).
    d. **Trisomy** (i.e., the presence of three rather than the normal two copies) **of the sex chromosomes produces a much less severe phenotype** than trisomy for any of the autosomes (see Chapter 2 II B).

C. **Genomic imprinting** is differential expression of a gene depending on whether it was inherited from the mother or the father. This is sometimes called a **parent-of-origin effect.**

1. In classic mendelian genetics (see Chapter 3 I), the parent from whom a gene was inherited has no effect on its expression.

2. **Imprinting reflects a functional change in a gene.** The DNA sequence is not altered, but expression of the affected gene is modified.

3. **Imprinting affects only a minority of genes.** For most genes, expression does not seem to be related to parent of origin.

4. Imprinting of affected genes **occurs soon after conception** and, once established, is usually **transmitted to all the descendants** of an imprinted cell.

5. A gene's **imprint is reversed or removed** when a cell passes through **gametogenesis.** The effect usually depends on whether oogenesis or spermatogenesis is occurring.

6. The **molecular mechanisms** involved in genomic imprinting are poorly understood.
   a. **Imprinted genes** are usually differentially **methylated.**
   b. An **alteration of chromatin structure** may also be involved.

7. **Clinical consequences of genomic imprinting**
   a. The phenotypic features associated with **small deletions** of some chromosomes are thought to be due, at least in part, to a lack of expression of essential imprinted gene(s) on the intact homologue.
      (1) A **deletion** of the proximal long arm of **chromosome 15** (15q11q13) on the chromosome inherited from the **father** produces the **Prader-Willi syndrome,** a condition characterized by mental retardation and obesity (see Chapter 2 III A 3 a).
      (2) A **cytogenetically identical deletion** on the chromosome inherited from the **mother** produces a clinically different condition, **Angelman syndrome.** Af-

fected children have severe mental retardation, ataxia, lack of speech, and sei-zures.

(3) The difference between these two phenotypes is thought to be due to the lack of expression of a maternally imprinted gene or genes in Prader-Willi syn-drome and the lack of expression of different paternally imprinted gene(s) in the same chromosome region in Angelman syndrome. In both instances, the deletion affects the chromosome that normally expresses these genes so there is no active copy in the cell.

b. The phenotypic features associated with **uniparental disomy** of some chromo-somes are thought to be due to a lack of expression of essential imprinted gene(s). Uniparental disomy is the inheritance of both chromosomes in a pair from the same parent rather than inheriting one from each parent, as normally occurs.

(1) In most cases of **Prader-Willi syndrome** (see Chapter 2 III A 3 a) in which there is no cytogenetic deletion, **maternal uniparental disomy for chromo-some 15** has been found (see Chapter 2 II D).

(a) The cause of Prader-Willi syndrome in association with maternal unipa-rental disomy 15 is thought to be as follows: When both copies of chro-mosome 15 are inherited from the mother, neither expresses the mater-nally-imprinted gene(s) in the Prader-Willi region.

(b) Even though there is no chromosome deletion, there is still no gene prod-uct and Prader-Willi syndrome occurs.

(2) Maternal **uniparental disomy for chromosome 7** has been found in some chil-dren with otherwise unexplained small stature. The poor growth in these chil-dren is thought to be caused by a lack of expression of a maternally im-printed gene or genes.

c. Absence of some kinds of tumor suppression can occur by loss of just one copy of the responsible gene (rather than loss of both copies, as is usually required) if the remaining copy is inactivated by imprinting (see Chapter 11 III B). This mecha-nism appears to be involved in the development of **Wilms tumor,** which is a childhood neoplasm of the kidney.

STUDY QUESTIONS

DIRECTIONS: Each of the numbered items or incomplete statements in this section is followed by answers or by completions of the statement. Select the ONE lettered answer or completion that is BEST in each case.

1. Which one of the following types of genetic disease occurs most frequently?

(A) Autosomal dominant
(B) Autosomal recessive
(C) X-linked
(D) Chromosome abnormality
(E) Multifactorial

2. The overall incidence among livebirths of genetic disease and other congenital anomalies apparent by 25 years of age is approximately

(A) 0.5%
(B) 1%
(C) 8%
(D) 15%

3. The proportion of adult hospital admissions that occurs for diseases that are due mostly or entirely to genetic factors is approximately

(A) 1%
(B) 10%
(C) 30%
(D) 50%
(E) 75%

4. High-resolution chromosome banding is best described by which one of the following statements?

(A) It permits identification of individual single-copy genes
(B) It uses chromosomes in the mid-metaphase stage of cell division
(C) It permits the resolution of 350 to 400 dark and light bands per haploid chromosome set
(D) It is used to demonstrate fragile sites
(E) It allows demonstration of small alterations of chromosome structure

5. Which one of the following lists contains the correct order of meiotic events?

(A) Separation of sister chromatids, recombination, formation of the synaptonemal complex, separation of homologous chromosomes
(B) Separation of homologous chromosomes, formation of the synaptonemal complex, recombination, separation of sister chromatids
(C) Recombination, formation of the synaptonemal complex, separation of sister chromatids, separation of homologous chromosomes
(D) Formation of the synaptonemal complex, recombination, separation of sister chromatids, separation of homologous chromosomes
(E) Formation of the synaptonemal complex, recombination, separation of homologous chromosomes, separation of sister chromatids

6. Which one of the following statements describes a difference between gametogenesis in males and females?

(A) Synaptonemal complexes are only formed in females
(B) Mitotic division of germ-cell precursors occurs only in males
(C) Dictyotene occurs during meiosis I in females but not in males
(D) Meiosis in males begins in the fetus, whereas female meiosis does not begin until puberty
(E) Oocytes do not complete mitosis until after fertilization, whereas spermatocytes complete mitosis before mature sperm are formed

DIRECTIONS: Each set of matching questions in this section consists of a list of four to twenty-six lettered options (some of which may be in figures) followed by several numbered items. For each numbered item, select the ONE lettered option that is most closely associated with it. To avoid spending too much time on matching sets with large numbers of options, it is generally advisable to begin each set by reading the list of options. Then, for each item in the set, try to generate the correct answer and locate it in the option list, rather than evaluating each option individually. Each lettered option may be selected once, more than once, or not at all.

Questions 7–11

Match each of the following cytogenetic features with the most appropriate structure.

(A) Chromatid
(B) Centromere
(C) Variable band
(D) Fragile site
(E) Satellite

7. A feature not visualized on routine chromosome preparations

8. One of the two replicated copies of the chromosome that separate during meiosis

9. The primary constriction that divides the long arm of the chromosome from the short arm

10. A structure that normally occurs only on acrocentric chromosomes

11. A structure surrounded by heterochromatin that is stained during C banding

Questions 12–16

Match each of the following statements with the appropriate epigenetic mechanism.

(A) Genomic imprinting
(B) X chromosome inactivation
(C) Both
(D) Neither

12. Occurs in normal males but not in normal females

13. Occurs in normal females but not in normal males

14. Randomly turns off genes from either the mother or the father

15. Creates a mosaic pattern of gene expression in tissues of normal individuals

16. Accounts for parent-of-origin effects in the expression of some genes

ANSWERS AND EXPLANATIONS

1. The answer is E [I C]. Multifactorial disorders are the most frequently occurring type of genetic disease, with an incidence of about 46/1000 by 25 years of age. As a group, single gene disorders occur less than 1/10 as often as multifactorial conditions. Chromosome abnormalities have an incidence less than 1/25 as great.

2. The answer is C [I C]. Although most individual genetic diseases are rare, genetic diseases and congenital anomalies as a group are quite common, affecting some 79/1000 individuals by age 25 years.

3. The answer is B [I D 2]. Approximately 10% of adult hospital admissions are for diseases that are caused largely or entirely by genetic factors. Some 30% to 50% of admissions to pediatric hospitals are for genetic conditions or congenital anomalies.

4. The answer is E [IV A 2 b, C 1 b (2)]. High-resolution chromosome banding is done on cells captured in prophase or prometaphase. The chromosomes in such preparations are more extended, and regions that comprise single bands in standard G-banded preparations can be resolved into sub-bands, permitting the identification of smaller cytogenetic alterations. High-resolution banding generally permits the identification of 800 or more bands in the haploid karyotype, but this resolution is still far too poor to distinguish single-copy genes. Demonstration of fragile sites requires the application of a different special technique.

5. The answer is E [III B 1]. In meiosis I, DNA replication is followed by pairing of homologous chromosomes and formation of the synaptonemal complex. Recombination occurs between the homologues, which subsequently begin to separate, forming chiasmata (crossovers). In the first meiotic metaphase, one chromosome from each homologous pair goes to each daughter cell. The sister chromatids separate in the second meiotic division.

6. The answer is C [III C 2]. Oocytes are arrested in the dictyotene of meiosis I until just prior to ovulation. Meiosis in males begins at puberty. Formation of synaptonemal complexes and recombination occur during meiosis in both males and females. Mitotic division of germ-cell precursors prior to the onset of meiosis takes place in both oogenesis and spermatogenesis.

7–11. The answers are 7-D [IV C 1 b (6)], **8-A** [IV C 2 a (1) (a)], **9-B** [IV C 2 a (1) (a)], **10-E** [IV C 2 a (1) (c)], **11-B** [IV B 2 a (2), C 1 a (5)]. Fragile sites can be visualized only under special culture conditions, such as folate deprivation. Mitotic chromosomes contain parallel sister chromatids that separate during cell division. The centromere is the primary constriction that separates the p (short) and q (long) of the chromosome. The centromere is surrounded by heterochromatin that stains specifically with the C-banding technique. Satellites occur at the tips of the short arms of the acrocentric chromosomes (numbers 13, 14, 15, 21, and 22).

12–16. The answers are 12-D [V B, C], **13-B** [V B 1, 2], **14-B** [V B 4], **15-B** [V B 5], **16-A** [V C]. X chromosome inactivation normally occurs in cells of females, turning off most of the genes on one of the two X chromosomes. The process is random, with the maternally derived X chromosome (X^m) being inactivated in some cells and the paternally derived X chromosome (X^p) being inactivated in other cells. X inactivation occurs early in embryogenesis; all of the cells descended from an embryonic progenitor with X^m inactivated will have an inactive X^m, and cells descended from an embryonic progenitor with X^p inactivated will have an inactive X^p. Consequently, normal female tissues are composed of a mosaic of cells, some with an inactive X^m and others with an inactive X^p.

Genomic imprinting occurs in both males and females. Imprinting is a functional difference in gene expression determined by whether the gene was inherited from the father or the mother.

Chapter 2

Chromosome Anomalies

Fred J. Dill
Barbara C. McGillivray

I. **GENERAL FEATURES.** Chromosome abnormalities may be suspected in a variety of clinical situations. Fifteen percent of recognized (or diagnosed) pregnancies result in a spontaneous abortion; half of those aborted fetuses are chromosomally abnormal. Later in gestation, 6% of stillborn infants and a similar percentage of neonatal deaths have chromosome anomalies (i.e., abnormalities, aberrations). The fetus with a chromosome abnormality is more likely to be undergrown, to have malformations, or to have hydrops. Similarly, the small or dysmorphic infant or child may have a chromosome abnormality. Inherited chromosome problems may be suspected in couples with infertility or recurrent spontaneous abortions, with or without stillborn or liveborn dysmorphic infants. When the diagnosis of a chromosome abnormality is made prenatally, the outcome may be difficult to predict. Most available information regarding the clinical consequences of chromosome problems comes from observation of children diagnosed because of problems after birth.

A. **Types of chromosome anomalies** may be numerical or structural.

1. **Numerical anomalies** can result in either aneuploidy or polyploidy.
   a. **Aneuploidy** is the addition or loss of one or, rarely, two chromosomes.
   b. **Polyploidy** is the addition of complete haploid sets of chromosomes.

2. **Structural anomalies** are rearrangements of genetic material within or between chromosomes. These may be either genetically **balanced,** in which there is no change in the amount of essential genetic material, or **unbalanced,** in which there is a gain or loss of essential chromosome segments.

B. **Frequency of chromosome anomalies**

1. Fifty percent of early spontaneous abortions, or more than 5% of all recognized pregnancies, are chromosomally abnormal.

2. **Approximately 0.5% (1/200) of newborn infants have a chromosome abnormality.** Table 2-1 summarizes the types of abnormalities and their time of diagnosis.
   a. **Sex chromosome aneuploidy** is responsible for 33% of chromosome abnormalities.
   b. **Autosomal aneuploidy** causes 25% of chromosome abnormalities.
   c. **Balanced autosomal structural rearrangements** account for 33% of chromosome abnormalities.
   d. **Unbalanced structural anomalies** cause 8% of chromosome abnormalities.

3. Only the balanced structural anomalies and some sex chromosome anomalies are compatible with a normal phenotype.

C. **Clinical spectrum of chromosome anomalies.** A chromosome abnormality may be suspected in the following clinical situations:

1. **The infertile couple**
   a. Two to four percent of infertile couples have an autosomal rearrangement. Either person of the couple may have an altered chromosomal number or a deletion involving sex chromosomes.
   b. Chromosome abnormalities can result in nonproduction of sperm or ova or implantation failure.

2. **Spontaneous abortion and stillbirth**

TABLE 2-1. Types of Chromosome Abnormalities

Chromosome Abnormality	Resultant Aberration	Presentation
Triploidy	Three copies of all chromosomes	Usually results in miscarriage
Monosomy		
Autosomal	Single copy of one autosome	Lethal in early pregnancy
X chromosome	Single sex chromosome	Usually lethal during pregnancy, may present during infancy, childhood, or adolescence
Trisomy		
Autosomal	Three copies of an autosome	Lethal during gestation for all autosomes except 13, 18, and 21, which present at birth
Sex chromosome	Extra sex chromosome	Usually presents in late childhood or adulthood
Deletion		
Autosomal	Partial monosomy of one autosome	Usually presents at birth or during early childhood
X chromosome	Partial monosomy of an X chromosome	Variable presentation from birth to adulthood
Duplication		
Autosomal	Partial trisomy	Presents from birth to early childhood

    a. Spontaneous abortions may be associated with an empty gestational sac, a growth-disorganized embryo, or a malformed embryo or fetus (first trimester losses). Fetal growth retardation is common.
    b. Aneuploidy is seen in 50% or more of spontaneous abortions. It also results in stillbirth, usually with malformations.

  3. Abnormal livebirths
    a. Common clinical features include malformations, developmental delay, poor physical growth, and reproductive failure.
    b. The **occurrence** is often secondary to aneuploidy or unbalanced structural rearrangements.

II. NUMERICAL ALTERATIONS

A. Trisomy

  1. Definition. Trisomy is the presence of three copies of a chromosome rather than the normal two copies. Trisomies for each of the autosomes (i.e., nonsex chromosomes) except chromosome 1 have been recorded.
    a. Most trisomic embryos are lost in early pregnancy. Trisomy is the most common finding in chromosomally abnormal embryos studied after a spontaneous abortion.
    b. Viability of embryos with specific trisomies is dependent on both the size of the genetic imbalance and the genetic content of the specific chromosomes involved.

With rare exceptions, only autosomal trisomies 13, 18, and 21 survive to term and are seen in the population.

c. Trisomy for sex chromosomes, such as XXX or XXY, have fewer deleterious effects on development; neither spontaneously aborted fetuses nor stillborn fetuses are likely to have XXX or XXY. Most of these trisomies result in term livebirths.

2. Clinical examples

a. Trisomy 21. Approximately 1 in 680 newborns has Down syndrome. The frequency is doubled at 10 to 12 weeks of pregnancy; trisomy 21 is a common finding in spontaneously aborted fetuses.

  (1) Prenatal. The abnormalities observed on ultrasound include nuchal thickening, cystic hygroma that proceeds to fetal hydrops if severe, duodenal stenosis or atresia ("double bubble" sign), and short femur lengths (a less reliable sign). **Low maternal serum α-fetoprotein levels** increase the possibility that a fetus is affected with Down syndrome (see Chapter 14 II F 1).

  (2) Infancy. The infant has a characteristic face with a flat nasal bridge, epicanthic folds, Brushfield spots, protruding tongue, small ears, and a flat occiput. Investigations may reveal hyperbilirubinemia, rare leukemoid reactions, or cardiac lesions (most common are atrial septal, ventricular septal, and atrioventricular canal defects).

  (3) Childhood and adulthood. All affected children have mental retardation, which is usually moderate. Other features include short stature, autoimmune abnormalities, and hearing loss. All males are infertile; females have reduced fertility and a 50% risk of having a trisomy 21 pregnancy. Older adults are more likely to develop an Alzheimer type of presenile dementia. The life span, once the individual has survived the first year, averages 50 to 60 years.

b. Trisomy 13. The newborn incidence is approximately 1 in 5000.

  (1) Prenatal. Most trisomy 13 fetuses spontaneously abort in the first trimester. During the second trimester, abnormalities observed on ultrasound include growth retardation, congenital heart lesions, midline brain and facial lesions (e.g., holoprosencephaly), and omphalocele.

  (2) Newborn. The newborn also has midline abnormalities (i.e., scalp cutis aplasia, brain malformations, central or unilateral facial clefts), omphalocele, and polydactyly. Almost all affected newborns have lethal cardiac anomalies. Mental retardation in survivors is profound.

c. Trisomy 18. The newborn incidence is approximately 1 in 3500.

  (1) Prenatal. Most trisomy 18 pregnancies result in spontaneous abortions or stillbirths. Abnormalities such as severe intrauterine growth retardation, congenital heart lesions, and diaphragmatic hernia are frequently detected by ultrasound.

  (2) Infancy. The newborn with trisomy 18 has a small facies with prominent occiput, small ears, overlapping fingers, and rocker-bottom heels. Almost all of these newborns have cardiac as well as other internal malformations. Newborns are more likely to be female, and they are profoundly handicapped.

d. Klinefelter syndrome (47,XXY). The incidence of Klinefelter syndrome is 1 in 800 males.

  (1) The **clinical presentations** include the:

   (a) Young boy with mild delay and behavioral immaturity

   (b) Older boy with small, soft testes

   (c) Adult male with a eunuchoid habitus, gynecomastia, and poor musculature

   (d) Normal-appearing male with infertility

  (2) Affected males have increased risks for breast cancer and schizophrenia.

  (3) Progressive hyalinization and fibrosis of the seminiferous tubules usually lead to inadequate testosterone production at puberty and in adulthood, requiring supplementation of testosterone on a long-term basis. Most males are infertile.

e. 47,XYY syndrome occurs with the same frequency as 47,XXY.

(1) Males with 47,XYY are not dysmorphic.

(2) The diagnosis may be made coincidentally at prenatal diagnosis or with new-born screening.

(3) **Clinical features** include tall stature and mild social problems, but the majority of affected males are thought to be normal with normal fertility. Although initially publicized as such, the diagnosis of 47,XYY is **not associated with increased aggressive tendencies or criminal behavior** involving violence.

f. **47,XXX.** The incidence rate is 1 in 800 females, and most are never diagnosed.

(1) The **majority of 47,XXX females have no clinical manifestations** and have normal fertility and produce normal offspring. A small number may present with radioulnar synostosis, oligomenorrhea, and premature menopause.

(2) There is an increased risk of psychiatric problems, specifically schizophrenia, in these women.

3. **Pathogenesis of trisomy and associated factors**

a. **Nondisjunction** is a failure of segregation of chromosomes or chromatids at cell division, which can occur during meiosis or mitosis (Figure 2-1).

(1) Nondisjunction during the **first division of meiosis** (meiosis I) results from failure of homologous chromosomes to segregate (see Figure 2-1B).

(2) Nondisjunction at the **second division of meiosis** (meiosis II) results from the failure of sister chromatids to segregate (see Figure 2-1C).

(3) Both events produce gametes that are disomic or nullisomic for specific chromosomes, and fertilization produces aneuploid zygotes, either trisomic or monosomic (see II A 1, B 1, respectively).

(4) **Mitotic nondisjunction in somatic cells,** like a meiosis II error, is the failure of sister chromatids to segregate at anaphase. This results in a trisomic and a monosomic cell.

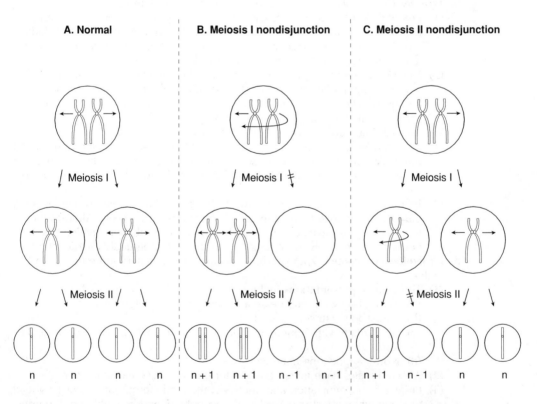

FIGURE 2-1. *(A)* Normal disjunction of a chromosome pair during meiosis I and II. *(B)* In meiosis I nondisjunction, it is the homologous chromosomes that fail to disjoin. *(C)* In meiosis II nondisjunction, it is the sister chromatids that fail to disjoin. Mitotic nondisjunction is equivalent to an error in meiosis II. The gametic chromosome number, which in humans is 23, is noted by *n*.

(5) Nondisjunction is a common event that appears to occur at a higher frequency in oogenesis than in spermatogenesis. Studies using cytogenetic and DNA polymorphisms (see Chapter 4 I B) have shown that in approximately 90% of the cases, the extra chromosome in Down syndrome patients comes from the mother. The majority of the extra chromosomes were derived from meiosis I errors.

(6) No **environmental agents,** such as low-level radiation, exogenous hormones, alcohol, or other drugs, have been shown to have a measurable influence on the rate of nondisjunction as measured by the frequency of trisomic infants born both to women exposed to these agents and to control mothers. (See Chapter 10 II for more information regarding environmental effects in pregnancy.)

(7) There is **no established genetic etiology** for primary nondisjunction in humans.

(8) The only clear influence on the rate of nondisjunction is the age of the mother.

b. Maternal age effect (see Chapter 7 II D 2). The occurrence of trisomy in livebirths and in spontaneous abortions increases with the age of the mother. Figure 2-2 indicates the rates for liveborn infants. The nature of the factors influencing chromosome segregation behavior as it relates to increasing age is unknown despite considerable research effort.

c. In trisomic cells during meiotic division, **secondary nondisjunction** occurs. For example, the female with Down syndrome produces either disomic or monosomic chromosome 21 gametes.

4. Recurrence risks. The occurrence rate of initial liveborn trisomy is correlated with maternal age (Table 2-2).

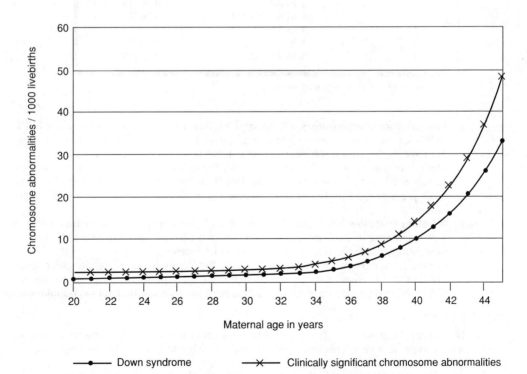

FIGURE 2-2. The influence of maternal age on the incidence per 1000 livebirths for Down syndrome and clinically significant chromosome abnormalities. The overall data include other trisomies, sex chromosome abnormalities, and unbalanced structural abnormalities. The occurrence of the latter is independent of maternal age. Therefore, the marked increase in the rate is due to numerical errors that are caused by nondisjunction.

TABLE 2-2. Chromosome Abnormalities in Newborns

Maternal Age at Birth	Risk for Newborn with	
	Down Syndrome	A Significant Chromosome Abnormality*
20	1 in 1420	1 in 500
21	1 in 1420	1 in 500
22	1 in 1330	1 in 500
23	1 in 1330	1 in 490
24	1 in 1250	1 in 480
25	1 in 1250	1 in 480
26	1 in 1210	1 in 480
27	1 in 1250	1 in 480
28	1 in 1210	1 in 460
29	1 in 1180	1 in 440
30	1 in 1140	1 in 420
31	1 in 1000	1 in 390
32	1 in 830	1 in 330
33	1 in 630	1 in 290
34	1 in 490	1 in 250
35	1 in 360	1 in 190
36	1 in 282	1 in 160
37	1 in 220	1 in 130
38	1 in 170	1 in 110
39	1 in 130	1 in 88
40	1 in 100	1 in 70
41	1 in 80	1 in 55
42	1 in 60	1 in 43
43	1 in 48	1 in 34
44	1 in 38	1 in 27
45	1 in 30	1 in 20

* Excludes unbalanced translocation and XXX.

   a. Trisomies for chromosomes 13, 18, and 21. The recurrence risk for trisomy is 1% to 2% for the mother whose first trisomic infant was born when she was younger than age 30 (in which the occurrence is less than 1 in 1200). If the mother is older than age 30 when the infant is born, the risk will be the same as her age-associated risk (e.g., if she was 37 years of age at the birth of the affected infant and is 39 years of age during her next pregnancy, her risk will be that of any 39-year-old).

   b. All other trisomies (excluding those for sex chromosomes) are rarely found late in a pregnancy or in livebirths. The diagnosis of a trisomic spontaneous abortion does not increase the risk for a liveborn with trisomy.

   c. Klinefelter syndrome, XYY, and XXX. Only the frequency of Klinefelter syndrome (47,XXY) is increased with advanced maternal age. The recurrence rate for these sex chromosome abnormalities is not higher than that for the general population.

B. Monosomy

   1. Definition. Monosomy is the presence of only one member of a chromosome pair in a karyotype. It is generally more detrimental to embryonic and fetal development than is the equivalent trisomy.

     a. Autosomal monosomies are not observed in livebirths or in early spontaneous abortions because they are lethal to the conceptus.

     b. Monosomy for the X chromosome (45,X) is common in chromosomally abnormal, spontaneously aborted embryos, but it is also seen in patients with Turner syndrome.

2. Clinical example. Among liveborn females, 1 in 2500 has Turner syndrome.

   a. First trimester. The majority of 45,X conceptuses are growth-disorganized embryos that spontaneously abort during the first trimester of pregnancy. These monosomies represent about 10% of early spontaneous abortions.

   b. Second trimester. Some 45,X fetuses are detected on ultrasound. The fetus has a cystic hygroma or a more generalized fluid collection (e.g., hydrops fetalis). Additional findings include preductal coarctation and horseshoe kidney. The majority of these fetuses are stillborn.

   c. Infancy. Infants with Turner syndrome may be normal, or they may have features such as residual neck webbing from the cystic hygroma, shield chest, coarctation, and edema of the hands and feet.

   d. Childhood. The presenting features during childhood are short stature or a cardiac murmur. Teenagers present with primary or secondary amenorrhea or lack of secondary sex characteristics because of streak ovaries. The majority are infertile. Turner syndrome females are mentally normal but may have spatial–perceptual abnormalities.

   e. Adulthood. Women with Turner syndrome who go untreated with replacement hormonal therapy have osteoporosis and earlier cardiovascular disease.

   f. Note that many females with the Turner phenotype may have karyotypes other than 45,X [e.g., X chromosome mosaicism (see II C 2 b), Xq isochromosome (see III C), or Xp deletion (see III A)]. However, the karyotype in spontaneously aborted fetuses and those with fetal hydrops is likely to be 45,X.

3. Pathogenesis. Monosomy may result from nondisjunction or chromosome lag. A chromosome may lag at anaphase and be excluded from a new nucleus. In males, lag of the Y chromosome at meiosis is thought to be a common cause of X chromosome monosomy (i.e., Turner syndrome).

4. Recurrence risks for 45,X or variations do not increase with advancing maternal age, and there is no increased risk after a pregnancy that results in a miscarriage, a stillbirth, or an infant with Turner syndrome.

C. Mosaic aneuploidy

1. Definition. Mosaicism is the presence of two or more cell lines with different karyotypes in a single individual.

   a. A normal diploid line commonly exists with an abnormal cell line. The abnormal line may have a numerical or a structural anomaly.

   b. Note that a specific cell line may be represented in all tissues or may be confined to single or multiple tissues.

2. Clinical features. The range of features for any mosaic situation depends on the specific chromosome involved and the proportions of normal and abnormal cell lines.

   a. Autosomal examples

   (1) Mosaic trisomy 8. Children are usually well grown with mild facial dysmorphism and are mentally retarded. Their fingers have flexion deformities, and there are deep creases on the palms and soles (Figure 2-3). Lymphocyte chromosomes are commonly normal, whereas fibroblast cultures demonstrate mosaicism for chromosome 8. Therefore, when the diagnosis is suspected, skin biopsy is necessary (see Chapter 1 IV C). Nonmosaic trisomy 8, like most other autosomal trisomies, is fatal.

   (2) Mosaicism for trisomies 13, 18, and 21 occurs in some patients. About 2% of those with trisomy 21 have normal and trisomic cells. Clinical features are usually similar to those in nonmosaic cases, but milder forms do not come to attention.

   b. Sex chromosome example: mosaic Turner syndrome. The clinical presentation of mosaic Turner syndrome is variable and depends on the proportions of the normal and aneuploid cell lines.

   c. Undiagnosed low-level mosaicism. A parent with low-level mosaicism or gonadal mosaicism may be clinically normal and escape attention. The condition may be diagnosed only when two or more offspring are noted to have the nonmosaic trisomy for the same chromosome.

FIGURE 2-3. A child with mosaic trisomy 8 exhibiting growth failure and flexion contractures of the fingers and toes. These children also exhibit deep palmar creases and are significantly handicapped.

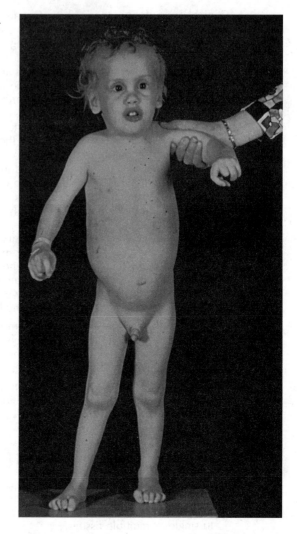

d. Confined chorionic mosaicism (confined placental mosaicism). In approximately 2% of chorionic villus sampling preparations, mosaicism confined to the chorion is detected. This may complicate prenatal diagnostic testing (see Chapter 14 II C 5 d).

3. Pathogenesis. Mosaicism arises from nondisjunction or chromosome lag in early cleavage or embryogenesis. Because cells are channeled into specific lineages in early development, the mosaicism can be confined to the placenta, the embryo, or a tissue within the embryo.

4. Recurrence risks. Parents of children with autosomal mosaicism do not have an increased risk for subsequent children to have mosaicism. However, parents of children with autosomal mosaicism have the same risks for future autosomal trisomic offspring as those with nonmosaic trisomic offspring.

5. Implications for offspring of mosaic individuals. All mosaic individuals, including those with undiagnosed low-level mosaicism, have an increased risk of having nonmosaic chromosomally abnormal offspring because of secondary nondisjunction (see II A 3 c). The risk depends on the proportion of trisomic germ-line (sex) cells to normal germ-line cells.

D. **Uniparental disomy (UPD)**

1. **Definition.** UPD is the presence in a diploid cell line of both chromosomes of a given pair from only one of the parents. This may occur by chromosome lag in a trisomic cell such that the remaining two chromosomes originated from one parent. As chromosome loss or lag from a trisomic cell could occur during cleavage or in a subsequent cell lineage, the resultant diploid cell line could have UPD.

2. **Possible consequences of UPD** include the following:
   a. **Imprinting of single genes or chromosome regions.** If genes may be expressed differently according to the parent of origin (see Chapter 1), then having both chromosomes from one parent may result in abnormal levels of gene product.
   b. **Homozygosity for mutant alleles** (see Chapter 3)

3. **Possible presentations of UPD**
   a. **Confined placental mosaicism.** If the zygote was originally trisomic, and one chromosome was lost secondary to lag, in one-third of cases, the resulting diploid fetus will have UPD for the chromosome involved in the trisomy.
   b. **Intrauterine growth retardation (IUGR).** UPD for chromosome 7 has been documented in Russell-Silver dwarfism, which is a syndrome involving unexplained IUGR, triangular facies, hemihypertrophy, and normal intelligence. It is possible that UPD may explain a proportion of other cases of IUGR as well.
   c. **Microdeletion syndromes demonstrating skewed parent of origin.** A proportion of children with Prader-Willi syndrome has UPD for chromosome 15 (maternal), whereas in children with Angelman syndrome, the UPD for chromosome 15 is paternal.

E. **Polyploidy**

1. **Two polyploid conditions occur in humans.**
   a. **Triploidy** is the instance of 69 chromosomes with XXX, XXY, or XYY sex chromosome complements.
   b. **Tetraploidy** is the instance of 92 chromosomes and either XXXX or XXYY sex chromosome complements.

2. **Clinical examples**
   a. **Triploidy** represents 20% of chromosomally abnormal spontaneous abortions and is occasionally encountered later in pregnancy.
      (1) **First trimester.** The placenta has focal trophoblastic hyperplasia and hydatidiform changes to the chorionic villi (partial hydatidiform mole). Unlike the true molar pregnancy, a small embryo is usually present.
      (2) **Second and third trimesters.** On ultrasound, growth retardation and progressive oligohydramnios are recognized. The fetus has a relatively large head, congenital heart lesions, and syndactyly. The placenta is small.
      (3) **Livebirths.** Rarely, liveborn infants survive for a brief period with clinical features like those in the fetus.
   b. **Tetraploidy** represents 6% of early chromosomally abnormal spontaneous abortions.
      (1) Most tetraploid fetuses are lost in the first trimester.
      (2) In the rare instance of an ongoing pregnancy, the fetus has marked growth retardation, microcephaly, and multiple malformations.

3. **The pathogenesis of triploidy and tetraploidy differ.**
   a. **Triploidy** results from a failure of meiosis in a germ cell or from a fertilization error such as dispermy. Meiotic failure could result in fertilization of a diploid egg with a haploid sperm or fertilization of a haploid egg with a diploid sperm.
   b. **Tetraploidy** is a consequence of a failure of the first cleavage division, which results in a doubling of the chromosome number immediately after fertilization.

4. **Recurrence risks.** Neither triploidy nor tetraploidy has an increased risk of recurrence.

III. **STRUCTURAL ALTERATIONS** result from breakage and fusion of chromosome segments in novel ways. Many new structures, such as acentric fragments of chromosomes and dicentric chromosomes, are very unstable at cell division, which leads to loss of chromosome material that may result in cell death. A variety of stable chromosome alterations occur in humans.

A. **Deletions** represent a loss of chromatin from a chromosome.

1. **Classification**
   a. **Terminal deletions** arise from one break. The acentric fragments that are formed are lost at the next cell division.
   b. **Interstitial deletions** arise from two breaks, fusion at the break sites, and loss of the interstitial acentric fragment.
   c. **Ring chromosomes** arise from breaks on either side of the centromere and fusion at the breakpoints on the centric segment. Segments distal to the breaks are lost so that individuals with chromosome rings have deletions from both the long arm (q) and short arm (p) of the chromosome involved.
   d. Deletions may also occur as a result of **segregation of a familial inversion or translocation** (see III D–F).

2. **Clinical examples.** Deletions of many segments of the karyotype are documented. A cytogenetically detectable deletion in euchromatin (see Chapter 1 IV B 1) results in an abnormal phenotype. Three well-characterized deletion syndromes are described below. In each, the recognizable clinical features are secondary to the loss of a critical area of the chromosome involved (usually a specific band or sub-band of the chromosome).
   a. **5p- (Cri du chat, or cat cry syndrome)**
      (1) **Features.** This syndrome was the first autosomal deletion to be described. The infants have round facies, a cat-like cry, which disappears with time, and cardiac defects. Infants with cat cry syndrome are severely mentally retarded.
      (2) Most children have a de novo deletion of a variable amount of the short arm of chromosome 5 (5p), with the critical area being 5p15.
   b. **4p- (Wolf-Hirschhorn syndrome)**
      (1) **Features.** The infants have prominent foreheads and a broad nasal root ("Greek warrior helmet"). The philtrum is short, and the mouth is downturned. These infants are severely mentally retarded. They commonly have cardiac defects and exhibit growth failure.
      (2) Ten to fifteen percent of the deletions are associated with **familial translocations**. The essential region involved is 4p16.
   c. **Ring chromosome 14.** The clinical features are dependent on the breakpoints, but commonly observed breakpoints are at 14p11 and 14q32. Children may have mild dysmorphic features; seizures are frequent, and the occurrence of mental retardation is variable.

3. **Microdeletion syndromes** result from small deletions that require high-resolution banding for cytogenetic diagnosis.
   a. **Prader-Willi syndrome.** The clinical features of Prader-Willi syndrome evolve after birth.
      (1) **Infancy.** The infant has profound hypotonia and poor feeding for the first year. The differential diagnosis includes sepsis, a metabolic abnormality, or a myopathy.
      (2) **Early childhood.** Between the second and third years, the child with Prader-Willi syndrome develops an insatiable appetite and truncal obesity; the hands and feet are small. The face has bifrontal narrowing and almond-shaped eyes; the hair color is fair (Figure 2-4). Most children have developmental delay.
      (3) **Late childhood.** Obesity increases without therapy. Behavioral problems and rage episodes develop with age.
      (4) **Chromosomes.** About 60% of children with Prader-Willi syndrome have cytogenetically visible deletions or rearrangements involving 15q11–13; an additional 15% are detected using fluorescent in situ hybridization (FISH) technol-

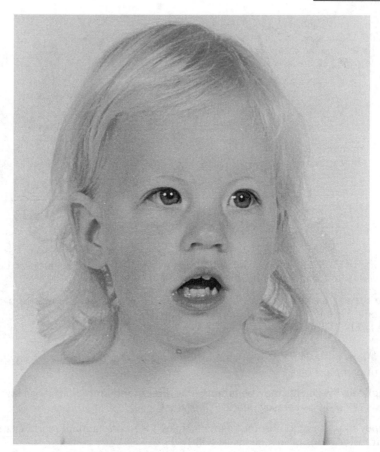

FIGURE 2-4. A young child with Prader-Willi syndrome in association with a 15q deletion. She exhibits bifrontal narrowing and is fair skinned.

ogy (see Chapter 1 IV C 1 b 9) to detect submicroscopic deletions (Figure 2-5). The remaining 25% of cases result from maternal UPD of chromosome 15 and have no deletion. In these cases, the cause of the Prader-Willi phenotype is failure of expression of imprinted genes in the critical region.

b. Miller-Dieker syndrome (agyria, lissencephaly). Lissencephaly, or smooth brain, may be found in a variety of conditions. Miller-Dieker syndrome refers to lissencephaly and dysmorphic features (e.g., microcephaly, a high forehead, furrow-

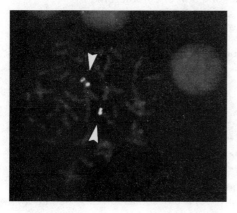

FIGURE 2-5. The bright rhodamine fluorescence *(arrows)* represents a hybridization signal for a Prader-Willi region probe and a chromosome 15 identifier probe. In this fluorescence in situ hybridization (FISH) example, the signal for the Prader-Willi region is present on only one chromosome 15, which indicates a submicroscopic deletion.

FIGURE 2-6. A pair of G-banded chromosomes 17 from a patient with Miller-Dieker syndrome. The normal chromosome 17 is on the *left,* and the chromosome with the p13.3 deletion is on the *right.* The breakpoint is indicated by the *arrow.*

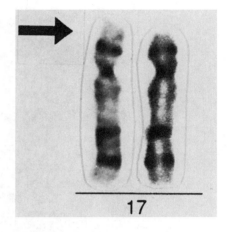

17

ing of the central forehead), which are associated with a deletion of 17p13.3 (Figure 2-6). Death occurs early.

4. The **recurrence risk** is negligible for these deletion syndromes unless a parent has a chromosome rearrangement (see III F). Therefore, parents must be investigated before the family is counseled.

B. **Duplications** represent a gain of chromosome material and result in trisomy for segments of chromosomes.

1. Duplicated segments may be arranged as **direct tandem repeats** or as **inverted repeats** of chromosome segments.

2. Duplications of chromosome segments may arise from familial rearrangements such as **translocations** or **inversions** (see III D–F).

3. The **risk of recurrence** is not high unless the duplication is part of a familial chromosome rearrangement.

C. **Isochromosomes.** One of the chromosome arms (p or q) is duplicated, and all material from the other arm is lost. The arm on one side of the centromere is a mirror image of the other.

1. **Clinical examples.** Isochromosomes for most autosomes incur a major genetic imbalance, which creates a lethal situation. However, isochromosomes for the q arms of some acrocentric chromosomes (see Chapter 1 IV C 2 a) are compatible with a normal phenotype provided they are the sole representative of the involved chromosome in the karyotype.

a. For example, in an isochromosome of the long arm of chromosome 21 [45,XX,i(21q)], the short arms of both 21 chromosomes are absent from the karyotype and the long arms are represented twice in one chromosome. This is similar to a robertsonian translocation carrier (see III E 1 a–c), in which loss of short-arm material for the involved acrocentric chromosomes has **no adverse effect on the phenotype**.

b. If a chromosome or area is imprinted, the uniparental disomy situation created with an isochromosome has clinical consequences. For example, maternal i(15q) leads to **Prader-Willi syndrome**.

c. For sex chromosomes, isochromosome Xq is seen in approximately 10% to 15% of females with **Turner syndrome**. These females have one normal X chromosome, and the Xq isochromosome. This is the functional equivalent of monosomy Xp. The clinical picture is identical to 45,X Turner syndrome (see II B 2).

2. **Pathogenesis.** Isochromosomes may arise from a centromere division error that is at right angles to the normal separation. Long-arm isochromosomes have, by definition,

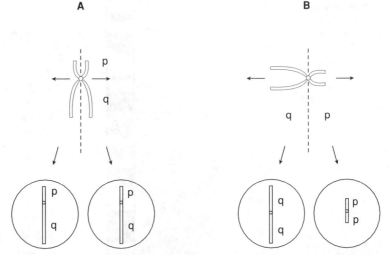

FIGURE 2-7. *(A)* Normal centromere division. *(B)* Centromere misdivision, creating a long-arm isochromosome on the *left* and a short-arm isochromosome on the *right*.

deletions of the short arm, and short-arm isochromosomes have deletions of the long arm (Figure 2-7). Other more complex mechanisms also result in isochromosomes or isodicentric chromosomes.

3. **Recurrence.** If a parent has an isochromosome for an autosome such as i(21q) the risk for trisomic offspring is 100%. Since the isochromosome can go to one gamete at meiosis, only disomic and nullisomic gametes can be produced. Fertilized nullisomic gametes are lethal monosomies. Fertilized disomic gametes are trisomic (chromosome 21).

D. **Inversions** are a reversal of the order of chromatin between two breaks on the chromosome. They are encountered as new mutations or may be present in multiple generations in families.

1. **Types of inversions**
   a. **Pericentric inversions** are the result of breaks and rearrangements on both sides of the centromere (Figure 2-8). An inverted chromosome often has a strikingly different morphology than the parental chromosome.
   b. **Paracentric inversions** are the result of breaks and rearrangements on the same side of the centromere. These inverted chromosomes have similar overall morphology to the parental chromosomes, but the band order is changed.

2. **Meiotic segregation**
   a. **Pericentric inversions**
      (1) Since carriers of inversion usually have one normal and one inverted chromosome, the pairing constraints at prophase of meiosis necessitate the **formation of a loop** (Figure 2-9).
         (a) A recombination event within the loop structure produces chromosomes with duplications and deletions of segments outside the breakpoints that formed the inversion.
         (b) Chromosome strands not involved in the recombination are similar to the parental chromosomes (one normal; one inverted).
      (2) Embryos receiving a **recombined chromosome** have **unbalanced karyotypes**. Survival to term depends on both the size of duplications and deletions and the chromosome involved.
   b. **Paracentric inversions**
      (1) As with pericentric inversions, meiotic pairing constraints lead to **loop formation** between the junctions of the inverted segment.

FIGURE 2-8. Example of a pericentric inversion in chromosome 6, with breakpoints at bands p22 and q25 indicated by *arrows*. A carrier of the inversion would have both a normal chromosome 6 *(6)* and an inverted chromosome 6 *(Inv 6)*.

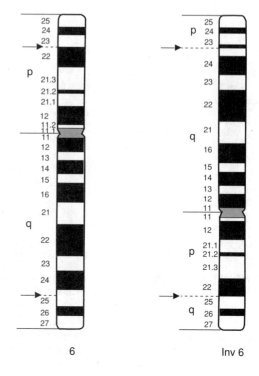

6   Inv 6

(2) A single recombination event within the loop produces **unstable recombinant chromosomes** (either dicentric or acentric), which are usually lethal and rarely seen in liveborn children of carriers. Most often, only the parental chromosomes (normal or inverted) are transmitted to clinically normal offspring.

3. **Clinical features**
   a. **Carriers** of either pericentric or paracentric inversions **are normal**.
   b. **Diagnosis** is based on the following:
      (1) Coincidental finding at prenatal diagnostic testing
      (2) Spontaneous abortions, with unbalanced products having large duplications and deletions
      (3) Stillbirths or livebirths, with small duplication and deletion products of the inversion

4. **Recurrence risks**
   a. If the ascertainment is through an **abnormal stillbirth or livebirth,** there is an overall 5% to 10% risk for recurrence of an abnormal livebirth.
   b. If the ascertainment is through **recurrent miscarriage,** the risk is low for an abnormal livebirth.
   c. If the finding is **coincidental** at prenatal diagnosis, the risk of recurrence is 1% to 3%.
   d. Each family needs to be considered individually.

E. **Robertsonian translocations** (centric fusions) result from fusion of whole arms of acrocentric chromosomes, which are chromosomes 13–15, 21, and 22 (Figure 2-10).

1. The **breakpoints** forming these rearrangements are at or near the centromeres of both chromosomes involved.
   a. Only the long-arm fusion chromosome product is usually recovered (the short-arm product is lost), so that **heterozygous carriers** for this class of rearrangements **have only 45 chromosomes**.
   b. These carriers of robertsonian translocations are normal, and the translocation is

A. Pericentric inversion segregation

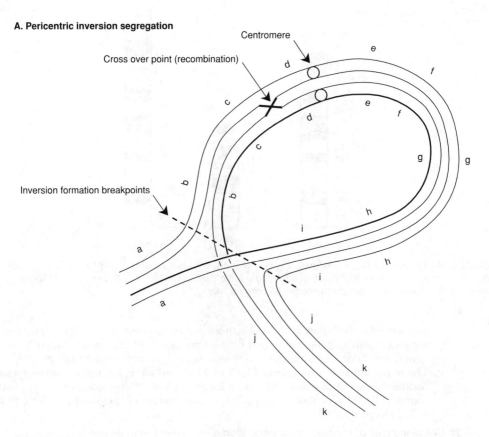

B. Segregation products

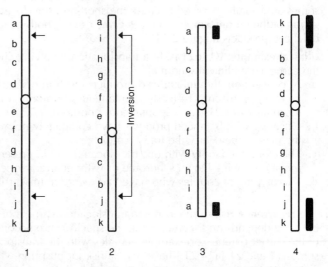

FIGURE 2-9. Pericentric inversion segregation. *(A)* The loop formed to accommodate homologous pairing of the inverted segment is shown here. Note that the centromere is within the loop. This example shows a single crossover event within the loop. *(B)* With a single crossover, two segregation products (*1* and *2*) will be like the parental chromosomes, normal or inverted, and two (*3* and *4*) will have duplications and deficiencies (indicated by the *black bars*). In *3*, segment *a* is duplicated and segment *jk* is absent; in *4*, the situation is reversed. Both products, *3* and *4*, will produce an abnormal embryo, fetus, or newborn. Note that if a crossover does not take place within the inversion loop, all products will be like the parental chromosomes.

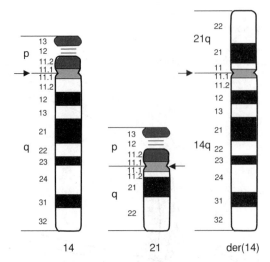

14   21   der(14)

FIGURE 2-10. Example of 14;21 robertsonian translocation, with breakpoints at 14p11 and 21q11 indicated by *arrows*. A carrier of this translocation would have single normal 14 *(14)* and 21 *(21)* chromosomes and the single derivative chromosome 14 product *[der (14)]*.

considered to be balanced because short-arm material on acrocentric chromosomes consists of genetically inert heterochromatin and ribosomal RNA (rRNA) genes, which occur in multiple copies on other acrocentric chromosomes.

   c. The **robertsonian translocation 45,XX or XY,t(13q14q) is the most common translocation found in humans** and has an incidence rate of approximately 1 in 1500 individuals. Translocation 14q21q is also common and is frequently a cause of familial Down syndrome.

2. **Consequences of meiosis in carriers.** Homologous segments of two translocation chromosomes pair at meiosis. However, in robertsonian translocations, three chromosomes are usually involved because the short-arm translocation product is lost. Segregation of the chromosome produces gametes with both genetically balanced and unbalanced products (Figure 2-11).

3. **Clinical example: t(14q21q).** In a translocation involving chromosomes 14 and 21, the carriers are clinically normal.

   a. At conception, the unbalanced products result in essentially trisomy 21 (likely to go to term), trisomy 14 (early spontaneous abortion), or monosomy of either chromosome 14 or 21 (early spontaneous abortion).

   b. Offspring with balanced products have completely normal chromosomes or, like the parent, they carry the translocation.

   c. Therefore, the family with this translocation could present with multiple family members having Down syndrome or with recurrent miscarriages.

   d. **Karyotyping** of couples who have had recurrent miscarriages should be considered.

4. The **recurrence risk** to robertsonian translocation carriers of all types for abnormal offspring depends on ascertainment, the specific chromosomes involved, and the sex of the carrier parent. For example, females with the translocation between chromosomes 14 and 21 [t(14;21)] have a 10% risk for offspring with Down syndrome, whereas the male carrier has a 2% risk (Table 2-3).

F. **Reciprocal translocation** results from breakage and exchange of segments between chromosomes. The points of exchange can be at any location along the chromosomes (Figure 2-12).

1. **Consequences of meiosis in carriers** (Figure 2-13)

   a. Homologous segments of the two chromosomes involved in a translocation undergo pairing to **form a four-part structure** (see Figure 2-13A).

A. Meiotic pairing complex

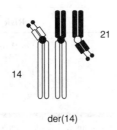

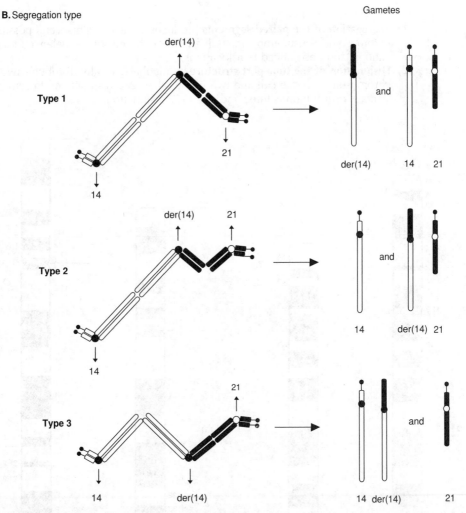

FIGURE 2-11. Robertsonian translocation segregation. *(A)* Meiotic pairing complex in a carrier of a t(14; 21)(p11;q11) robertsonian translocation. The complex is shown as a three-part structure with homologous segments of the involved chromosomes paired. *(B)* Segregation is one of the three possibilities *(1–3)*. In type *1*, the derivative *[der(14)]* chromosome segregates from chromosomes 14 and 21. Fertilization of the resulting gametes produces a balanced translocation karyotype or a normal one. Both gametes produce a normal phenotype. In segregation types *2* and *3*, all of the gametes are abnormal and will result in long-arm (q) trisomy or monosomy of either chromosome 21 or 14. Only one of the gametes from type *2* [der(14) and 21] will produce viable offspring after fertilization. These children will have Down syndrome (trisomy 21q).

TABLE 2-3. Risks of Carriers for Having Liveborn Offspring with Unbalanced Karyotypes

Abnormality	Risk
Robertsonian t(14;21)	10% (female)
	2% (male)
Isochromosome i(21q)	100%
Reciprocal translocations	≤ 30%–40%*
Inversions	≤ 5%–10%*

* Risks for reciprocal translocations and inversions vary among individual anomalies. Those that produce a large chromosome imbalance usually have a lower risk since they are lethal to the embryo and result in miscarriage.

(1) **Segregation of the paired segments** produces gametes with several possible chromosome constitutions, including normal chromosomes, balanced translocations, and unbalanced translocations.

(2) **Disjunction of the four-part structure** at anaphase usually distributes two chromosomes to one cell and two to the other (2:2 disjunction). In some instances, distribution is three and one (3:1 disjunction).

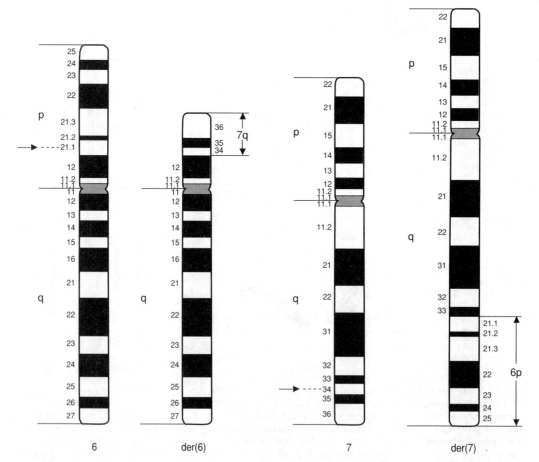

6   der(6)   7   der(7)

FIGURE 2-12. Example of a 6;7 reciprocal translocation with breakpoints at 6p21 and 7q34 indicated by the *arrows*. A carrier of this translocation would have single normal chromosomes 6 and 7 and the two derivative chromosomes *[der(6) and der(7)]*.

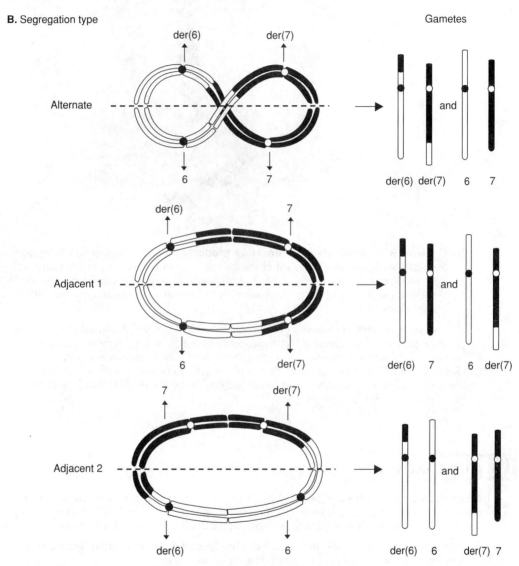

A. Meiotic pairing complex

der(6) 7

6 der(7)

B. Segregation type

Gametes

der(6) der(7)

Alternate

6 7

der(6) der(7) 6 7

der(6) 7

Adjacent 1

6 der(7)

der(6) 7 6 der(7)

7 der(7)

Adjacent 2

der(6) 6

der(6) 6 der(7) 7

FIGURE 2-13. Reciprocal translocation segregation. *(A)* Meiotic pairing complex in a carrier of t(6;7)(p21; q34) reciprocal translocation. The complex shows a four-part structure with homologous segments of the involved chromosomes paired. *(B)* Segregation is one of three types (alternate or adjacent centromeres to the spindle pole at anaphase). Gametes from alternate segregation have a balanced translocation or are normal. Gametes from adjacent 1 and 2 segregation are all abnormal, with both duplications and deficiencies. For most translocations, abnormal clinical outcomes usually result from adjacent 1 segregation, as many of the unbalanced products produce viable abnormal offspring or result in recognized pregnancy loss. Most adjacent 2 segregation products have large duplications and deficiencies and would be lost before implantation. Note that segregation may result in movement of three chromosomes to one pole and one chromosome to the other, unlike the 2:2 segregation described in III F 1. For most translocations, this would be associated with major lethal imbalances. However, for a subset of reciprocal translocations, usually involving a small acrocentric chromosome (e.g., chromosome 21), viable 3:1 unbalanced products occur.

FIGURE 2-14. An X chromosome from a male with fragile X mental retardation showing the Xq27.3 fragile site *(arrow)*.

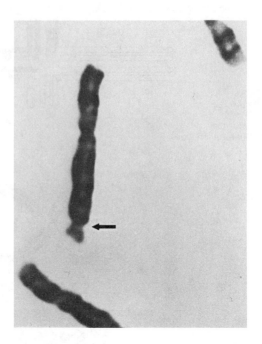

    b. Gametes with unbalanced translocation products from 2 : 2 disjunction have both duplications and deficiencies for chromosome segments involved in the translocation (see Figure 2-13B). Those from 3 : 1 disjunction may have duplications or deficiencies of segments of both chromosomes or be nullisomic or disomic for either chromosome.

  2. The **recurrence risks** to carriers of reciprocal translocations for abnormal offspring depend on previous reproductive history, ascertainment, predicted type of segregation, and the likely survival potential of zygotes with a specific chromosome imbalance. Generally, for those translocations that could result in chromosomally abnormal viable offspring, the risk for carriers is rarely greater than 20% to 30% and is likely to be lower (see Table 2-3).

IV. OTHER ANOMALIES

  A. **Chromosome fragile sites** are gaps or breaks in chromosomes that can be visualized if the cell cultures are provided with specific conditions [see Chapter 1 IV C 1 b (6)]. They are genetically transmitted traits and are specific to the location on chromosomes.

    1. There are over 100 fragile sites reported. One type, the **folate-sensitive group,** is now known to be the location of expanded trinucleotide repeats.

    2. Folate-sensitive sites have been found on **autosomes** and on the **X chromosome.** Only two sites on the X chromosome are associated with a clinical phenotype, the most common being **fragile X mental retardation.**

      a. Fragile X mental retardation exhibits a fragile site on the X chromosome at Xq27.3 (Figure 2-14).

      b. The clinical presentation and the details of inheritance are described in Chapter 3.

  B. **Marker chromosomes** are derived from structural rearrangements and are commonly found as extra chromosome pieces.

    1. The mechanism of formation and the chromosome of origin are unknown. Most chromosomes presenting as constitutional markers (as compared to tumor-cell–marker chromosomes) are commonly smaller than chromosome 22. They may be in the form of a ring or a bisatellite chromosome, or they may have metacentric morphology.

2. **Small markers** may exhibit mitotic instability and may have a mosaic form. Various amounts of heterochromatin or euchromatin may be present.

3. **Many markers are compatible with normal development and normal intelligence**, and they may be inherited with no phenotypic consequence. Others, such as inverted-duplication chromosome 15 markers, can have associated phenotypic abnormalities.

4. **Identification** of many markers can now be done using fluorescence in situ hybridization technology [see Chapter 1 IV C 1 b (7)].

5. The **clinical implications** depend on the origin and content of the marker itself.

C. **Chromosome breakage.** Chromosome breaks result in apparently random visible lesions in metaphase chromosomes. They can lead to structural changes such as deletions and translocations.

1. **Induction of lesions.** Lesions resulting from chromosome breaks may be induced by a variety of sources, including faulty DNA repair or synthesis, environmental insults such as radiation, or chromosome-breaking chemicals. Cell cultures from normal individuals exhibit chromosome breakage in low frequency. In a number of single gene syndromes, individuals have an intrinsically high incidence of breakage.

2. **Clinical examples.** These conditions are characterized by hematologic abnormalities and malformations in addition to chromosome breakage. Some of these are also associated with an increased risk for malignancy.
   a. **Fanconi anemia (Fanconi pancytopenia)**
      (1) **Clinical features**
         (a) Children may present with a variety of external and internal malformations. The most diagnostic malformations are radial and thumb abnormalities, patchy pigmentation over the trunk, congenital heart disease, and renal malformations.
         (b) In time, children develop pancytopenia from **bone marrow hypoplasia**. They may ultimately develop **leukemia** and require a bone marrow transplant.
      (2) **Confirmation of diagnosis** is achieved by demonstrating an elevated frequency of chromosome breakage in cultured lymphocytes. The frequency of breakage is increased markedly over that in controls with the use of the alkylating agent **diepoxybutane (DEB)**.
   b. **Bloom syndrome**
      (1) **Clinical features.** Affected children exhibit growth retardation and abnormal skin with telangiectases involving the face. All have an increased risk for developing malignancies. An increased frequency of chromosome breakage and homologous chromosome exchanges can be detected in cultured cells.
      (2) **Diagnosis** can be made by observing sister chromatid exchanges in cultured lymphocytes at up to 12 times the normal value.
   c. **Ataxia-telangiectasia**
      (1) **Clinical features.** In this condition, children present with progressive ataxia and telangiectasia involving the ears, conjunctiva, and other facial areas. Survival is poor with death resulting from chronic infections and malignancies.
      (2) **Diagnosis.** Cell lines are sensitive to ionizing radiation. Chromosomes from children with ataxia-telangiectasia exhibit increased breakage frequency under normal culture conditions.

STUDY QUESTIONS

DIRECTIONS: Each of the numbered items or incomplete statements in this section is followed by answers or by completions of the statement. Select the ONE lettered answer or completion that is BEST in each case.

1. A family seeks their physician's advice. The woman is pregnant, and she is concerned because her brother has Down syndrome. The physician ascertains that the affected brother lives in a local group home. Of the following methods of investigating and counseling, which one would be most appropriate?

(A) Review the family history
(B) Confirm the diagnosis in the affected brother
(C) Karyotype the affected brother
(D) Karyotype the woman coming for counseling

2. A newborn female is noted to have dorsal edema of the hands and feet as well as a cardiac murmur. The clinical suspicion is Turner syndrome, and a karyotype is quickly arranged. The results show that the infant is mosaic; 50% of the cells are 45,X and 50% of cells are 46,XY. The physician should advise the parents to take which one of the following actions with their child?

(A) The child has a Y chromosome and should be raised as a boy, which requires surgery and male hormones to help the process
(B) The child has a variant of Turner syndrome and will be short, is likely to have a congenital heart lesion, needs cardiac assessment, and should be raised as a female
(C) The child should be raised as a female but will require a gonadectomy because of the risk of malignancy

3. Of the following clinical situations, which one warrants a karyotype?

(A) A woman with one spontaneous abortion
(B) The parents of a child with trisomy 21
(C) The sister of a boy with Prader-Willi syndrome demonstrated to have the common deletion
(D) A couple with a stillbirth and three spontaneous abortions
(E) The maternal uncle of an infant with a maternally derived t(21;21)

DIRECTIONS: The set of matching questions in this section consists of a list of four to twenty-six lettered options (some of which may be in figures) followed by several numbered items. For each numbered item, select the ONE lettered option that is most closely associated with it. To avoid spending too much time on matching sets with large numbers of options, it is generally advisable to begin each set by reading the list of options. Then, for each item in the set, try to generate the correct answer and locate it in the option list, rather than evaluating each option individually. Each lettered option may be selected once, more than once, or not at all.

Questions 4–9

For each chromosomally abnormal pregnancy, assess the recurrence risk for future pregnancies.

(A) Increased
(B) Decreased
(C) Unchanged

4. A spontaneous abortion with triploidy

5. A stillbirth with triploidy

6. A spontaneous abortion with 45,X

7. A spontaneous abortion with trisomy 18

8. A liveborn with trisomy 21 (mother, age 23)

9. A liveborn with trisomy 21 (mother, age 40)

ANSWERS AND EXPLANATIONS

1. The answer is A [II A 2 a]. If there is a history of recurrent miscarriages, difficulties conceiving, or other family members with Down syndrome, the physician should consider the additional history as well as the possibility of a translocation accounting for the Down syndrome individual. If the mother was older than 35 years of age at the birth of the brother affected with Down syndrome, then trisomy would be the suspected cause. Since the affected brother is available, he could either be examined or the diagnosis could be documented. However, the question of a familial translocation would not be answered without karyotyping. The physician should arrange for blood to be sent to the local cytogenetic laboratory. By karyotyping the affected person first, the physician is able to offer information to the whole family. If the diagnosis is confirmed as a trisomy, the physician can reassure the family that the risk of Down syndrome is the same as the general population risk. If a translocation is discovered, the physician will need to karyotype the parents of the affected individual.

2. The answer is C [II B 2 c]. Although this infant does have a variant of Turner syndrome, it would be insufficient to offer the usual counseling. The parents need to be aware that a cell line with a Y chromosome is present, as this will put the gonads at increased risk for gonadoblastoma development. The child has presented as a female and, athough there is a Y chromosome line, it is not appropriate to rear her as a male. Although surgical conversion is possible, it would be extremely difficult to create a normal-appearing male surgically, and sexual function would be lacking. If an infant presents as a male (i.e., if traits such as unilateral testis or hypospadias are present), consideration may be given to raising him as such. Males with mixed gonadal dysgenesis may do well, but most often have short stature, and the gonads must be carefully watched.

3. The answer is D [III A 3 a, E, F; Table 2-2; Table 2-3]. The couple who experienced a stillbirth and three miscarriages has a history suggestive of translocation. In couples having three or more miscarriages, 1% to 3% have such a rearrangement. A woman who had one miscarriage is not at an increased risk statistically to have a translocation. The parents of a child with trisomy 21 are not necessarily candidates for karyotyping because the risk of recurrence depends on the maternal age, and the chromosomes of the parents would be expected to be normal. If the boy with Prader-Willi syndrome has the common interstitial deletion, it is not secondary to a familial rearrangement. Therefore, a karyotype of other family members is not necessary. A mother with a translocation resulting in t(21;21) is most likely to have chromosomally normal parents and siblings. If a parent of her own had the rearrangement, she would have had Down syndrome herself. Her brother also would be unlikely to carry the translocation.

4–9. The answers are: 4-C [II A 2 a; Table 2-1], **5-C** [II A 2 a], **6-C** [II C 2; Table 2-1], **7-C** [II A 2 c (1)], **8-A** [II A 2 a; Table 2-2], **9-C** [II A 2 a; Table 2-2]. Triploidy is a common cause of early spontaneous abortions; it is a sporadic event, and it is not associated with an increased risk in future pregnancies.

A spontaneous abortion with 45,X is also a common finding in early miscarriages. Turner syndrome is not known to be associated with increased maternal age, nor is there an increased risk in subsequent pregnancies.

Data suggest that trisomies ending in early miscarriages do not increase the risk for a subsequent liveborn with a trisomy. Data confirm that the recurrence risk of trisomy 21 to a mother at or below 30 years of age is increased to 1% to 2%. The same data show no increased risk (beyond that already existing with age) for an older mother.

Chapter 3

Single Gene Alterations

Barbara McGillivray
Michael R. Hayden

I. PATTERNS OF INHERITANCE

A. **Single gene (mendelian) inheritance** describes those conditions in which single mutant genes have a significant effect on human health and in which simple patterns of inheritance are seen. In 1866, Mendel called the characteristics that were transmitted either entirely or almost unchanged by hybridization as dominant, whereas those that became latent in the process were called recessive. Genes are recognized by the physical characteristics or traits that they determine. Pedigree analysis is essential in determining the mode of inheritance of many traits.

1. **Definitions.** The mode of inheritance for single gene conditions depends on whether the specific phenotype is seen in the heterozygote (dominant) or only in the homozygote (recessive).

   a. **Gene.** This term describes the hereditary factor that interacts with the environment to determine a trait.

   b. **Alleles** are alternative forms of a gene at a given locus. There may be multiple normal and abnormal alleles of any particular gene.

   c. A **locus** is the specific physical location of a gene on a chromosome. Since human chromosomes are paired, individuals have two alleles at each locus (the exceptions are genes on the Y chromosome and the X chromosome in males).

   d. **Genotype** describes the genetic constitution of an individual, which is the specific allelic makeup of an individual.

   e. **Phenotype** describes the end result of both the genetic and environmental factors giving the clinical picture or the observed expression of the gene. Genotype–phenotype correlation studies seek to define whether certain clinical features of a condition are seen with a specific mutation to the gene.

   f. If the alleles at a single locus are identical, the individual is said to be **homozygous.** The alleles can be either normal or abnormal.

   g. If the alleles at a single locus are different, the person is said to be **heterozygous.** The term usually refers to having one normal and one abnormal or mutant allele. Such heterozygous individuals are also referred to as carriers.

   h. A **dominant** condition is seen in both the heterozygote and the homozygote. This implies that a single copy of the mutant allele is enough for the condition to be expressed.

   i. A **recessive** condition is seen only in the homozygote, which means that the mutant allele must be present on both chromosomes. Dominant and recessive refer to the expression of the clinical conditions, not to the genes themselves.

   j. **Autosomal** refers to the autosomes, which are the nonsex chromosomes. An autosomal condition results from mutant alleles on an autosome.

   k. **X- or Y-linked** refers to genes having loci on either the X or Y chromosome. With X-linked alleles, both recessive and dominant inheritance may be seen. The term **sex-linked** is also used to represent X-linked inheritance.

   l. A **compound heterozygote** is an individual with two different mutant alleles at one locus. β-Thalassemia may be caused by inheritance of different abnormal mutations of the normal β-globin gene from each parent. With the availability of mutation analysis, many individuals with autosomal recessive conditions have been shown actually to be compound heterozygotes, not true homozygotes.

   m. A **double heterozygote** is an individual with two mutant alleles, each at a different locus.

2. **Pedigree symbols and construction.** The pattern of inheritance of many single gene traits has been deduced from examination of the family history. When the history is

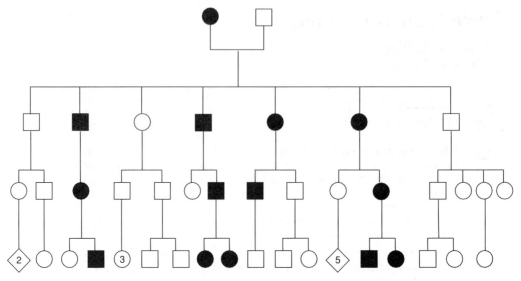

FIGURE 3-1. Pedigree typical of dominant inheritance.

taken, the pedigree is a shorthand or graphic representation of the details. Individuals are characterized according to their sex, their generation, and their biologic relationship to each other. In Chapter 13 I B, the steps involved in constructing pedigrees are explained. Figure 13-1 illustrates the most commonly used symbols, with an example pedigree.

B. Autosomal dominant inheritance. More than half of the currently described traits are inherited in a dominant fashion: approximately one-third as recessive and one-tenth as X-linked. Dominant implies that the disease allele need be present only in a single copy (as in the heterozygote) to result in the phenotype.

1. The **criteria** of autosomal dominant inheritance include the following.
   a. The transmission of the trait is from generation to generation without skipping. In a typical dominant pedigree (Figure 3-1), there can be many affected members in each generation.
   b. Except for a new mutation, every affected child will have an affected parent.
   c. In the mating of an affected heterozygote to a normal homozygote (the usual situation), each child has a 50% chance to inherit the abnormal allele and be affected and a 50% chance to inherit the normal allele.
   d. The two sexes are affected in equal numbers. Since the loci are on the autosomes (i.e., nonsex chromosomes), a sex differential is not seen unless the mutant allele involves a sex-limited structure such as the uterus.

2. **Features.** To provide the most accurate counseling, a number of potential complicating factors are important to consider in autosomal dominant inheritance. Each of the following may alter the idealized dominant pedigree.
   a. **New mutations.** An isolated case of a dominant disorder may be the result of a new mutation, but other causes (e.g., genetic heterogeneity or a minimally affected parent) and nonpaternity should also be considered.
      (1) A new mutation is seen more often with diseases that are so severe that people who are affected by them are less likely to reproduce than normal. The majority of cases of achondroplasia are the result of new mutations.
      (2) Increased paternal age is associated with an increase in new mutations at some loci. It has been suggested that the increase in new dominant mutations may be related to the accumulation of cell divisions undergone by the sperm with time.
      (3) The rate of new mutations is available for some dominant conditions and is useful for counseling.

b. **Reduced penetrance.** Penetrance refers to expression of the mutant phenotype and is an all-or-nothing phenomenon. It is expressed as the percentage of individuals who have the mutant allele and are actually affected. If the frequency of expression of a genotype is less than 100%, reduced penetrance exists. **Nonpenetrance** refers to the situation in which the mutant allele is inherited but not expressed.

(1) In a particular disorder, penetrance would be calculated by determining the total number of individuals expressing the disease divided by the total number of individuals inheriting the disease allele. A common autosomal dominant condition, polydactyly, is expressed in 65% of those inheriting the responsible allele.

(2) Penetrance is a clinical term and may be influenced by factors including age (e.g., Huntington disease) or better detection methods (e.g., magnetic resonance imaging for signs of tuberous sclerosis).

c. **Variable expressivity.** Expressivity refers to how or to what degree a particular allele is expressed in an individual.

(1) Variable expression is common in **dominant disorders,** which means that all family members should be examined carefully, with the features of the condition kept in mind.

(2) **Affected individuals** who are capable of reproducing are generally less severely affected. More severe expression may be seen in their children (i.e., they may express the full spectrum of the syndrome), and such expression may be unexpected by the parents.

d. **Observer fallibility.** Before counseling a family, the geneticist should consider how the diagnosis was made and whether the diagnosing individual has sufficient expertise to make a reliable genetic diagnosis. The danger lies in basing the counseling on another physician's or the family's diagnosis. As much information as possible should be obtained to corroborate a diagnosis.

e. **Variation in age of onset.** Adult polycystic kidney disease (APKD) is an autosomal dominant condition, but the renal cysts appear with time. Before the advent of molecular testing (see Chapter 6), the diagnosis could not be reliably ruled out in a young person. In some cases, heterozygous individuals may die of other causes before any renal problems manifest.

f. **Mosaicism.** If a parent is mosaic for a disease allele because of a postzygotic mutation, he or she may appear clinically unaffected. If the mosaicism involves the gonad (and therefore the germ cells), an increased recurrence risk for what appears to be a new dominant mutation may occur. For example, most cases of lethal osteogenesis imperfecta (type II) are dominant mutations. The observed recurrence risk is 6%, not the low expected risk. Demonstration of mosaicism for the collagen mutation has been observed in sperm from the father of two affected children.

g. **Genetic heterogeneity.** Different mutations, at the same locus or at different loci, may result in a similar clinical picture. Heterogeneity causes difficulties in counseling two unrelated, but similarly affected, individuals (e.g., a man and a woman who both have sensorineural deafness and wish to have children). In addition, the conditions may be inherited in different manners (e.g., retinitis pigmentosa may be inherited as an autosomal dominant, autosomal recessive, or X-linked trait).

h. **A phenocopy** is a mimic of a phenotype usually produced by a specific genotype. The phenocopy may be caused by an environmental factor. For example, an infant may present in a similar clinical fashion with warfarin embryopathy (i.e., the mother used a blood thinner while she was pregnant) or Conradi syndrome, which is a single gene condition.

i. **Variation in severity dependent on sex.** The severity of a dominant condition may depend on the sex of the affected parent. In Huntington disease, those with early severe disease are more likely to have an affected father; in myotonic dystrophy, those with early onset are usually born to affected mothers.

3. **Clinical examples**

a. **Huntington disease** is an autosomal dominant, adult-onset disease involving selective cell death within the caudate nuclei. The clinical presentation includes a choreic movement disorder, mood disturbances, and progressive loss of mental activity. The course from onset to death is usually 15 years and begins in the fourth decade. (There is less frequent juvenile onset when the affected parent is the father.) The gene location is the short arm of chromosome 4 (4p), with the most common mutation being an unstable triplet repeat (see II F 3).

   b. **Marfan syndrome** is a disorder of connective tissue with variable expressivity involving the skeletal system (e.g., abnormal proportions, scoliosis, arachnodactyly), cardiovascular system (e.g., mitral and atrial valve prolapse, aortic dilatation leading to aortic dissection), and ocular system (e.g., lens dislocation). The diagnosis is made on clinical grounds, with involvement in at least two systems. The molecular basis of Marfan syndrome is mutation of a structural gene (fibrillin) on chromosome 15q.

C. **Autosomal recessive inheritance.** The phenotype is usually observed only in the homozygote, and the typical pedigree demonstrates affected male and female siblings with normal parents and offspring. Recessive inheritance is suspected when parents are consanguineous; it is considered proven when corresponding enzyme levels are low or absent in affected individuals and are at half-normal values in both parents.

1. **Criteria**
   a. If the trait is rare, parents and relatives other than siblings are usually normal.
   b. In the mating of two normal heterozygotes, the segregation frequency with each pregnancy is 25% homozygous normal, 50% heterozygous normal, and 25% homozygous affected.
   c. If the recessive genes are alleles, all children of two affected parents are affected.
   d. Both sexes are affected in equal numbers.
   e. If the trait is rare, parental consanguinity is increased.

2. **Features.** A number of features are important to keep in mind before counseling families regarding autosomal recessive inheritance.
   a. **Heterozygote frequency.** Affected individuals are almost always the offspring of normal heterozygotes (not homozygotes). The relationship of gene frequency to different genotypes at one locus is described by the Hardy-Weinberg law (see Chapter 7 I). The homozygote frequency (q^2) is usually known [e.g., the number of individuals in the country with cystic fibrosis (CF)], and the heterozygote frequency can be calculated from 2pq. The trait is maintained in the much more frequent heterozygote. Carrier frequencies range from 1 in 10 individuals for hemochromatosis to fewer than 1 in 200 people for rare disorders. Calculating the carrier frequency is important for designing screening programs.
   b. **Carrier state.** Carriers are assumed to be unaffected, but some may show half-normal enzyme levels (e.g., the level of hexosaminidase A in Tay-Sachs disease heterozygotes) or minimal clinical features. The majority of carriers are clinically normal, however.
   c. **Consanguinity.** In the classical description of the rare autosomal recessive trait alkaptonuria, 60% of affected children had parents who were cousins. Consanguineous individuals have a proportion of their genes in common by descent. First cousins have one-eighth of their genes in common, whereas siblings have one-half of their genes in common. Consanguinity may arise in counseling in several situations:
      (1) Couples concerned that they are related by descent
      (2) Religious isolates, such as the Amish in North America
      (3) Geographic isolates, such as in the Lac St. Jean area in Canada or areas of the Appalachian mountains
   d. **Autosomal recessive phenotypes in the local population.** It is important to know an area's population when counseling because there may be particular racial groups in which a disease allele is carried more frequently because of the founder effect (see IV C) or heterozygote advantage. Knowledge of the local population allows appropriate screening and counseling. Examples of this include:
      (1) Sickle cell anemia in blacks
      (2) Tay-Sachs disease in Ashkenazi Jews

(3) CF in northern European Caucasians

e. Heterogeneity. Clinically similar individuals may have genetic causes for their condition but have mutant alleles at different loci. Albinism, sensorineural deafness, and congenital hypothyroidism may all be recessively inherited but have different loci involved in different families. If two affected parents with deafness have different loci involved, their children will have normal hearing but will be double heterozygotes.

3. **Clinical examples**
   a. **Galactosemia**
      (1) Clinical aspects. Affected infants present with cataracts or hepatomegaly and may die of sepsis. Abnormal or absent galactose-1-phosphate uridyl transferase results in an inability to use lactose. Female survivors have ovarian failure, perhaps due to intrauterine damage.
      (2) Treatment involves dietary restriction of lactose-containing products. Untreated survivors suffer mental deficiency.
      (3) Genetic background. The condition is heterogeneous, with a number of allelic variants described, such as the Duarte allele.
   b. **Homocystinuria**
      (1) Clinical aspects. Individuals with homocystinuria may be mistakenly diagnosed as having Marfan syndrome because they have an abnormal body habitus (i.e., long limbs) and may have dislocated lenses. Two-thirds of people with homocystinuria are mentally handicapped or have psychiatric problems. Deficient cystathionine β-synthetase results in increased levels of homocystine and methionine, the latter thought to cause the problems in the condition.
      (2) Treatment of homocystinuria involves a low methionine diet. Sudden death is common in untreated patients because of thromboembolic phenomena. Individuals with other metabolic defects causing their homocystinuria are less likely to respond to dietary manipulation.
      (3) Genetic background. Homocystinuria is an autosomal recessive amino acid disease that results from an inability to convert homocysteine to cystathionine.
   c. **Cystic fibrosis**
      (1) Clinical aspects. Approximately 1 in 5000 infants in northern European populations have CF and present with chronic respiratory infections, malabsorption, or failure to thrive. Secretions of the gut and lung are thick in these children, and their sweat is altered, with high sodium and chloride levels ("salty kisses"). The chronic pulmonary disease begins before 1 year of age and is the cause of 90% of deaths in patients with CF.
      (2) Treatment. Currently, the best treatment includes regular chest physiotherapy to loosen secretions, antibiotics, and replacement of digestive enzymes.
      (3) Genetic background. The gene has been localized to chromosome 7q; it codes for a chloride transport factor (CFTR) and multiple alleles are described.

D. **X-linked inheritance** can be either recessive or dominant, although in patients with a recessive X-linked condition, the phenotype is usually only observed in the male. X-linked inheritance is suspected when several male relatives in the female line of a family are affected. Because males have only one X chromosome, they are hemizygous, not heterozygous, for X-linked genes.

1. **Criteria**
   a. If the trait is rare, parents and relatives (except maternal uncles and other male relatives in the female line) are usually normal.
   b. Hemizygous affected males have neither affected sons nor daughters. All daughters of affected males are obligate heterozygotes (i.e., they do not show a mutation clinically but carry the mutant allele). There is no male-to-male transmission.

c. Female heterozygous carriers are clinically normal but will transmit the trait to sons (i.e., hemizygous affected) 50% of the time. Daughters of carrier mothers are normal heterozygotes 50% of the time and normal homozygotes 50% of the time.

d. Most often, affected daughters are produced only by matings of heterozygous females with affected males.

e. Except for those with new mutations, every affected male is born of a heterozygous female.

f. If the trait is dominant, all female offspring of affected males will themselves be affected. On average, 50% of either male or female offspring of an affected female heterozygote will be affected. Unlike autosomal dominant pedigrees, there is no male-to-male transmission.

2. Features. Some specific features of X-linked inheritance that cause problems are important to keep in mind.

a. The sporadic case. If a male is affected but there are no other affected family members, the question is whether the condition is the result of a new mutation or whether the mother is heterozygous.

(1) Heterozygous females may be detected by subtle clinical features, intermediate enzyme levels, or molecular methods. In approximately two-thirds of cases of X-linked recessive diseases that are lethal in childhood and in which there is only one affected male in the family, the mother is a heterozygote. In one-third of cases, the son has a new mutation.

(2) Bayesian methods (see Chapter 13) using other information about the family can further qualify the risk of X-linked inheritance.

b. Heterogeneity. Diseases with similar clinical features may be inherited through differing mechanisms.

(1) Albinism is usually inherited as an autosomal recessive condition, with involvement of eyes, hair, and skin.

(2) An X-linked form, **ocular albinism,** primarily involves the eyes, with little skin and hair involvement. The condition may be misdiagnosed in a blond child and incorrect counseling provided.

(3) A good clinical examination and family history are essential.

c. Affected females. Dosage compensation (Lyon hypothesis; see Chapter 1 V B) occurs as a consequence of random X chromosome inactivation at the late blastocyst stage in females. The net effect is hemizygosity for the majority of the X chromosome. Females who are heterozygous for X-linked conditions have clones of cells in which one allele or the other is active. X-linked conditions affecting females can be explained by the following mechanisms.

(1) Random inactivation. By chance, the normal X chromosome is inactivated more often than the abnormal, resulting in a situation similar to that in a hemizygous affected male, with the majority of cells expressing the mutant X chromosome.

(2) Heterozygous mother and an affected father. The risk for affected female offspring (i.e., homozygous for the mutant allele) would be 25% with each pregnancy.

(3) 45,X Turner syndrome inheriting a mutant allele on the single X chromosome. An affected female exhibits hemizygosity for X-linked genes, as does a male.

(4) 46,XY females with sex reversal syndromes (e.g., androgen insensitivity) can also inherit an X-linked disorder.

(5) An **affected male** can produce an affected female offspring if there is a new mutation in the X chromosome from the normal mother.

(6) A **heterozygous female** can produce an affected female offspring if there is a new mutation in the X chromosome from the normal father.

(7) Nonrandom X inactivation. In Turner syndrome with an isochromosome X, the isochromosome is nonrandomly inactivated. If a mutant allele is present on the normal X, it will be expressed as in the hemizygous male (see Chapter 2 II C 2; III C 1 b). Nonrandom X inactivation may also be seen in **X;auto-**

some **translocations,** where the X chromosome involved in the translocation is not inactivated. If the X chromosome has a mutant allele or the translocation itself produces a mutation, the female will be affected.

   d. **X-linked lethal conditions.** If the condition is lethal in males, any affected males would die before or at birth. Heterozygous females would be normal, but half of their male offspring would not survive. The end result would be an altered sex ratio for the condition with two females to every male.

3. **Clinical examples**
   a. **Duchenne muscular dystrophy (DMD)**
      (1) **Clinical aspects.** The incidence of DMD is approximately 1 in 3600 males, with onset in the first year of life. Characteristics include progressive weakness and muscle wasting, hypertrophy of calf muscles, and death, with cardiac or respiratory failure in the late teens to twenties.
      (2) **Genetic background.** Gene localization pinpointing Xp21 was accomplished by studying affected females with X;autosome translocations and affected males with X chromosome deletions. The normal gene product was identified as the muscle protein, dystrophin, which perhaps acts as a fiber protector. Approximately 60% of affected males have detectable deletions, allowing direct molecular techniques [see Chapter 6 II A 2, 3 a (3)] for analysis, and the remainder of families require linkage analysis [see Chapter 5].
   b. **Fragile X syndrome**
      (1) **Clinical aspects.** Mental retardation is more common in males, suggesting the existence of X-linked mutations. The most common cause of inherited mental retardation is fragile X syndrome, which occurs in 1 in 1500 males. Affected males have large ears, a prominent chin, megalotestes, and mild-to-moderate mental retardation. As children, they present with speech delay or autistic features. Unlike most X-linked syndromes, females are affected (usually more mildly than males) in one-third of cases. The probability of mental retardation in a family is increased by the number of generations through which the mutation passes (Sherman paradox).
      (2) **Genetic background.** The diagnosis was initially made with specialized chromosome-culturing methods, which depleted folate and led to expression of a fragile site at Xq27.3 in a proportion of the cells. More recently, the mutation was found to be an unstable triplet expansion (CGG) involving the gene FMR-1 at Xq27 (see II F). In fragile X families, the expansion may be moderate in size (premutation) or extremely large (full mutation). Males and females inheriting a premutation are unaffected. Males inheriting a full mutation are affected, whereas females have a variable clinical picture depending on X inactivation.
      (3) The **gene** follows a pattern of X-linked inheritance, but the dynamic nature of the mutations is responsible for the following complications.
         (a) A premutation is not altered in size with father-to-daughter transmission. Therefore, all daughters of a transmitting male are unaffected.
         (b) Progression from premutation to full mutation occurs only in offspring of females, and the risk of expansion varies with the size of the premutation in the mother.
         (c) If a mother is affected (i.e., she has a full mutation), all sons and 50% of the daughters inheriting the mutant allele will be affected.
         (d) Females inheriting the fragile X allele from a normal mother have a 30% chance of being affected.
         (e) Males who receive the mutant allele from a normal mother have an 80% chance of expressing the disease phenotype and a 20% chance of being a normal transmitting male.

E. **Mitochondrial inheritance.** Human cells have hundreds of mitochondria dispersed throughout the cytoplasm, each containing a number of circular DNA molecules. Muta-

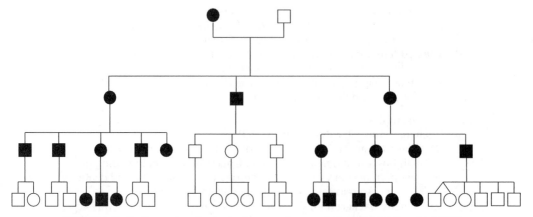

FIGURE 3-2. Pedigree showing typical maternal transmission of mitochondrial DNA.

tions involving the mitochondrial DNA are now known to account for a small number of genetic conditions.

1. Criteria

    a. Each mitochondrion contains a number of copies of the circular genome. Mitochondrial enzymes are usually encoded by nuclear genes, but some of the cytochrome oxidase enzymes are derived solely from mitochondria.

    b. Almost all mitochondrial DNA is maternally inherited. Pedigrees with mitochondrial inheritance should show that all children of an affected mother are affected and all children of an affected father are normal (Figure 3-2).

    c. Specific tissues have different proportions of mitochondria. Rich areas include striated and cardiac muscle, the kidney, and the central nervous system (CNS). Therefore, mitochondrial diseases are commonly myopathies, neurologic syndromes, and cardiomyopathies.

2. Clinical examples

    a. Kearns-Sayre syndrome is a sporadic condition with onset before 20 years of age. Characteristics include progressive external ophthalmoplegia, retinal pigment abnormalities, heart block, and cerebellar ataxia. Studied patients exhibit deletions of muscle-derived mitochondrial DNA.

    b. Leber's optic neuropathy. Optic atrophy, occasional movement disorder, and electrocardiographic (ECG) abnormalities characterize this disorder, which is transmitted exclusively by women to children of both sexes. The disorder is secondary to mutations of one of the genes coding for subunits of complex I in the electron transport chain.

II. TYPES AND MECHANISMS OF MUTATION. The development of DNA technology has allowed the delineation of mutations at the level of DNA sequence. In the human genome, there are many different types and mechanisms of mutations, including major gene rearrangements and point mutations. These mutations may affect transcription and/or translation and may alter expression or function of the protein product.

A. Major gene rearrangements

    1. Deletions are easily detected using recombinant DNA technology (see Chapter 6 II A) and are indicated by the absence or altered size of a DNA fragment. Gene deletions are uncommon causes of mutation in the human genome except for a few diseases.

        a. α-Thalassemia is caused by deletion of the α-globin gene cluster, which are four highly related sequences in close proximity to each other.

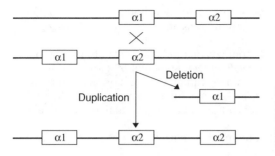

FIGURE 3-3. The α-globin gene comprises two pairs (α1 and α2) of highly related sequences in close proximity. Mispairing during meiosis can result in one chromosome with a deletion of an α-globin gene.

(1) Because of the sequence similarity of these genes, mispairing of chromosomes may occur during meiosis.

(2) After mispairing and crossing over, one product contains a deficiency of genetic material (Figure 3-3).

(3) Unequal crossing over in the region of the α-globin gene cluster has resulted in chromosomes that lack functional α-globin genes. These chromosomes are common in Southeast Asian populations.

(4) Fetuses that lack all α-globin genes usually die of generalized edema either during the pregnancy or shortly after birth.

 b. Growth hormone deficiency is another disorder that commonly results from deletions.

  (1) Like the α-globin gene cluster, the growth hormone gene cluster also consists of similar DNA sequences in close proximity to each other.

  (2) Mispairing and unequal crossing over in meiosis again causes deletions of the growth hormone gene, with the resultant effect of dwarfism in homozygotes.

 c. Familial hypercholesterolemia (FH), which results from defects in the low-density lipoprotein (LDL) receptor gene (see Chapter 6 II A 3 c), can also be caused by deletions due to unequal crossing over involving the highly repetitive *alu* sequences. Deletions occur in this situation after mispairing of homologous *alu* sequences with deletions of part of the gene for this protein.

2. Duplications of DNA sequences are common in evolution and may be caused by mispairing between homologous DNA sequences in close proximity, with duplication of genetic material that is contained within the gene (see Figure 3-3). The mechanism of duplication is similar to that seen in α-thalassemia. Duplications may alter the reading frame. FH and DMD are examples of genetic disorders that may be caused by duplications.

3. Insertions are rare causes of mutation in the human genome. However, **transposition of DNA** is not an uncommon occurrence in the human genome, although it usually does not involve the coding sequence. When transposition does occasionally disrupt a gene, defective gene expression may result.

 a. The **long interspersed repetitive sequence (LINE)** and ***alu* (or SINE) sequence** [see Chapter 1 II A 2 c (1)] are examples of sequences that can insert within genes.

 b. Hemophilia is an example of a disease that has resulted from an insertion of a LINE in the factor VIII gene disrupting its function. Similarly, neurofibromatosis has arisen as a result of insertion of an *alu* sequence.

B. **Point mutations. Single nucleotide substitutions** similar to those seen in bacteria and viruses are the most common cause of mutagenesis in the human genome. If codons are affected by a single nucleotide substitution, these point mutations are called **missense mutations.** Disorders that have clearly been shown to be caused by many different point mutations include β-thalassemia, cystic fibrosis, phenylketonuria (PKU), and Tay-Sachs disease.

1. **β-Thalassemia** was the first disease to be clearly defined as being caused by different point mutations, which may affect transcription, translation, and RNA cleavage, or RNA splicing and translation.
   a. **Clinical aspects.** Children born with homozygous β-thalassemia are usually not anemic at birth because of the high levels of fetal hemoglobin. However, the disease usually manifests at 1 to 2 years of age with anemia, pallor, and failure to thrive. Hepatosplenomegaly results from extramedullary hematopoiesis. In addition, bone marrow proliferation results in frontal bossing. Sexual and physical development is retarded.
   b. **Treatment.** Blood transfusion and bone marrow transplantations are currently the only feasible methods of treatment.

2. **Cystic fibrosis.** See Chapter 5 II B 3 for a full explanation of the clinical and genetic aspects of cystic fibrosis.

3. **Phenylketonuria**
   a. **Genetic aspects.** PKU is inherited as an autosomal recessive trait caused by different mutations in the enzyme phenylalanine hydroxylase, which converts phenylalanine to tyrosine.
      (1) In patients with PKU, phenylalanine cannot be degraded and thus accumulates, which causes damage to the CNS and mental retardation.
      (2) Mutations other than point mutations [e.g., translation mutations (see II D)] that cause PKU have been defined.
   b. **Treatment.** In many instances, neonatal screening for PKU is performed so that appropriate treatment can begin early to prevent mental retardation. CNS damage and mental retardation can be avoided to a large extent by dietary changes to prevent phenylalanine accumulation.
   c. **Clinical aspects.** See Chapter 8 II B 2 a for a discussion of the metabolic and clinical aspects of PKU.

4. **Missense mutations** can result in the following:
   a. **An altered codon for a particular amino acid residue** [e.g., a single nucleotide change at the sixth position of the β-globin chain of hemoglobin causes a glutamic acid to valine substitution, which results in sickle cell anemia; see Chapter 6 II B 2 b (2)]
   b. **An altered protein function,** which may occur via different mechanisms, including:
      (1) A mutation directly involving crucial residues, such as at a catalytic site
      (2) A mutation altering the three-dimensional structure of the protein such that its function is compromised

C. **Transcription mutations** may occur 5′ to the start codon in the DNA sequence that is critical for regulating transcription. For example, different mutations have been found in the **TATA box,** a region located about 30 nucleotides upstream from the initiation codon. In addition, there are residues at the 3′ end of the β-globin gene, which are also important in regulating transcription. Mutations in these distal promoter elements might cause decreased transcription with decreased production of the β-globin protein.

D. **Translation mutations.** Mutations affecting translation have frequently been seen in β-thalassemia and have also been described in other diseases, such as lipoprotein lipase deficiency and PKU.

1. **Nonsense mutations** affect translation via nucleotide substitution, which produces a premature stop codon (see Chapter 1 II A 3 g). These substitutions result in truncated proteins, which are frequently unstable and degraded.

2. **Frameshift mutations** are either deletions or insertions of one or a few nucleotides in the coding region of the gene. These mutations change the triplet code for all the codons that follow and thus completely alter the sequence of amino acids. In some cases, frameshift mutations lead to premature termination of the protein by creating a stop codon.

E. RNA mutations

1. **RNA cleavage and stability mutations** can result in inappropriate cleavage of the growing RNA, which causes cleavage to occur at sequences downstream. The result is RNA that is abnormally large, appears to be unstable, and is rapidly degraded.

2. **RNA splicing mutations.** RNA splicing is critical to normal gene expression because introns must be precisely removed to produce appropriate messenger RNA (mRNA) for translation into protein. Mutations may affect splicing, either by altering normal splice sites at intron and exon junctions or by creating new splice sites within introns or exons.

   a. Potential splice sites that are not used are termed **cryptic splice sites.** RNA is not normally spliced at these sites.

   b. The 5′ exon/intron junction is called the **donor splice site,** and the 3′ intron/exon junction is the **acceptor splice site.**

   c. The **5′ end** of the intron always begins with nucleotides **GT,** and the **3′ end** of the intron always has the nucleotides **AG.**

   d. **Mutations that alter either the AG or GT splice junctions** lead to complete absence of normal splicing, which results in an unstable mRNA that is rapidly degraded.

      (1) People with these mutations have **no functional protein product.**

      (2) Many mutations that cause **β-thalassemia** affect RNA splicing by one of the following mechanisms.

         (a) Mutations can **affect the normal donor or acceptor splice site** and prevent normal splicing of RNA, resulting in a molecule that is unstable and rapidly degraded.

         (b) Mutations can **affect nucleotides** that are important for creating new splice sites, which results in an abnormal, unstable RNA product that is rapidly degraded.

   e. **The end result of a mutation** is alteration of the function of a gene.

      (1) Mutations in the coding region result in a **protein with altered function,** while mutations in regulatory sequences of a gene may result in either **increased or decreased amounts of the protein.**

      (2) The net effect of these mutations is usually **loss of normal function** (common in recessive illnesses) or, less frequently, gain of a **new biologic function with resultant disease** (typical in some autosomal dominant traits).

F. **Dynamic mutations.** In the past few years, a new mechanism of human mutation has been described that is caused by expansion of a trinucleotide repeated sequence in novel genes. These trinucleotides may be present in the 5′ untranslated region of the gene, the coding region of the genes, or the 3′ untranslated region of the gene.

1. Very great expansion of a sequence of **repeated CGG** units in the 5′ end of the gene to more than 200 CGG repeats is associated with fragile sites on the chromosome. When this occurs in a gene on the X chromosome, it is associated with loss of function of that gene and the fragile X syndrome.

2. A **CTG repeat expansion** in the 3′ end of the gene leads to myotonic dystrophy, which is the most common cause of muscular dystrophy in adults.

3. Another category for dynamic mutations results from small expansions, usually more than 35 but fewer than 150, that occur due to amplification of a **CAG repeat** in the coding region of the gene. This results in five separate neurodegenerative conditions, including Huntington disease, spinocerebellar ataxia, spinobulbar muscular atrophy (SBMA), dentatorubro-pallidoluysian atrophy, and Machado-Joseph disease.

   a. These diseases generally are associated with a later age of onset and selective neuronal death in particular tissues. Patients present with neurologic and psychiatric symptoms. Besides SBMA, which is X-linked, all of these disorders are autosomal dominant.

   b. It has also been suggested that other forms of cerebellar ataxia, and possibly other disorders such as schizophrenia and manic depressive illness, might also be caused by a CAG repeat amplification in a novel gene. Currently, it is not known how these CAG expansions cause disease.

4. **Anticipation** is the occurrence of a genetic disease with greater severity or with an earlier age of onset in more recent generations of a family.
   a. Anticipation is **characteristic of dynamic mutations** caused by expansion of trinucleotide repeats.
   b. Anticipation results from the **enlargement of the trinucleotide repeated region** as the dynamic mutation passes through meiosis and early embryonic development.
   c. In conditions that are caused by dynamic mutations (e.g., fragile X syndrome, myotonic dystrophy, Huntington disease), there is a **good correlation between the size to which the trinucleotide repeated sequence has expanded and the disease severity or age at onset.**

G. Dominant negative mutations

1. Mutations that exert a **dominant effect** may do so because the **body cannot produce enough of the gene product** if only one allele at the locus is functioning normally. FH provides one example of such a locus (see Chapter 6 II A 3 c).

2. Other mutant genes exert a dominant effect because they produce an **abnormal product that interferes with the function of the normal allele's product.** Mutations of this kind are said to have a **dominant negative effect.**
   a. In one form of **dominantly inherited isolated growth hormone deficiency,** a mutation of one allele produces a product that binds to the normal peptide encoded by the other allele, which prevents the growth hormone from being secreted.
   b. The severity of the phenotype in **osteogenesis imperfecta** is usually much greater if the disease is caused by a mutation in the *COL1A1* gene that alters the structure of the resulting procollagen peptide than if the disease is caused by a *COL1A1* mutation that decreases the amount of the procollagen produced.
      (1) In the former case, the *COL1A1* **mutation alters the stability of type I collagen,** which is a trimer composed of two procollagen peptides produced by the *COL1A1* gene and one procollagen peptide produced by the *COL1A2* gene. This is a **dominant negative mutation.**
      (2) When a mutation of the *COL1A1* gene is present that just decreases the amount of procollagen produced, the patient will make less type I collagen, but it will have normal structure and stability.

H. Ethnic distribution of specific mutations. Various mutations may exhibit strikingly different frequencies in different populations.

1. **Frequency in specific populations.** Several genetic diseases occur at high frequency in certain populations. Examples include the following.
   a. **Sickle cell anemia** is carried by 1 in 10 blacks.
   b. **Tay-Sachs disease** is carried by 1 in 25 Ashkenazi Jews.
   c. **FH** affects 1 in 100 French Canadians.

2. **Selective advantage** may explain the high frequency of a particular genetic trait within certain populations.
   a. For example, the geographic distribution of sickle cell anemia closely parallels that of malaria, and it has now been shown that the **sickle-globin gene protects an individual against malaria.**
   b. Therefore, persons living in Africa who have the sickle cell trait have a selective advantage, which results in an increased frequency of this trait within that population.

3. **Founder effects** are another cause of a high frequency of specific mutations in certain populations.
   a. The **Afrikaner population** of South Africa is descended from a few Dutch ancestors (founders) who arrived in South Africa in the middle of the seventeenth century. One of these early settlers carried the gene mutation for porphyria variegata.

As a result, this genetic disease has its greatest frequency in the world in the Afrikaner.

  b. **Porphyria variegata** is inherited as an autosomal dominant trait and predisposes individuals to photosensitivity and episodes of severe abdominal pain and shock after exposure to certain drugs, including anesthetics.

4. **Identical mutations** occurring in more than one population can be attributed to at least two possibilities.

  a. Mutations may have occurred before ethnic divergence and are observed in different ethnic groups.

  b. Mutations may have occurred independently in different population groups. Certain sequences, such as the CG dinucleotides, are particularly prone to single nucleotide substitutions. CG substitutions may produce both nonsense and missense mutations and represent mutation hotspots in humans.

5. **Chromosome haplotypes.** One way to determine whether similar mutations have arisen independently or share a common origin is to determine the pattern of RFLPs on the chromosome with the particular mutation. This pattern has been termed a chromosome haplotype.

  a. **Mutations that have arisen independently** may occur on different background chromosomal haplotypes.

  b. **Mutations that have a common origin** usually have the same background chromosomal haplotype.

  c. For example, **similar mutations causing β-thalassemia are present in both blacks and Chinese.** However, these same mutations occur on different β-globin gene haplotypes, which suggests independent origins of these alleles in these two population groups.

III. **IN VIVO MODELS FOR STUDYING GENES.** After genetic mutations in a particular gene are found and associated with a specific disease, the next challenge is to understand how these mutations cause the disease. One approach is to study the pattern of expression of the gene product in the tissue in which disease occurs. Another approach is studying the biochemical properties of the gene and its product in vitro. Understanding the biologic function of any gene is also significantly hastened by studies in live organisms.

A. **Study methods.** In an effort to study the normal function of a gene for which no function is known or to reproduce a disease that is caused by loss of function of a particular gene, a strategy called **gene targeting** is now available.

1. **Homologous recombination approach.** Gene targeting can make use of the process of **homologous recombination** to insert a sequence into a particular gene so that the gene is no longer translated. The result is a loss of the particular gene product and its function.

  a. **Targeting construct.** The gene to be studied is disrupted by creating a targeting construct, which contains an interruption within the coding region of the gene.

  b. The construct is introduced into **mouse embryonic stem cells,** which have the potential to reconstitute an embryo after introduction into a blastocyst.

  c. **Homologous recombination** occurs as a result of the introduced DNA molecules recombining by virtue of their sequence identity with DNA of the cell. The interruption of the gene contained in the targeting construct is then introduced into the endogenous gene and results in an interruption of the gene within the embryonic stem cell.

  d. The embryonic stem cell is then **introduced into a blastocyst,** which is then allowed to develop into a transgenic animal that has some normal genes and some interrupted genes.

  e. **Transgenic animals.** The germline of these animals is chimeric and can be bred to produce offspring that are homozygous for the introduced mutation. By doing this, an animal can be created that has complete deletion of a particular gene product.

2. **Nonhomologous recombination approach.** Another approach for assessing the function of an unknown gene or for producing an animal model for a particular illness is to create a construct that contains either the coding sequence or the coding and noncoding sequences for a particular gene.

   a. Complementary DNA (cDNA), cosmids, or YAC clones that encompass the gene of interest are **introduced into a fertilized mouse egg,** which is then transferred into a pseudopregnant mother.

   b. The animal that is born is called a **founder** and is bred to produce more animals with the same extra genes.

   c. Using this method, the **inserted DNA usually randomly integrates into the genome** by a nonhomologous recombination event.

   d. To achieve stable inheritance of the introduced DNA fragment, **integration must occur** in a cell type that gives rise to functional germ cells, such as oocytes or sperm.

B. **Benefits**

1. **Homologous recombination approach.** This approach has been taken to produce animal models for **cystic fibrosis and FH,** both of which result from **loss of function** of a particular gene.

2. **Nonhomologous recombination approach.** This approach has been used to create transgenic animal models of **Alzheimer disease** and to study the effects of **overexpression** of various particular proteins on the physiology of the animals. Novel insights concerning the interaction of the particular protein with other proteins and insights into its normal function have been obtained.

3. These models have been **crucial for defining the molecular and cellular mechanisms underlying genetic illnesses** and also serve as useful models for new therapies.

STUDY QUESTIONS

DIRECTIONS: The numbered item or incomplete statement in this section is followed by answers or by completions of the statement. Select the ONE lettered answer or completion that is BEST.

1. X-linked ichthyosis is a skin disorder often caused by deletion of the gene for steroid sulfatase (STS), which is located between repeat sequences on the short arm of the X chromosome (Xp). The most likely reason for this deletion is the presence of which one of the following mutations?

(A) A missense mutation
(B) A nonsense mutation
(C) Recombination between repeat sequences
(D) A mutation affecting RNA splicing
(E) A high frequency of CG dinucleotides in the STS gene

DIRECTIONS: Each set of matching questions in this section consists of a list of four to twenty-six lettered options (some of which may be in figures) followed by several numbered items. For each numbered item, select the ONE lettered option that is most closely associated with it. To avoid spending too much time on matching sets with large numbers of options, it is generally advisable to begin each set by reading the list of options. Then, for each item in the set, try to generate the correct answer and locate it in the option list, rather than evaluating each option individually. Each lettered option may be selected once, more than once, or not at all.

Questions 2–6

Match the type of mutation that is most commonly associated with the following genetic diseases.

(A) Deletions
(B) Insertions
(C) Duplications
(D) Point mutations
(E) Frameshift mutations

2. Cystic fibrosis (CF)

3. α-Thalassemia

4. β-Thalassemia

5. Duchenne muscular dystrophy (DMD)

6. Growth hormone deficiency

Questions 7–11

Match each condition described below with the term that best defines it.

(A) Allelic heterogeneity
(B) Variable expressivity
(C) Nonpenetrance
(D) Consanguinity
(E) Locus heterogeneity

7. A man shows no detectable signs of Marfan syndrome (an autosomal dominant disorder of connective tissue), although his father and two daughters are affected

8. Retinitis pigmentosa (a type of retinal degeneration) occurs in an autosomal dominant, an autosomal recessive, and an X-linked form

9. Tay-Sachs disease is seen in high frequency in the Chicoutimi area of Quebec, where most individuals are descended from a few early French settlers

10. Duchenne muscular dystrophy (DMD) is the consequence of either a deletion involving the dystrophin gene or a point mutation of the same gene

11. In a family with myotonic dystrophy, the father has frontal balding, severe weakness, and cardiac arrhythmia; his sister has early-onset cataracts; and his child has electromyographic abnormalities

ANSWERS AND EXPLANATIONS

1. The answer is C [II A 2]. The gene for steroid sulfatase (STS) is located between repeat sequences, and mutations often arise as a result of mispairing of homologous repeat sequences with deletions of part of this protein. The presence of these repeat sequences on either side of the gene would not, in any way, favor a missense or nonsense mutation or affect RNA splicing. There is no particularly high frequency of CG dinucleotides in the STS gene.

2–6. The answers are: 2-A [II B 2], **3-A** [II A 1], **4-D** [II B], **5-A** [I D 3 a], **6-A** [II A 1 b]. The most common mutation underlying cystic fibrosis (CF) is a deletion of a phenylalanine residue at position 508 of the CF gene that accounts for about 70% of all CF alleles. Major deletions or rearrangements detectable by Southern blot analysis have not been detected, but numerous other types of mutations including nonsense and missense mutations have been defined.

The most common mutation underlying α-thalassemia is a deletion as a result of the crossing over in the region of the α-globin gene cluster resulting in chromosomes lacking functional α-globin genes.

Point mutations are the most common cause of β-thalassemia. Many of these mutations decrease the abundance of normal β-globin mRNA either by causing a defect in the regulatory region or by affecting RNA splicing.

More than 60% of all mutations underlying Duchenne muscular dystrophy (DMD) are deletions. These mutations are not random but are clustered to certain regions of the gene.

Growth hormone deficiency is most often caused by unequal crossing over resulting in deletion for this particular hormone's gene.

7–11. The answers are: 7-C [I B 2 b], **8-E** [I B 2 g, C 2 e, D 2 b], **9-D** [I C 2 c], **10-A** [I B 2 g, C 2 e, D 2 b], **11-B** [I B 2 c]. A disorder is said to be nonpenetrant when there is no clinical evidence of a mutant allele in an individual known to have inherited the gene. When the gene is expressed, the form of expression may be highly variable, with some family members being severely affected, and others having few signs of the disorder. This is common with autosomal disorders and is called variable expression. Different mutations of either the same gene (i.e., at the same locus) or different genes may give a similar clinical picture. Consanguineous individuals have a proportion of their genes in common by inheritance from a common ancestor. In some villages originated by a few settlers, disease alleles may be in higher frequencies, and a particular recessive disorder may be more common in that community as a result.

Chapter 4

Genetic Polymorphism

J. M. Friedman
Barbara C. McGillivray

I. POLYMORPHISMS AND GENETIC MARKERS

A. **Definitions**

1. **Genetic polymorphism** is the occurrence in a population of two or more alleles at a locus in frequencies greater than can be maintained by mutation. Polymorphisms are genetic **differences that provide variation within a species**.
   a. In practice, it is difficult to know what frequency of an allele can be maintained by mutation, so an operational definition of polymorphism is often used: **A polymorphism is said to exist if the most common allele at a locus has a frequency of less than 99%**.
   b. **Polymorphisms are ubiquitous,** particularly in noncoding regions of DNA.

2. A **genetic marker** is a simply inherited genetic trait with readily recognizable alleles. In other words, a genetic marker is a **polymorphism that can easily be detected**.
   a. The marker may or may not be part of an expressed gene.
   b. In general, the most valuable genetic markers are those that are most polymorphic; that is, those for which an individual is most likely to exhibit two different forms and for which many different variants exist with appreciable frequencies in the population.

B. **Polymorphisms.** All polymorphisms **ultimately reflect alterations of DNA sequence** that may be **demonstrated via DNA technology**. Altered proteins, enzymes, or antigens and abnormal physical features can all indicate polymorphisms. Polymorphisms can be classified by their method of detection.

1. **DNA polymorphisms** are identified by direct detection of altered DNA sequence.
   a. **Restriction fragment length polymorphisms** (RFLPs) are inherited variations in DNA sequence that result in the gain or loss of a site recognized by a restriction endonuclease (e.g., *Eco*RI, *Taq*I). RFLPs may also result in alteration of the number of nucleotides between such sites (Figure 4-1).
      (1) RFLPs are transmitted as **simple codominant traits**.
      (2) RFLPs can be detected by the **Southern blot** (see Chapter 6 I A) or by analysis of DNA fragments generated by **polymerase chain reaction** (PCR) [see Chapter 6 I B].
      (3) RFLPs have been widely used in **gene linkage and mapping studies** (see Chapter 5 I and II, respectively).
   b. Approximately 10% of the genome is composed of **tandemly repeated DNA sequences.** These sequences are sometimes called "satellite" DNA. (The terminology has nothing to do with the satellites seen cytogenetically on chromosomes 13, 14, 15, 21, and 22.) Satellite DNA is named because of how it separates on density-gradient centrifugation. Two categories of tandemly repeated sequences are particularly **useful as genetic markers**.
      (1) **Short tandem-repeat polymorphisms (STRPs),** which are sometimes called **microsatellites** or simple sequence repeats (SSRs), are **extremely polymorphic** DNA segments that are usually less than 1 kb long and are composed of tandemly repeating units of 2, 3, or 4 nucleotides. An example is the $(CA)_n$ repeat, which is composed of the nucleotides cytosine (C) and adenosine (A). The sequence . . . CACACACACACA. . . . may have 10 to 60 CA units.
         (a) STRPs are present in **numerous copies throughout the genome**. For example, there are approximately 50,000 different $(CA)_n$ repeat loci in humans.

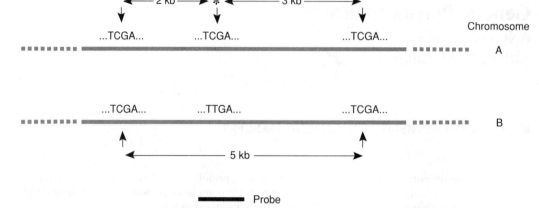

Chromosome

A

B

Probe

FIGURE 4-1. In this figure, action of the restriction enzyme *Taq*I is denoted by the *asterisk*. *Taq*I recognizes TCGA as a cutting site, so treatment of chromosome A produces two fragments—one measuring 2 kilobases (kb) and one measuring 3 kb. Treatment of chromosome B produces a single 5-kb fragment since *Taq*I does not recognize the sequence TTGA as a restriction site. The probe enables the corresponding piece of the chromosome to be recognized. (Reprinted with permission from Gelehrter TD, Collins FS: *Principles of Medical Genetics.* Baltimore, Williams & Wilkins, 1990, p 78.)

These loci can be distinguished using **PCR** (see Chapter 6 I B) because the DNA sequences flanking each tandem repeat are different.
- **(b)** STRPs are transmitted as **simple codominant traits**.
- **(c)** STRPs are particularly useful as genetic markers in **gene linkage and mapping studies**.

- **(2) Minisatellites** are extremely polymorphic tandem repeats between 1 kb and 30 kb in length. The repeated sequence is longer and more complex in minisatellites than in STRPs.
  - **(a)** Minisatellites may occur at only one site in the genome (single locus minisatellites) but similar repeated sequences frequently occur at many different sites (multilocus minisatellites).
  - **(b) Variable number of tandem repeats** (VNTRs) are minisatellite markers that can be identified because they contain, or are flanked by, sites recognized by a restriction endonuclease. VNTRs are a special kind of RFLP as well as a special kind of minisatellite.
  - **(c)** VNTRs are often detected by **Southern blot** analysis (see Chapter 6 I A), but these and other minisatellite markers can also be identified by **PCR**.
  - **(d)** Minisatellites are transmitted as **simple codominant traits**, but this is often not apparent when multilocus minisatellites are analyzed on Southern blot gels because of the complexity of the pattern produced.
  - **(e)** The extreme polymorphism and complexity of multilocus minisatellites makes them especially valuable for **forensic applications**. However, the complexity of the pattern produced with multilocus minisatellites has also led to controversy in their forensic use because of difficulty in determining allele frequencies in populations.
  - **(f) DNA fingerprinting,** which usually involves testing for minisatellite markers, has been used to establish paternity, determine zygosity, and identify a specific individual on the basis of a small sample of blood, semen, hair, or other tissue.

2. Many polymorphisms are detected by identifying **altered gene products**.
  - **a. Inherited enzyme variants** have an altered protein structure. This may be demonstrated by alteration of enzyme activity, electrophoretic mobility, thermostability, or other physical properties. **Examples** include the electrophoretic and activity variants of glucose-6-phosphate dehydrogenase (G6PD), which are common in people of African or southern European origin.

b. **Antigenic variants** may also reflect alterations of protein structure. They are usually demonstrated by serologic tests, such as red-cell agglutination or antibody-mediated cytotoxicity. The ABO and Rh blood groups and the human leukocyte antigen (HLA) system (see II C 2, 3, D) are important examples of polymorphic antigenic variants.

3. Some polymorphisms are observed as **alterations of physical features** (e.g., the dominantly inherited postaxial polydactyly that is common in African-Americans).

4. **Chromosome heteromorphisms** are heritable differences in chromosomal appearance. These polymorphisms may require special cytogenetic techniques (e.g., Q-banding) for their demonstration (see Chapter 1 IV C 1 b).
   a. The **most common types of chromosome heteromorphisms** include the following:
      (1) Variations in the size of the long arm of the Y chromosome
      (2) Variations in the size of the centromeric heterochromatin
      (3) Variations in cytogenetic satellite size and structure
      (4) The occurrence of fragile sites
   b. Chromosome heteromorphisms can be used to **distinguish chromosomes of maternal origin from those inherited from the father**. Chromosome heteromorphisms have, therefore, been used to determine the parental origin of aneuploidy and chromosomal rearrangements, although molecular studies are generally preferred now.

II. CLINICAL IMPORTANCE OF POLYMORPHISMS.

Most polymorphisms produce no clinical phenotype. Regardless of whether a clinical effect is produced, polymorphisms are useful as **genetic markers.**

A. **Disease genes.** Some disease genes occur with polymorphic frequencies.

1. **This is true for heterozygous carriers of relatively common autosomal recessive diseases.** Examples include the heterozygous states of sickle cell disease among people of African origin, thalassemia among people of Mediterranean or Southeast Asian origin, and cystic fibrosis among people of northern European origin.

2. In some instances, **mild disease manifestations occur in heterozygous carriers,** whereas **severe disease is seen among homozygotes** for the same gene (e.g., familial hypercholesterolemia and β-thalassemia).

3. Polymorphic genes may produce disease only when the individual carrying them is exposed to certain chemicals. Examples of such **pharmacogenetic predispositions** include G6PD deficiency and malignant hyperthermia (see Chapter 9 II B 1, 2).

B. **Genetic markers** can be used to determine the **likelihood of associated disease genes present within a family or individual** (see Chapter 5 I; Chapter 13 II B). They can also be used to determine the **relationship of individuals to each other** and to determine the **genetic similarity of blood, semen, or tissue to an individual.**

1. **Twins**
   a. From a genetic perspective, there are **two kinds of twins**.
      (1) Monozygotic (MZ), or identical, twins have all of their genes in common. MZ twins are derived from a single zygote that produces two separate embryos.
      (2) Dizygotic (DZ), or fraternal, twins have half of their genes in common, on average. DZ twins develop from two separate zygotes and bear the same genetic relationship to each other as do any siblings.
   b. **Genetic markers can be used to determine zygosity.**
      (1) MZ twins have identical alleles at all loci tested.
      (2) DZ twins differ from each other at a substantial number of loci.

(3) Genetic markers can be used in a similar fashion to determine zygosity within sets of **triplets or higher multiple births**.

(4) Genetic markers **do not need to be used to distinguish twins of unlike sex** who are almost always DZ twins.

2. Paternity testing

a. Paternity testing **requires samples from the child, the mother, and the putative father**.

b. In general, **paternity can be confidently excluded, but not proven with certainty**, using genetic markers. Two kinds of exclusions are possible.

(1) Paternity is excluded if neither of the putative father's two alleles at a locus is present in the child. For example, if the putative father is homozygous for a genetic marker that the child does not have, paternity is excluded.

(2) Paternity is excluded if the putative father lacks an allele that is present in the child but not in the mother. If a child has a marker that neither the mother nor the putative father has, paternity is excluded.

c. The more markers tested and the less common the alleles seen, the more likely that a wrongly accused man can be excluded as the father of a child.

d. A **probability of paternity** can be calculated based on the number of markers tested and the frequency of the alleles for which the child is informative. With **DNA fingerprinting**, which employs extremely polymorphic markers [see I B 1 b], probabilities of paternity that are very high can usually be obtained when a child is compared with the biologic father.

3. Other forensic uses of genetic markers include the following:

a. Determining the origin of blood, semen, or tissue specimens obtained at a crime scene. Small amounts of DNA can be used to test for specific genetic markers characterizing a victim or suspect. For example, DNA fingerprinting can be performed on specimens from a crime scene and compared with samples obtained from a suspect. A match provides strong evidence that the specimen obtained at the scene came from the suspect.

b. Identifying missing persons. Genetic markers of the missing person and his or her parents or other family members can be compared to establish true biologic relationships.

C. **Blood typing** is important for the prevention of transfusion reactions. **Blood groups** reflect cell-surface antigens coded by polymorphic genes that are usually inherited in a simple mendelian fashion. These antigens are most often identified by **serologic tests**.

1. The **MN blood group** consists of **two alleles** that are **codominantly expressed** (Table 4-1). Therefore, the genotype can be determined directly from the phenotype. The MN blood group is not usually important for blood transfusions or for determining maternal–fetal compatibility.

2. The **ABO blood group** plays an important role in **blood transfusions**.

a. The ABO blood group consists of **three major alleles**.

(1) The **A allele is expressed codominantly**. People who have an A allele express A antigen on the surface of their red blood cells. **People who do not have A allele spontaneously make antibody to A antigen.**

(2) The **B allele is expressed codominantly**. People who have a B allele express B antigen on the surface of their red blood cells. **People who do not have B allele spontaneously make antibody to B antigen.**

TABLE 4-1. MN Blood Group

Phenotype	Genotype
M	MM
N	NN
MN	MN

TABLE 4-2. ABO Blood Group

Phenotype	Genotype
O	*oo*
A	*Ao* or *AA*
B	*Bo* or *BB*
AB	*AB*

    (3) The **o allele is recessive** to the A and B alleles. **The o allele does not produce a corresponding cell-surface antigen.**

  b. The genotypes and phenotypes of the ABO blood group are shown in Table 4-2. The antigens and antibodies that occur with the various blood types appear in Table 4-3.

  c. Rules of blood transfusion

    (1) Blood cells expressing an antigen should be transfused only into persons who also have that antigen. For example, AB blood may be given to individuals of type AB, but not to individuals of type A, B, or O.

    (2) Blood cells lacking an antigen may be transfused into persons who have that antigen. For example, O blood may be given to individuals of type A, B, or AB, as well as to those of type O.

3. The **Rh blood group** contains an allele (usually called *D*) that produces a major cell-surface antigen. Individuals whose cells carry this major antigen are referred to as being **Rh-positive (Rh$^+$)**. Individuals whose cells lack the major Rh antigen are said to be **Rh-negative (Rh$^-$)**. The phenotypes and genotypes for the major Rh antigen are shown in Table 4-4.

  a. Rh$^-$ individuals are capable of making an antibody to the major Rh antigen but do not do so unless they have been exposed to Rh$^+$ blood. Sensitization of an Rh$^-$ woman usually occurs because of pregnancy with an Rh$^+$ fetus or because of transfusion with Rh$^+$ blood.

  b. Hemolytic disease of the newborn (erythroblastosis fetalis) is caused by **destruction of fetal red blood cells by maternal antibody.** The most common cause of severe hemolytic disease of the newborn is **Rh incompatibility.**

    (1) The "setup" for Rh hemolytic disease of the newborn occurs when the **mother is Rh$^-$ and the father is Rh$^+$.**

    (2) If the father's genotype is *DD*, all of the mother's pregnancies by him are at risk. If the father's genotype is *Dd*, only half of the mother's pregnancies by him are at risk, on average.

    (3) Rh hemolytic disease of the newborn usually does not occur in the mother's first pregnancy because sensitization is required before she begins to make anti-Rh antibody. Once hemolytic disease of the newborn occurs, however, it **tends to become worse** in each subsequent affected pregnancy.

TABLE 4-3. Antigens and Antibodies of the ABO Blood Group

Blood Type	Antigens on Red Blood Cells	Antibody in Serum
O	Neither A nor B	Both anti-A and anti-B
A	A	Anti-B
B	B	Anti-A
AB	Both A and B	Neither anti-A nor anti-B

TABLE 4-4. Rh Blood Group

Phenotype	Genotype
Rh$^+$	*DD* or *Dd*
Rh$^-$	*dd*

(4) Rh hemolytic disease of the newborn is usually preventable by avoiding sensitization of Rh$^-$ girls and women. This can be done by avoiding transfusion with Rh$^+$ blood and by treating Rh$^-$ pregnant women with **anti-Rh antibody (RhoGAM) injections**.

c. The Rh blood group is complex. The gene is duplicated, and, in addition to the major antigen (D) encoded by the *RHD* locus, there are **other minor Rh antigens** (called C and E) that are encoded by an adjacent locus. These minor Rh antigens can occasionally be of clinical significance.

D. **Tissue typing** is necessary for successful organ or tissue transplantation.

1. **The major histocompatibility complex (MHC)** is the most important genetic region for determining tissue types for transplantation. In humans, the MHC is called the **HLA complex**.
   a. The HLA complex is composed of **several closely linked genetic loci on chromosome 6**.
      (1) **Class I HLA loci** include **HLA-A, HLA-B, and HLA-C.** These loci function in the recognition of foreign antigens by cytotoxic T lymphocytes. Class I antigens are particularly important in graft rejection.
      (2) **Class II HLA loci** include **HLA-DR, HLA-DP, and HLA-DQ.** These loci are involved in recognition of foreign antigens by helper-T (Th) lymphocytes, which are a component of the humoral immune response.
      (3) **Class III HLA loci** code for some of the **components of the complement cascade.**
      (4) A few **other genes** with functions unrelated to the immune response also lie within the HLA complex, such as the gene for 21-hydroxylase, which is deficient in the most common form of congenital virilizing adrenal hyperplasia (see Chapter 12 II C 3).
   b. Most class I and class II HLA loci are **highly polymorphic.**
   c. Because the HLA loci are closely linked, all of the alleles in the complex are **usually transmitted as a unit** to the next generation. This unit, called a **haplotype,** comprises the set of alleles contained in the HLA complex of one chromosome 6.
   d. Most HLA genes produce **cell-surface antigens** that can be detected by serologic tests or other methods. The HLA genes themselves can be identified by direct DNA testing (see Chapter 6 II).
   e. HLA alleles are transmitted as **simple codominant traits**.

2. A general rule in organ transplantation is **the greater the similarity between HLA types of the donor and recipient, the better the chance for avoiding rejection.**
   a. **MZ twins make ideal donor/recipient pairs** for transplantation because they are completely identical with respect to their HLA types. MZ twins are also identical with respect to other loci outside of the HLA complex that influence the success of transplants.
   b. **A parent and child are usually haploidentical**, which means they share one (and only one) HLA haplotype.
   c. **Siblings usually have a 25% chance of being HLA identical**, a 50% chance of being haploidentical, and a 25% chance of being completely different with respect to the HLA complex.

III. **ETHNIC FACTORS IN GENETIC DISEASE.** The human population began as a relatively small population that gradually split into small breeding groups. The term "ethnic" often refers to these resultant groups, which may differ by culture, religion, race, or linguistic tradition. Comparison of mitochondrial polymorphisms has allowed investigators to conclude that because mitrochondria are maternally derived, all humans are derived from a common maternal ancestor or, at least, a small number of ancestors.

A. **Genetic differences.** With the exception of monozygous twins, every human is genetically different.

1. **Polymorphism is the rule**, particularly regarding the level of DNA variation. Extragenic regions (i.e., noncoding regions between genes) tend to be highly polymorphic.

2. The concept of the "wild type," which is frequently used in genetic studies of experimental organisms, is **not applicable to humans**. The wild type of an organism is homozygous for the normal allele at all loci. Studies in humans indicate that virtually every person carries some alleles that could cause (or predispose to) disease under the appropriate circumstances.

B. **Human populations differ genetically.**

1. **Physical differences** include the obvious traits that humans have traditionally used to define ethnic groups (e.g., body size, skin and hair pigmentation, facial structure).

2. **Medically important differences.** The frequency of many diseases differs among populations. Some examples of ethnicity of disease are provided in Table 4-5.

TABLE 4-5. Ethnic Distribution of Disease

Disease	Populations with High Disease Frequency
α-Thalassemia	Southeast Asians Africans
Anencephaly	Irish
β-Thalassemia	Italians Southeast Asians Greeks Africans
Cleft lip and cleft palate	Japanese Native Americans Mexicans
Congenital nephrosis	Finns
Congenital adrenal hyperplasia	Alaskan Eskimo
Cystic fibrosis	Northern Europeans
Diabetes mellitus	Ashkenazi Jews Polynesians Native Americans Mexicans
Glucose-6-phosphate dehydrogenase (G6PD) deficiency	Italians Greeks Africans Chinese
Hypertension	Africans
Nasopharyngeal cancer	Chinese
Sickle cell anemia	Africans
Tay-Sachs disease	Ashkenazi Jews

    a. Differences in disease frequencies among populations are most often apparent for multifactorial and recessive conditions.

    b. Differences in disease frequencies among populations may also be due to differences in diet or social practices.

3. Natural selection is responsible for some genetic differences among populations. Examples of natural selection include the following.

    a. Light skin and hair color among people of northern European descent probably evolved as an adaptation to a climate in which sunlight was less readily available to form vitamin D in the skin.

    b. The genes for diseases such as sickle cell anemia, G6PD deficiency, and thalassemia have become common in some populations because these genes confer resistance to malaria. In a broad periequatorial belt, the carrier frequency can be as high as 25% to 40% for sickle cell hemoglobin (HbS).

4. Genetic differences among populations arise because **mating is not random within the human species as a whole.**

    a. Genetic isolation. Populations in which members only mate with other members of the same group are said to be genetically isolated. Genetic isolation may arise because of geographic factors or religious or cultural practices.

        (1) Finland is comprised mainly of immigrants originally (prior to 1000 B.C.) from the Baltic region. Settlement spread slowly with a mainly rural population.

        (2) Within the present Finnish population are several otherwise rare or unknown recessive disorders (e.g., congenital nephrotic syndrome, Finnish type; congenital chloride diarrhea; early infantile ceroidfuscinosis).

    b. Small, genetically isolated populations encounter **phenomena that create genetic differences** and can be important determinants of gene frequencies.

        (1) Genetic drift refers to changes in gene frequencies that occur by chance. If one allele fails to be inherited, it will not be seen in descendants of that individual.

        (2) Founder effects (see Chapter 3 II G). If by chance a particular abnormal gene was present among the small group of founders (i.e., the initial frequency of the gene in the population was high), the frequency tends to remain high unless selection against the gene is strong.

5. Differences in gene frequencies among human populations are usually relative, not absolute.

    a. Some populations have higher frequencies and some have lower frequencies of various genes, but there are very few genes that are unique to one particular population. An example of a disease caused by a gene that is unique to a population is cerebro-osteonephrodysplasia, which is only described in siblings in the inbred Hutterite population.

    b. The number of generations that humans have gone through as a species is relatively small (approximately 85,000).

    c. Not many human populations have remained genetically isolated for more than a few generations. Mating between previously isolated populations often occurs as a result of migration, conquest of one group by another, or changes in cultural practices.

STUDY QUESTIONS

DIRECTIONS: Each of the numbered items or incomplete statements in this section is followed by answers or by completions of the statement. Select the ONE lettered answer or completion that is BEST in each case.

1. Which one of the following statements regarding genetic polymorphisms is correct?

(A) A polymorphism that occurs in noncoding regions of DNA is a genetic marker
(B) Polymorphisms resulting from alteration of the protein structure of a restriction endonuclease are restriction fragment length polymorphisms (RFLPs)
(C) Chromosome heteromorphisms are usually detected by DNA fingerprinting
(D) Genetic polymorphisms are variations in DNA sequence that occur commonly
(E) Blood groups are short tandem-repeat polymorphisms (STRPs)

2. Genetic polymorphisms are clinically important because

(A) they can be used as genetic markers in family studies
(B) they often cause chromosome rearrangements
(C) they usually cause disease when homozygous
(D) they are valuable vectors in gene therapy
(E) they cause variable number tandem repeats (VNTRs) that are important in tissue transplantation

3. A female patient with chronic renal failure has five people who are willing to serve as donors for a renal transplant: her husband, her identical twin, her half-brother, her sister, and her son. Based on the likelihood of HLA identity, the correct arrangement of individuals in order of decreasing suitability as a renal transplant donor is

(A) twin, husband, sister, son, half-brother
(B) husband, twin, sister, son, half-brother
(C) twin, son, sister, husband, half-brother
(D) twin, sister, half-brother, son, husband
(E) twin, sister, son, half-brother, husband

4. Which one of the following statements about genetic differences among human populations is correct?

(A) Genetic differences rarely affect genes for multifactorial diseases
(B) Genetic differences arise because of genetic isolation among groups
(C) Genetic differences are selected against by evolution
(D) Genetic differences are of no medical significance
(E) Genetic differences often are reflected by genes that occur only within a particular group

DIRECTIONS: The set of matching questions in this section consists of a list of four to twenty-six lettered options (some of which may be in figures) followed by several numbered items. For each numbered item, select the ONE lettered option that is most closely associated with it. To avoid spending too much time on matching sets with large numbers of options, it is generally advisable to begin each set by reading the list of options. Then, for each item in the set, try to generate the correct answer and locate it in the option list, rather than evaluating each option individually. Each lettered option may be selected once, more than once, or not at all.

Questions 5–9

For each patient listed, select the blood type that would be appropriate for a transfusion.

(A) A Rh$^-$ or O Rh$^-$ blood
(B) B Rh$^+$ or O Rh$^+$ blood
(C) O Rh$^-$, A Rh$^-$, B Rh$^-$, AB Rh$^-$, O Rh$^+$, A Rh$^+$, B Rh$^+$, or AB Rh$^+$ blood
(D) AB Rh$^+$ blood
(E) None of the above

5. A patient who is B Rh$^-$

6. A patient who is A Rh$^+$

7. A patient who is AB Rh$^-$

8. A patient who is O Rh$^-$

9. A patient who is AB Rh$^+$

ANSWERS AND EXPLANATIONS

1. The answer is D [I A 1, 2, B 1 a (1), 4].
Genetic polymorphisms are commonly occurring variations in a DNA sequence. Genetic markers are readily identifiable, simply inherited polymorphisms found throughout the genome. Variations of DNA sequence that result in the gain or loss of a restriction endonuclease site or in alteration of the number of nucleotides between restriction sites are called restriction fragment length polymorphisms (RFLPs). Chromosome heteromorphisms are recognized under the microscope in cytogenetic studies. Short tandem-repeat polymorphisms (STRPs) are highly polymorphic tandem repeats of two to four nucleotides. Most STRPs exist outside of gene-coding regions.

2. The answer is A [I A 2, B 1 b; II B]. Polymorphic genetic markers are widely used in genetic family studies. Chromosome heteromorphisms can be used to identify the origin of chromosomal rearrangements but are generally not involved in their causation. Most polymorphisms do not affect the function of genes and are not directly related to any genetic disease. Polymorphisms are variants, not vectors, and their use in gene therapy is only to mark a gene that is being manipulated. Variable number tandem repeats (VNTRs) are a highly polymorphic kind of restriction fragment length polymorphism (RFLP); they are not involved in the antigenic variation that is critical to tissue transplantation.

3. The answer is E [II D 2]. The identical twin must be human leukocyte antigen (HLA) identical to the patient, so she is the most suitable donor. The sister is the next best choice because she has a 25% chance of being HLA identical and a 50% chance of being haploidentical to the patient. The son has almost no chance of being HLA identical to his mother but must be haploidentical to her. The patient's half-brother also has almost no chance of being HLA identical; he has only a 50% chance of being haploidentical. It is un-

likely that the patient's husband shares any HLA haplotypes with her.

4. The answer is B [III B 4, 5]. Differences in gene frequencies among populations arise largely because of nonrandom mating between them. Multifactorial and autosomal recessive diseases most commonly exhibit different frequencies in different populations. Certain genes may become common in particular groups because of natural selection. Genetic differences among populations are important medically because they predispose some patients to different diseases more than other patients. Genetic differences among populations are usually relative rather than absolute because it is very uncommon for human populations to remain genetically isolated for more than a few generations.

5–9. The answers are: 5-E, 6-A, 7-A, 8-E, 9-C
[II C 3]. A patient who is B Rh$^-$ should not be given blood containing either the A or Rh$^+$ antigen. This eliminates the blood in (A), (B), (C), and (D).

A patient who is A Rh$^+$ should not be given blood containing the B antigen, but may be given either Rh$^+$ or Rh$^-$ blood. The blood in (A) is, therefore, satisfactory. Type O blood does not display a surface antigen that is recognized by individuals who lack it.

A patient who is AB Rh$^-$ may be given type O, A, B, or AB blood but should not be given Rh$^+$ blood. Only the blood in (A) is satisfactory.

A patient who is O Rh$^-$ can only be given O Rh$^-$ blood because the patient will have or will form antibodies against any blood with the A, B, or Rh$^+$ antigen.

A patient who is AB Rh$^+$ may receive a transfusion with blood of any ABO or Rh type. The patient will not form antibodies to any of these antigens, because all are present on the patient's own red blood cells. Responses (A), (B), (C), and (D) are all correct, but (C) is the best answer because an AB Rh$^+$ patient has no antibodies to the ABO or Rh antigens.

Chapter 5
Linkage and Mapping
J. M. Friedman

I. **LINKAGE** is the occurrence of two or more genetic loci in such close physical proximity on a chromosome that they are more likely to assort (or segregate) together rather than independently during meiosis (Figure 5-1). Linkage occurs because crossing over does not usually take place between loci that are close to each other.

A. Concepts of genetic linkage

1. **Linkage refers to loci, not to alleles.**
   a. For example, consider a genetic marker locus M that is linked to the locus for a dominantly inherited disease, D. If locus M has two allelic forms, M^a and M^b, then some families may carry the mutant D allele on the same chromosome as M^a, and others may carry the mutant D allele on the same chromosome as M^b. In either case, the allele at the marker locus and the D allele at the disease locus will usually be transmitted together at meiosis.
   b. The process of determining which allele at one locus is carried on the same chromosome as a given allele at another locus is called **determining the phase of the linkage.**
      (1) Thus, if a person is known to be heterozygous M^a/M^b at a marker locus and heterozygous D/d at a disease locus, **two possibilities exist**: The chromosome that carries the mutant allele at the disease locus may carry M^a at the marker locus, or it may carry M^b.
      (2) **Family studies are necessary** to establish which of these two possibilities in fact exists.

2. **The specific alleles present at linked loci in a given individual or family are irrelevant** as long as they are informative for testing.

B. **Measurement of genetic linkage can take place only in family studies.** Meiosis, which is required to demonstrate linkage, occurs only during gametogenesis. Therefore, only family members can be studied to determine if linkage of genes has occurred.

1. The unit used to express how close two linked genes are is the **centimorgan (cM)**, or **percent recombination**.
   a. Loci that are separated by crossing over in 1% of gametes are 1 cM apart.
   b. Loci that are so close that they are almost never separated by crossing over are linked at a genetic distance of 0 cM.
   c. Unlinked loci are separated by a genetic distance of 50 cM, because a given allele at one locus has a 50% chance of being transmitted with either allele at an unlinked locus.

2. The usual statistical method of measuring linkage in family data is calculation of the **lod score.**
   a. Lod is an acronym for "logarithm of the odds." The lod score is the $\log_{10}$ of the odds in favor of finding the observed combination of alleles at the loci being studied if they are linked at a given distance rather than being unlinked.
   b. **A lod score of +3 or greater** at a recombination distance of less than 50 cM between two loci is considered to be **strong evidence of linkage** (1000:1 odds for linkage).
   c. **A lod score of −2 or less** is considered strong evidence that there is **no linkage** (100:1 odds against linkage).

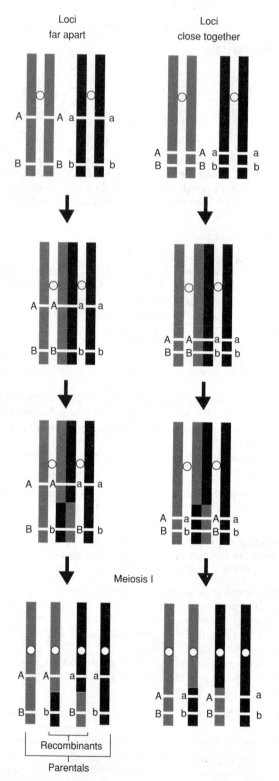

FIGURE 5-1. When loci are on different chromosomes or are far apart on the same chromosome (*left column*), the alleles segregate independently at meiosis, and parental and recombinant products are equally frequent. When the loci are close enough to be linked (*right column*), alleles on the same chromosome are usually not separated by crossing over, and parental products are more common than recombinant products. (Reprinted with permission from Gelehrter TD, Collins FS: *Principles of Medical Genetics.* Baltimore, Williams & Wilkins, 1990, p 203.)

C. **Two related concepts distinguished from linkage**

1. **Linkage disequilibrium** is the tendency for **certain alleles** at two linked loci to **occur together** more often than expected by chance.
   a. For example, if marker locus M with alleles M^a and M^b is linked to disease locus D at a genetic distance of 5 cM, and if it is found that the mutant allele at D occurs on the same chromosome as M^b more often than expected within a certain population, linkage disequilibrium exists.
   b. Linkage disequilibrium is **measured in a population, not in a family,** and often varies in different populations.

2. **Synteny** is the **occurrence of two loci together on the same chromosome**. Syntenic loci may not be linked if they are so far apart that crossing over usually occurs between them.

D. **Clinical applications of linkage**

1. Linkage is clinically useful because it may permit:
   a. **Determination of the likely genotype** of an individual at a disease gene locus on the basis of readily identifiable linked markers
   b. **Determination of the pattern of inheritance** or specific form of a disease that exhibits genetic heterogeneity (see III)
   c. **Gene mapping** by defining the order and recombination distance between loci on a chromosome (see II)

2. **Clinical uses of linkage** (see also Chapter 6 III) include:
   a. **Prenatal diagnosis** of genetic diseases, such as phenylketonuria (PKU)
   b. **Carrier detection** in autosomal or X-linked recessive diseases, such as Duchenne muscular dystrophy
   c. **Presymptomatic diagnosis** of late-onset autosomal dominant diseases, such as familial breast cancer
   d. **Elucidation of genetic factors in genetically heterogeneous conditions or multifactorial diseases,** such as insulin-dependent diabetes mellitus

3. The clinical use of linkage **always requires obtaining information on other family members** besides the one whose genotype is being determined.

4. The use of a linked marker to provide information about a disease gene **always involves some uncertainty** because recombination may occur between the loci for the marker and the disease.

II. **GENE MAPPING** is the assignment of genes to specific chromosome locations. More than 6000 genetic loci have been mapped to specific human chromosomes. Most of these loci are **short tandem-repeat polymorphisms (STRPs)** [see Chapter 4 I B 1 b (1)], which are excellent markers because of their extreme polymorphism and ease of testing by **polymerase chain reaction** (**PCR**) [see Chapter 6 I B]. The total also includes more than 450 genes. The average distance between mapped markers is less than 1 cM. Many additional loci are mapped each month as part of the Human Genome Project (see IV).

A. **Several methods** of gene mapping are available. The results of one method often complement those of another.

1. **Family studies** are used to demonstrate linkage between loci. If linkage between the loci can be shown to exist, both must reside on the same chromosome. The **frequency of recombination** between linked markers is a measure of **genetic distance** and can be used to place them in **linear order**.

2. **Somatic cell genetic methods** are used to demonstrate **synteny** or to show that an unmapped locus resides on a given chromosome. In general, somatic cell genetic methods involve the demonstration of loss of a given gene from cells that lack a specific

chromosome segment and retention of the gene in cells that retain that chromosome segment.

3. **Cytogenetic techniques,** especially fluorescent in situ hybridization (FISH) [see Chapter 1 IV C 1 b (7)], can be used to visualize a gene directly on a specific chromosome.

4. **Gene dosage studies** are an indirect means of identifying the location of genes.
   a. These studies are based on the concept that the amount of DNA or protein product specific for a given gene is directly proportional to the number of copies of that gene present in an individual or cell.
   b. For example, if a cell with trisomy for chromosome 21 exhibits 1.5 times as much of a certain protein as a normal cell and 3 times as much of the protein as a cell with monosomy 21, the implication is that the gene for that protein is on chromosome 21.

B. There are several **kinds of gene maps** that contain different, but complementary, information. In approximate order of increasing fine scale, these are:

1. The **cytogenetic map,** which places genes into specific cytogenetic bands of the karyotype

2. The **linkage map** (sometimes called a **genetic map**), which orders genes and markers by **recombination distances** (i.e., cM)

3. The **physical map,** which orders genes or markers along the DNA strand of a particular chromosome (The distance between markers on a physical map is measured in megabases, kilobases, or base pairs.)

4. The **DNA sequence,** which can also be thought of as a map because it represents a linear array of all the genes and markers it encodes

C. Importance of gene mapping

1. **The gene map is the anatomy of the human genome.** Just as knowledge of anatomy is necessary to understand the function of the human body, knowledge of the gene map is necessary to understand the function of the human genome.

2. **Analysis of the heterogeneity and segregation of human genetic diseases** is substantially enhanced by a detailed gene map.

3. Improved knowledge of genomic organization is necessary **to develop optimal strategies for gene therapy**.

4. Gene mapping provides information regarding **linkage** that is **clinically useful** (see I D 2).

III. **GENETIC HETEROGENEITY is the production of the same phenotype by more than one genotype.**

A. There are **two kinds** of genetic heterogeneity that are important clinically.

1. **Locus heterogeneity** is the production of similar phenotypes by mutations at different genetic loci. For example, tuberous sclerosis, an autosomal dominant condition that may produce mental retardation, seizures, and characteristic cutaneous lesions, can result from mutation of a gene on the long arm of chromosome 9 or from mutation of a gene on the short arm of chromosome 16.
   a. Locus heterogeneity **can confound linkage studies**.
   b. Locus heterogeneity can account for the fact that parents who both have an autosomal recessive disease sometimes have unaffected children. (One would ordinarily expect all such children to be affected because both parents are homozygous for the mutant gene.) This is seen most often in autosomal recessive deafness, a

disease that exhibits substantial locus heterogeneity. If two deaf parents are homozygous for *different* recessive genes, all their children will have normal hearing. Each child will be heterozygous at both deafness loci, but none of the children will be homozygous at either locus.

    c. Locus heterogeneity is the rule in **multifactorial diseases** (see Chapter 9 III C), in which genetic factors at many different loci may operate, and different loci may be involved in disease pathogenesis in different individuals.

  2. Allelic heterogeneity is the production of similar phenotypes by different mutant alleles at a single locus. For example, many different mutations of the *NF1* gene can produce neurofibromatosis, which is an autosomal dominant condition associated with a variety of cutaneous, central nervous system, and other lesions. All these mutations occur at the *NF1* locus, which therefore represents a series of mutant alleles.

    a. Allelic heterogeneity has been found for most genetic diseases that have been studied at the molecular level.

    b. So-called homozygotes for autosomal recessive diseases are actually compound heterozygotes in most cases, unless the parents are consanguineous. **At a molecular level, most people with autosomal recessive disease have two different mutant alleles.**

    c. Allelic heterogeneity can complicate identification of mutations by **direct DNA analysis** (see Chapter 6 II). In the case of large genes with extensive allelic heterogeneity, mutation identification may be impractical clinically, and other methods of molecular diagnosis may be required.

B. **Genotype–phenotype correlation** is the association of specific alterations of the genome with specific clinical features of a genetic disease. Many genetic diseases exhibit substantial variability in expressivity or incomplete penetrance (see Chapter 3 I B 2 b, c). The causes of such differences between affected people vary from disease to disease and probably from person to person. Possible causes of clinical variability include:

  1. Locus heterogeneity

  2. Allelic heterogeneity

  3. Somatic alteration of the mutant allele, which occurs commonly in some diseases (e.g., fragile X syndrome) that are caused by the expansion of trinucleotide repeats (see Chapter 3 II F)

  4. Epistatic effects, which are the effects of genes at other loci that are sometimes collectively called the "genetic background"

  5. Epigenetic effects that alter the expression of genes without changing their sequence [e.g., genomic imprinting (see Chapter 1 V C)]

  6. Nongenetic factors, such as environmental exposures or diet

  7. Chance

IV. **THE HUMAN GENOME PROJECT** is a collaborative international effort to identify and map all the genes and determine the DNA sequence of the entire human genome. The project has the goal of completion within 15 years of its formal inception in 1990.

A. It is estimated that the human genome contains about **3,000,000,000 base pairs of DNA** and **50,000 to 100,000 genes.** The Human Genome Project is by far the largest project ever undertaken in biology or medical science.

B. The **components** of the Human Genome Project include:

  1. Mapping and sequencing the human genome

2. Mapping and sequencing the **genomes of model organisms,** such as the bacterium *Escherichia coli,* the yeast *Saccaromyces cervisiae,* and the nematode *Caenorhabditis elegans,* as well as the fruit fly *Drosophila melanogaster,* and the mouse (These studies help to develop the essential technology and permit the comparative evolutionary and functional analyses necessary to understand the meaning of the human genomic sequence.)

3. Development of **informatics,** which are sufficiently powerful computer algorithms and software to permit efficient storage, retrieval, and analysis of the immense amount of data that is being accumulated

4. Study of the **ethical, legal, and social issues** raised by the scientific knowledge gained through the project

5. **Training of scientists** necessary to complete the project and apply its results effectively

6. **Development of new and improved technologies** required to complete the project on time with available resources

7. **Technology transfer** to facilitate application of the knowledge gained as rapidly and efficiently as possible

C. **Importance of the Human Genome Project**

1. Better understanding of the human genome produced by this project is expected to have major **benefits for medicine, the biotechnology and pharmaceutical industries, and agriculture.** Some of these benefits are already being seen as a result of the greatly improved genetic maps that have been developed since the project's inception.

2. Society will have to deal with a series of **profoundly important ethical issues** related to privacy, confidentiality, discrimination, individual freedom, and social responsibility arising from the knowledge gained through the Human Genome Project.

3. If the Human Genome Project succeeds scientifically, **it will raise more fundamental questions than it answers**. Knowledge of the sequence of the human genome by itself will not tell us how all the genes function, how they are regulated, how they interact with each other or with the environment, or how to treat serious genetic diseases more effectively. However, detailed understanding of the human genome should provide approaches of unprecedented power that can be brought to bear on these important questions.

STUDY QUESTIONS

DIRECTIONS: Each of the numbered items or incomplete statements in this section is followed by answers or by completions of the statement. Select the ONE lettered answer or completion that is BEST in each case.

1. Which one of the following statements regarding gene mapping is true?

(A) Most genes in the human genome have been mapped
(B) Family studies are necessary for gene mapping
(C) Distance on a physical map is usually expressed in centimorgans (cM)
(D) Gene mapping can be used to show genetic heterogeneity within a disease
(E) Short tandem-repeat polymorphisms (STRPs) are useful markers for mapping because they are not polymorphic

2. Allelic heterogeneity is best described by which one of the following statements?

(A) It can complicate the use of linkage for prenatal diagnosis of genetic disease
(B) It can preclude direct mutation identification as a practical means of molecular diagnosis
(C) It is rare among genetic diseases that have been studied molecularly
(D) It occurs when similar phenotypes are produced by mutations at different genetic loci
(E) It accounts for differences in the expression of autosomal recessive diseases between twins

DIRECTIONS: Each of the numbered items or incomplete statements in this section is negatively phrased, as indicated by a capitalized word such as NOT, LEAST, or EXCEPT. Select the ONE lettered answer or completion that is BEST in each case.

3. Both members of a couple are carriers of β-thalassemia, an autosomal recessive disease caused by a defect in the β-globin gene. The couple has only one child, a son, who is neither affected nor a carrier of β-thalassemia. DNA analysis using a β-globin probe gives the following phenotypes for a very closely linked polymorphic restriction site [1 and 2 are alternate alleles for this restriction fragment length polymorphism (RFLP)]:

Mother: *1,2*
Father: *1,2*
Son: *1,1*

All of the following statements about this family are true EXCEPT

(A) the mother's mutant β-globin allele is probably on the same chromosome as her *2* allele at the marker locus
(B) the father's mutant β-globin allele is probably on the same chromosome as his *2* allele at the marker locus
(C) a fetus of this couple found to have a *1,2* genotype for the marker locus on prenatal

testing is likely to be a heterozygous carrier of β-thalassemia
(D) if this woman has a pregnancy by an unrelated man who also is a carrier of β-thalassemia, the child is likely to have homozygous β-thalassemia if found to have a *2,2* genotype

4. All of the following statements regarding genetic linkage are true EXCEPT

(A) linkage refers to genetic loci, not to alleles
(B) family studies are necessary to demonstrate linkage
(C) lod scores are used to measure the likelihood that particular genes are linked
(D) if two genes are linked, the genetic distance between them is less than 50 centimorgans (cM)
(E) genetic linkage can be defined as the occurrence of two genes together on the same chromosome

DIRECTIONS: Each set of matching questions in this section consists of a list of four to twenty-six lettered options (some of which may be in figures) followed by several numbered items. For each numbered item, select the ONE lettered option that is most closely associated with it. To avoid spending too much time on matching sets with large numbers of options, it is generally advisable to begin each set by reading the list of options. Then, for each item in the set, try to generate the correct answer and locate it in the option list, rather than evaluating each option individually. Each lettered option may be selected once, more than once, or not at all.

Questions 5–10

For each of the following items related to gene mapping, select the most appropriate term.

(A) Physical map
(B) Genetic map
(C) Linkage
(D) Linkage disequilibrium
(E) Synteny

5. Usually identified by a lod score of +3 or greater at a recombination distance of less than 50 centimorgans (cM)

6. Orders loci with distances measured in base pairs or kilobases

7. Orders loci according to the frequency of meiotic recombination between them

8. Often differs among populations

9. Occurs when specific alleles at two loci are found together more often than expected by chance

10. Uses family studies to determine the order of genes on a chromosome

ANSWERS AND EXPLANATIONS

1. The answer is D [II A–C]. If a genetic disease is shown to map to different loci in different families, locus heterogeneity is established. Only a small proportion of genes in the human genome have currently been mapped. Family studies are an important method of gene mapping, but a variety of other techniques are also used.

Physical maps order loci on the physical strand of DNA. Distances on a physical map are, therefore, measured in base pairs (or kilobases or megabases). Short tandem-repeat polymorphisms (STRPs) are useful markers for mapping because they are highly polymorphic and because they are so frequent and widely distributed throughout the genome.

2. The answer is B [III A 1, 2]. Allelic heterogeneity is the production of similar phenotypes by different mutant alleles at a single locus. In contrast, locus heterogeneity occurs when two or more different loci produce a similar phenotype. Locus heterogeneity, not allelic heterogeneity, confounds clinical use of linkage. Allelic heterogeneity does, however, complicate molecular diagnosis by direct mutation analysis. For some large genes, such as that for neurofibromatosis type I, extensive allelic heterogeneity precludes direct mutation identification as a practical means of molecular diagnosis.

Allelic heterogeneity is very common; most disease genes studied molecularly have been shown to exhibit substantial allelic heterogeneity. Allelic heterogeneity can account for phenotypic differences among patients with a genetic disease, but this would not apply to identical twins who have all of their genes in common (see Chapter 9 III D 1).

3. The answer is D [I A 1, 2]. The marker restriction fragment length polymorphism (RFLP) is closely linked to the β-globin locus, but the phase of the linkage (i.e., which allele at the marker locus is carried on the same chromosome as the mutant allele at the disease locus) varies from individual to individual. The couple's son is homozygous normal at the β-globin locus, and he is homozygous for allele *1* at the marker locus. This means that in both of his parents, the *1* allele at the marker locus

is likely to be on the same chromosome as the normal allele at the β-globin locus, and the *2* allele at the marker locus is likely to be on the same chromosome as the mutant β-globin allele.

Because the disease locus and the marker locus are closely linked, a fetus of this couple found to be *1,2* at the marker locus is likely to be a heterozygous β-thalassemia carrier. A fetus found to be *2,2* at the marker locus is likely to have homozygous β-thalassemia. A fetus found to be *1,1* at the marker locus is likely to be homozygous normal at the β-globin locus.

If this woman has a child by another man who is also a carrier of β-thalassemia, his mutant β-globin gene may or may not be on the same chromosome as a *2* allele at the marker locus. Although the marker locus and the β-globin locus are linked in all members of the population, linkage does not imply anything about which allele at one locus is associated with a particular allele at the other locus (unless linkage disequilibrium also exists). In some individuals, the mutant β-globin allele may be carried on the same chromosome as a *1* allele at the marker locus, or a normal β-globin allele may be carried on the same chromosome as a *2* allele at the marker locus. In addition, the new father might not be informative at this marker locus. For example, he might be homozygous *2,2* so that all of his children inherit a *2* allele from him regardless of whether or not they inherit the mutant allele at the β-globin locus. It may be possible to use linkage to infer whether a fetus has inherited a mutant allele at the β-globin locus from the new father, but *only* if the new father is shown to be informative at the marker locus *and* the phase of the linkage is determined to be appropriate in him.

4. The answer is E [I A–C]. Linkage is the occurrence of two or more genetic loci in such close physical proximity on a chromosome that they are more likely to assort together rather than independently at meiosis. Linkage refers to loci, not to alleles at those loci. Different specific alleles at two linked loci may be in coupling in different families.

Linkage can only be identified and measured within a family because the effects of meiosis are only apparent within a family. Logarithm of the odds (lod) scores are usually used to measure linkage. A lod score is the logarithm of the ratio of the likelihood that two loci *are* linked to the likelihood that the loci are *not* linked, given a particular set of data.

Unlinked loci are separated in meiosis approximately 50% of the time. Two linked loci are separated at meiosis less than 50% of the time, and their genetic distance is, therefore, less than 50 centimorgans (cM). Some genes that lie on the same chromosome are unlinked because they are far enough apart that crossing over occurs between them half of the time, on average. Loci that lie on the same chromosome are said to be syntenic but may or may not be linked.

5–10. The answers are: 5-C [I B 2 b], **6-A** [II B 3], **7-B** [II B 2], **8-D** [I C 1 b], **9-D** [I C 1], **10-B** [II B 2]. Lod scores are the usual statistical method of measuring linkage. Loci that are separated by recombination less than 50% of the time are said to be linked. This recombination fraction corresponds to a genetic distance of 50 centimorgans (cM).

Physical maps array loci along a DNA strand; distances between loci are measured in base pairs. In contrast, genetic or linkage maps line up loci according to their behavior during meiosis (i.e., whether they segregate independently). Linkage maps are constructed by family studies because only this method permits analysis of the results of meiosis. Distances on a genetic map are measured in percent recombination or cM.

Linkage describes the close physical proximity of two or more loci on a chromosome, but the specific alleles present at each locus are irrelevant to the identification of linkage. If a certain allele at one locus is found more often than expected by chance with a certain allele at another linked locus, linkage disequilibrium is said to be present. Linkage disequilibrium is specific for a given population and often differs among populations.

Synteny occurs when two or more loci are on the same chromosome. Syntenic loci may or may not be linked, but linked loci are always syntenic. Syntenic loci may be far enough apart on a chromosome for crossing over to occur between them frequently. By definition, linked loci are so close that recombination usually does not occur between them.

Chapter 6

DNA Diagnosis

Michael R. Hayden

I. **TECHNIQUES FOR DNA ANALYSIS.** In the past, the diagnosis of genetic disorders was based on the recognition of a secondary product or the cellular effect of a mutant gene. However, recent progress in technology and an enhanced understanding of the structure and function of human genes have provided the opportunity to investigate and diagnose genetic disease at the level of the abnormal gene itself. Several methods of recombinant DNA technology that have important application to clinical genetics are discussed in this section.

A. **Southern blot**

1. **Method.** This technique combines **gel electrophoresis with the use of specific probes** (Figure 6-1).
   a. **Obtaining DNA.** Usually DNA is obtained from white blood cells. Approximately 5–10 μg of DNA are treated with a restriction enzyme that makes sequence-specific cuts. The resulting DNA fragments are separated by gel electrophoresis.
   b. **Denaturing DNA.** The DNA is denatured to separate the strands, which are then transferred to a membrane.
   c. **Labeling DNA.** A radiolabeled DNA or RNA probe is added to the DNA on the membrane. The probe recognizes and hybridizes with the complementary DNA sequence, thus allowing the specific fragment of interest to be detected.

2. **Applications.** The Southern blot is a very common approach to DNA diagnosis. This method takes advantage of the fact that sequences within a DNA probe recognize similar sequences in digested human DNA (i.e., the principle of molecular hybridization). Many genetic diseases for which DNA diagnosis is possible can be detected using Southern blot analysis. Examples of the use of this technology for specific diseases are given later in this chapter (see II A 3).

3. **Limitations.** Significant amounts of DNA are needed for the Southern blot. The technique is also labor intensive and may take 7–14 days to achieve a result. Southern blotting usually involves the use of radioactive material, which requires special training and safety precautions for laboratory personnel.

B. **Polymerase chain reaction (PCR)** is a powerful technique for selective and rapid **amplification** of target DNA or RNA sequences.

1. **Method.** The technique is based on the enzymatic amplification of a DNA fragment that is flanked by two stretches of nucleotide primers, which hybridize to opposite strands of the sequence being investigated (Figure 6-2).
   a. **Heat separation of DNA strands and hybridization of primers.** The technique works by using heat to separate the two strands of DNA, which allows primers to bind to their complementary sequence.
   b. **Amplification.** The segment between the primers is amplified in the presence of *Taq* polymerase and deoxynucleotides.
   c. **Temperature increase.** Further increases in temperature stop the reaction, which begins again when the temperature is lowered.
   d. **Cycle continues.** The amount of amplified DNA increases rapidly each time the cycle occurs.

2. **Applications.** PCR is extremely important because of its sensitivity, specificity, and speed. PCR has revolutionized genetic analysis and detection of disease pathogens. For example, PCR is used to identify specific disease-causing mutations (e.g., in sickle-cell disease; see I D), to type DNA markers for linkage studies [see Chapter 5 I], and to provide a rapid test for atypical mycobacteria.

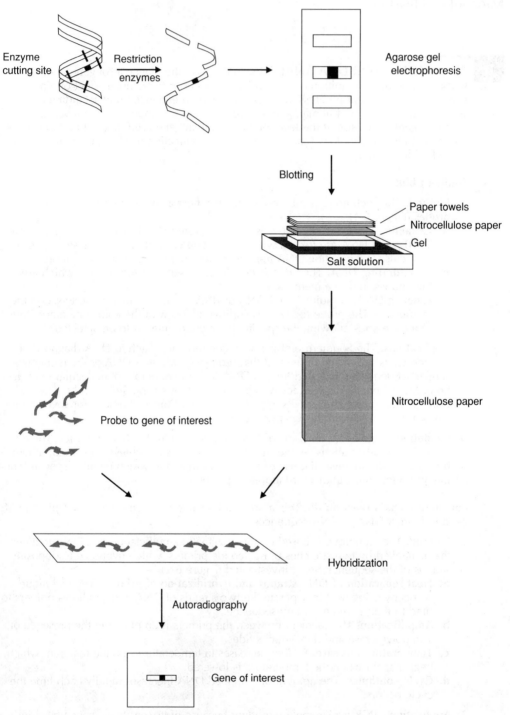

FIGURE 6-1. Southern blot analysis.

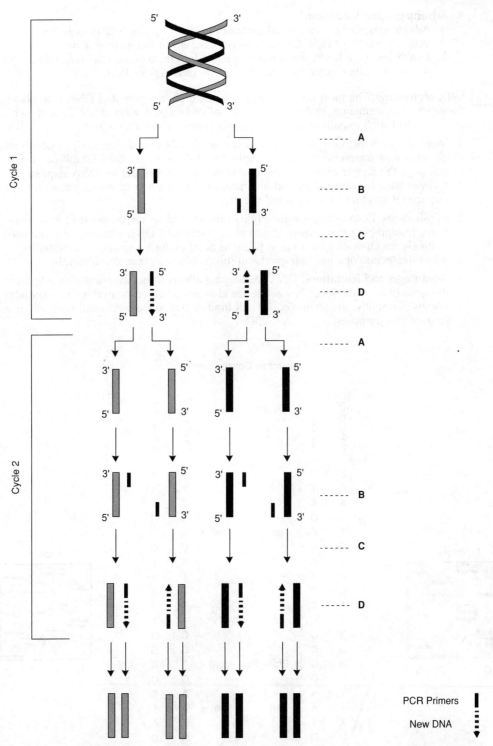

FIGURE 6-2. Polymerase chain reaction (PCR) is based on the amplification of a DNA fragment flanked by two primers that are complementary to opposite strands of the sequence being investigated. In each cycle, *(a)* heat denaturation separates the strands of the target DNA. *(b)* Primers are added in excess and hybridized to complementary fragments. *(c)* Deoxynucleotides and *Taq* polymerase are added while the temperature increases. *(d)* The primer is extended in the 3′ direction as new DNA is extended in the 5′ direction.

3. Advantages and limitations
a. Advantages. Only a very small amount of DNA (1 μg or less, or only a single cell) is needed for PCR. Often, results are achieved in less than 1 day.

b. Limitation. One limitation is that sequence information must be available to synthesize the oligonucleotide primers that are essential for PCR.

C. **DNA sequencing.** The most precise way to characterize a segment of DNA is to obtain the exact DNA sequence. In this way, abnormal variations can be identified and then used to detect such mutations in family members and others (Figure 6-3).

1. Methods.
Two methods are used for determining DNA sequence, both of which rely on separating fragments in which lengths vary by one nucleotide. Established methods (e.g., the Sanger method and the Maxam-Gilbert method) for DNA sequence analysis have been modified and incorporated into automated systems that allow sequence information to be gathered rapidly.

2. Applications.
DNA sequencing methods can be used on the products of PCR reactions, resulting in rapid sequencing of these fragments. DNA sequencing is not used routinely for DNA diagnosis but is likely to be of major importance in the future, when the technology has improved and the cost has decreased sufficiently.

3. Advantages and limitations.
DNA sequencing allows direct assessment of whether the gene of the patient has any sequence changes when compared with a normal control. Currently, the technology is still limited and, therefore, is still primarily used for research purposes.

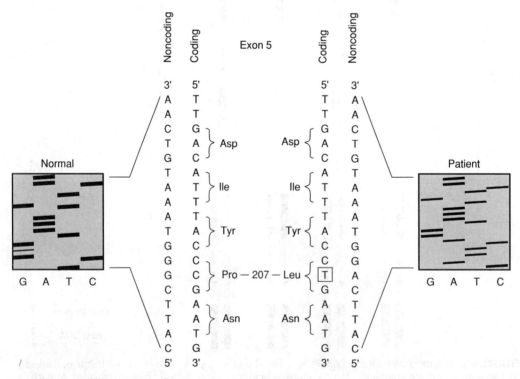

FIGURE 6-3. DNA sequencing allows precise identification of the abnormal variation in an abnormal patient's DNA. Note the difference in the boxed nucleotides between the abnormal patient and the normal control. (Reprinted with permission from Ma Y, Henderson HE, Murthy V, et al: A mutation in the human lipoprotein lipase gene as the most common cause of familial chylomicronemia in French Canadians. *N Eng J Med*, 324:1761–1766, 1991.)

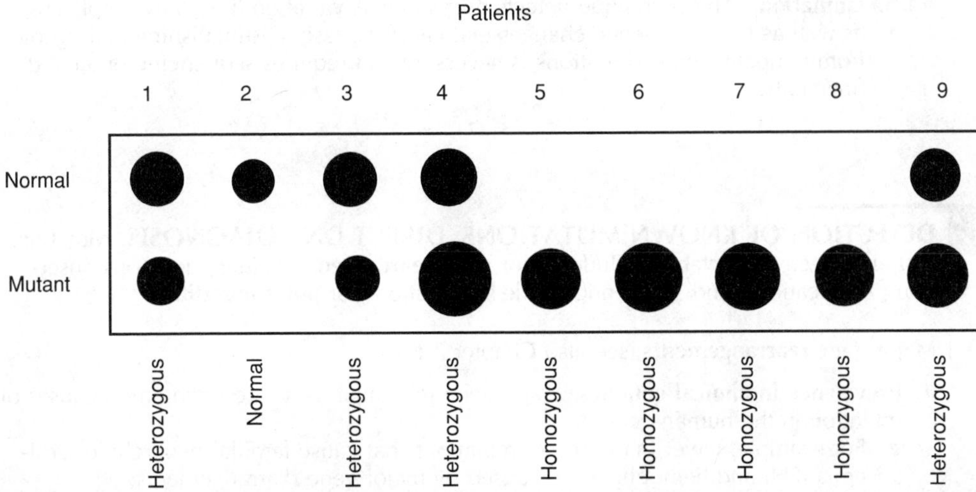

Patients

FIGURE 6-4. Allele-specific oligonucleotide (ASO) hybridization allows detection of both the normal gene and the abnormal gene that causes a particular disease. In this case, the patient has a recessive disorder, and the people who are homozygous and heterozygous for the mutation can be detected. Results show that only patient 2 is normal. Patients 1, 3, 4, and 9 are heterozygous carriers. Patients 5–8 are homozygous for the mutant gene and, therefore, are affected.

D. Allele-specific oligonucleotide (ASO) probe analysis

1. **Method.** This technique uses two synthetic oligonucleotide probes: one probe specific for a normal gene and the other probe specific for a known genetic mutation. The ASO probes for the normal and mutant genes are used as hybridization probes to determine whether a patient has two copies of a normal gene or a mutation responsible for a particular disease (Figure 6-4).

2. **Applications.** Oligonucleotide analysis is most helpful for diagnosing genetic diseases that typically arise from a single predominant mutation (e.g., sickle cell disease, α_1-antitrypsin deficiency).

3. **Advantages and limitations**
   a. **Advantage.** ASO probe analysis can be used on DNA that has been selectively amplified by PCR, which allows rapid and accurate DNA-based diagnosis.
   b. **Limitations.** ASO probe analysis is possible only with precise knowledge of the structure of the normal gene and of the molecular basis of the mutation. Also, the method is limited in that, for many diseases, there is a separate and specific mutation in each family.

E. Electrophoresis of single-stranded or denatured DNA

1. **Method.** Under appropriate conditions, this technique allows the identification of differences between DNA sequences from a patient with a particular disease and from a normal control. These differences are detected by shifts in the bands that are elicited.

2. **Application.** Electrophoresis of single-stranded or denatured DNA detects normal DNA variation or polymorphisms as well as DNA sequence changes that cause disease. DNA sequencing of the altered fragment must be performed to identify whether the change detected is a mutation causing a specific genetic disease.

3. **Advantages and limitations**
   a. **Advantages.** This technique allows rapid screening of a particular gene for possible mutations. This approach is most useful for screening DNA fragments of genes that have been amplified by PCR for variations.

    b. Limitations. This technique detects normal DNA variation (i.e., polymorphisms) as well as DNA sequence changes that cause disease. Distinguishing pathogenic from nonpathogenic alterations is necessary and requires sequencing of altered fragments.

II. DETECTION OF KNOWN MUTATIONS: DIRECT DNA DIAGNOSIS.

Mutations that are directly detectable include **major gene rearrangements** (e.g., deletions, insertions, duplications) and single-nucleotide substitutions, or **point mutations.**

A. Major gene rearrangements (see also Chapter 3 II A)

1. **Prevalence in clinical genetics.** Major gene rearrangements are uncommon causes of mutation in the human genome.
   a. For example, fewer than 10% of mutations that cause familial hypercholesterolemia (FH) and hemophilia are caused by major gene rearrangements.
   b. However, **more than 50% of cases of α-thalassemia, Duchenne muscular dystrophy (DMD), and Becker muscular dystrophy (BMD) are caused by deletions.** A deletion of the α-globin gene causes α-thalassemia, whereas DMD and BMD are often caused by deletions in the dystrophin gene (see Chapter 3 II A 1).

2. **Strategy for detection.** To perform direct DNA-based analysis of a genetic disease caused by a major rearrangement, the normal gene must be cloned and available for use as a probe. If the rearrangements are large enough, and if the gene sequence surrounding the rearrangements are known, major gene rearrangements are easily detected using Southern blot analysis or PCR.

3. **Examples of disorders caused by major gene rearrangements**
   a. **Duchenne muscular dystrophy**
      (1) **Clinical features.** DMD is an X-linked inherited disorder that presents during early childhood with delay in walking and general development. DMD leads to generalized weakness with pseudohypertrophy of the calves.
         (a) **Life expectancy.** People affected with DMD live approximately 17 years. Death is primarily due to cardiorespiratory problems.
         (b) **Incidence.** DMD occurs in about 1 of every 4000 male births and very rarely in females.
      (2) **Genetic background**
         (a) DMD has been shown to be caused by **multiple different defects in the dystrophin gene,** which maps to the short arm of the X chromosome (i.e., Xp).
         (b) A **frameshift mutation** (see Chapter 3 II D 2), which interrupts the coding of the protein, is more likely to result in DMD than BMD.
      (3) **Diagnosis.** DMD can be diagnosed using DNA technology either by detecting the high frequency of deletions in the disorder or by using polymorphic DNA markers within and around the gene.
      (4) **Clinical example of direct DNA diagnosis of DMD.** A 6-year-old boy was recently diagnosed with DMD. The boy's maternal aunt is planning a pregnancy and wishes to know her risk of having a child with DMD (Figure 6-5). There are no other family members with DMD. In this case, DNA analysis revealed that this boy had a large deletion in his dystrophin gene. His mother had a similar deletion and was a carrier for DMD. DNA testing of the boy's aunt revealed that she did not have the deletion in the DMD gene. Therefore, her offspring would not be at increased risk of having DMD.
   b. **Becker muscular dystrophy**
      (1) **Clinical features** of BMD are similar to those of DMD but much milder.
      (2) **Genetic background**
         (a) BMD has been shown to be **allelic to DMD,** with defects also in the dystrophin gene that result in the milder presentation of symptoms.

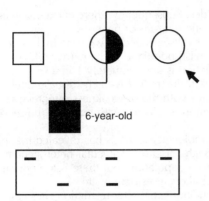

FIGURE 6-5. The proband, the affected person who brought the family to medical attention, is indicated by an *arrow*. The proband's aunt does not carry the deletion for Duchenne muscular dystrophy (DMD); therefore, her offspring are not at risk of having this disease.

6-year-old

       (b) BMD is most often due to a mutation that does not alter the rest of the coding sequence of the dystrophin gene.
   (3) Diagnosis. BMD can also be diagnosed by detecting the high frequency of deletions in the disorder.
  c. Familial hypercholesterolemia
   (1) Clinical features. In people with FH, low-density lipoprotein (LDL) cholesterol is not appropriately removed from the circulation because of mutations in the LDL receptor. LDL levels are therefore increased, which results in blood-vessel–wall damage and premature atherosclerosis.
       (a) Incidence. In the general population, FH occurs in approximately 1 in 500 people, except in certain parts of the world (e.g., Quebec, Canada; South Africa) where FH occurs in approximately 1 in 100 people.
       (b) Life expectancy. Screening for FH is important, as FH does result in a high frequency of premature heart attacks and early death.
       (c) Treatment is directed to lowering cholesterol levels, which can reduce the risk for later atherosclerotic events.
   (2) Genetic background. FH most often results from defects in the LDL receptor gene. The condition is inherited as an autosomal dominant trait.
       (a) FH is caused by a different mutation in most families (i.e., the same mutation does not cause FH in all families affected by FH).
       (b) Major rearrangements do not account for a very large number of mutations underlying FH (see Chapter 3 II A 1 c), except in the French Canadian population, in which a major deletion accounts for approximately 65% of FH patients.
       (c) In the French Canadian and South African Afrikaner populations, a single founder was known to have introduced this defective LDL receptor gene into the population's gene pool centuries ago. Subsequent expansion of the population has caused the frequency of this gene to increase.

B. **Point mutations**

  1. Prevalence in clinical genetics. Point mutations represent the most common type of mutations underlying genetic disease (see Chapter 3 II B).

  2. Some point mutations are **missense mutations**; others are **nonsense mutations** (see Chapter 3 II B).
   a. Strategy for detection. Direct DNA diagnosis requires that the normal gene be cloned and available for use as a probe. Southern blot analysis or PCR amplification and digestion with the appropriate enzyme may reveal an altered pattern of restriction fragments between normal and affected persons.
   b. Examples of disorders caused by point mutations that frequently alter restriction sites
    (1) Tay-Sachs disease
      (a) Clinical features. Tay-Sachs disease is characterized by defective lyso-

somal degradation of gangliosides. Subsequently, there is excessive accumulation of the gangliosides in the neurons of patients.

(i) **Incidence.** Infantile Tay-Sachs disease occurs with the highest frequency in the Ashkenazi Jewish population. The carrier rate for Tay-Sachs disease in this population is approximately 1 in 25.

(ii) **Life expectancy.** Children with infantile Tay-Sachs disease often present at about 5 months of age with motor weakness; progressive motor and mental deterioration results in death between the second and fourth years of life.

(b) **Genetic background.** Detailed molecular analysis has revealed that many different mutations cause Tay-Sachs disease. Molecular heterogeneity occurs even in the Ashkenazi Jewish population, but there is a predominant mutation in this population that alters a restriction site.

(2) **Sickle cell anemia.** Similar point mutations that alter restriction sites can aid in the diagnosis of sickle cell anemia.

(a) In this hereditary disease that is common in people with African ancestry, the mutation in the β-globin gene changes the amino acid glutamine to valine by changing the codon GAG to GTG. This also abolishes a particular enzyme-cutting site.

(b) Persons with sickle cell anemia have an abnormally large DNA fragment detected after hybridization with β-globin DNA that is digested with the appropriate enzyme (Figure 6-6).

3. **Point mutations may not directly alter restriction sites.** An example of a disease with a predominant mutation in this category is cystic fibrosis (CF).

a. **Clinical features.** Intestinal obstruction and infection are the most life-threatening manifestations of CF.

(1) **Incidence.** CF affects white populations with an incidence of approximately 1 in every 2500 births. Approximately 1 in 20 whites are carriers of CF.

(2) **Life expectancy.** Average life expectancy for a person with CF is 20 years.

b. **Genetic background.** CF is a common autosomal recessive disease. The gene for CF has now been cloned, and more than 250 different mutations have been defined.

(1) Approximately 70% of white patients with CF have been shown to have a 3-base pair (3 bp) deletion that does not alter a restriction site.

(2) **ASO probe analysis** provides a rapid and simple way to screen for common CF mutations in the general population.

(3) Based on knowledge of the frequency of specific mutations underlying CF in white people of Western European descent, it is possible to detect approximately 90% of carriers with CF.

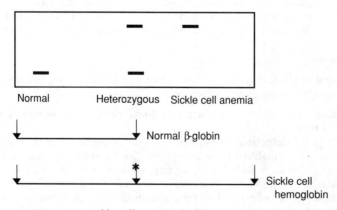

FIGURE 6-6. The mutation causing sickle cell anemia abolishes a restriction site. Thus, patients with sickle cell anemia have a larger band than the normal fragment for β-globin detected by a particular DNA probe.

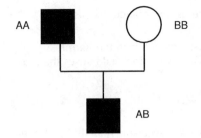

FIGURE 6-7. In this family, the son has inherited marker A from his father and has also inherited the gene for an autosomal dominant disease. The DNA marker is linked to the gene causing this disease, which means that the A marker cosegregates with the mutant allele.

III. DETECTION OF UNKNOWN MUTATIONS: INDIRECT DNA DIAGNOSIS.

Most of the approximately 4000 inherited diseases are caused by unknown mutations. In some instances, these disorders can be diagnosed indirectly, using markers for the mutant gene. These "tags" are variations in DNA that do not cause the disease but have been demonstrated to be close to or linked to the gene or mutation of interest.

A. Limitations of indirect DNA diagnosis

1. Numerous family members are needed to determine the form of the marker that segregates with the mutant gene in that family.

2. The distance between the marker and the mutant gene limits the accuracy of indirect DNA diagnosis.
   a. For each distance of 1 million bp between the marker and gene, there is a 1% chance of recombination during each meiosis, which can render the results incorrect.
   b. For example, if it has been shown that in a particular family an autosomal dominant disease is segregating with marker A, any offspring who inherits marker A from an affected person whose DNA has markers AB is highly likely to have also inherited the mutant gene (Figure 6-7). The accuracy of the assessment largely depends on the distance between the marker and the mutant gene.

3. **Genetic heterogeneity.** When using an indirect approach to DNA diagnosis, it is important to know the likelihood of genetic heterogeneity (i.e., whether mutations underlying a particular disease may occur at different loci in different families). **Polycystic kidney disease (PKD)** and **Alzheimer disease** are examples of diseases that demonstrate genetic heterogeneity.
   a. The gene underlying PKD has now been identified. PKD has been found to be caused by mutations in a gene on chromosome 16 in most families. However, some people with PKD have a causative mutation on another chromosome.
   b. If a DNA marker near the gene on chromosome 16 is used in all instances to determine the risk of someone having the mutant gene, the results of DNA testing will likely be incorrect in families who have the causative gene on another chromosome.
   c. **The discovery of genetic heterogeneity has made DNA diagnosis of PKD difficult.** In each case, the likelihood that the mutant gene in this patient is on chromosome 16 must be determined before additional DNA analysis can be used to assess risk for the disease.

B. Special applications for indirect DNA diagnosis: diseases involving a known gene

1. **When the causative gene is identified but the specific mutation in a particular family is unknown,** variations in noncoding regions within the gene that alter a restric-

tion site can help mark the abnormal gene and trace its inheritance. In this case, blood from family members is needed.

2. The accuracy rate will be very high, because the distance between the harmless DNA variation that alters a restriction site and the DNA variation that causes the mutation is likely to be small.

C. Clinical examples of indirect DNA approaches

1. General indirect DNA approach

a. Presentation of patient (Figure 6-8). The proband is a 30-year-old man (III-1) who requests predictive testing for multiple endocrine neoplasia type 1 (MEN1), an autosomal dominant genetic disorder with variable expressivity and age of onset. His father (II-1) died of the disease, which was confirmed at autopsy, and the proband (III-1) wants to know whether he has or has not inherited the abnormal gene. Also, he is considering having children and wishes to know his risk status before reproducing.

b. Testing. DNA markers closely linked to the abnormal gene have been identified. After initial counseling, blood is collected from several appropriate affected and unaffected family members for DNA testing. The DNA analysis reveals that the proband (III-1) inherited the marker that was segregating with the gene.

c. Results. The proband is given a 98% risk of having inherited the gene.

d. Discussion. In this case, blood from numerous relatives was needed to perform the analysis. Risk assessment was possible because numerous DNA markers were available and because there is a very low risk of genetic heterogeneity in this illness. The proband's first cousin (III-2) also requested predictive testing and was found to have markers AA. Because marker A is not inherited with the disease, the proband's cousin was given a very low risk of having inherited the illness.

2. Indirect DNA approach: diagnosis of phenylketonuria (PKU)

a. Presentation. A couple in their mid-twenties has a 5-year-old girl with PKU, which is an autosomal recessive disorder caused by a defect in the gene for phenylalanine hydroxylase. The affected child is on a special diet and has mild devel-

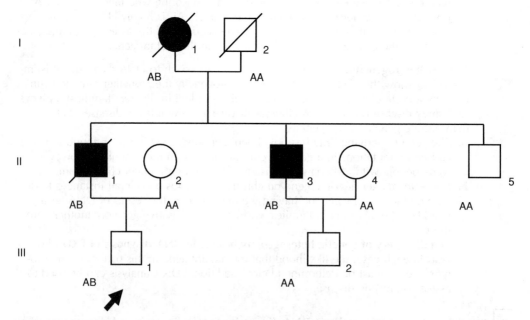

FIGURE 6-8. The *arrow* indicates the proband. In this pedigree for multiple endocrine neoplasia type 1 (MEN I), an autosomal dominant disease with variable expressivity, the gene is segregating with the B marker. III-1 has inherited the B marker from his father and has a high risk; whereas III-2 (the proband's cousin) has inherited the A marker from his father and has a low risk of inheriting MEN I.

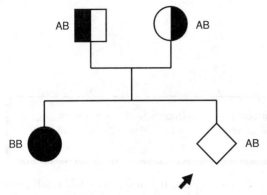

FIGURE 6-9. The *arrow* indicates the proband in this family with phenylketonuria. The mutation is segregating with the B marker. In this case, the fetus *(diamond)* has inherited an A marker from one parent and a B marker from the other and, therefore, is a carrier.

opmental delay. The couple recently discovered that they are expecting another baby, and they wish to know whether the second child will have PKU.

b. Testing. In this case, the gene for phenylalanine hydroxylase has been cloned, but the specific mutation underlying PKU in the 5-year-old is not known. However, variations in the noncoding regions of the PKU gene can be used to determine whether the fetus is likely to be affected by PKU, to be a carrier for PKU, or to have two normal phenylalanine hydroxylase genes. Both the mother and father have AB markers.

c. Results. DNA analysis reveals that the affected child inherited a B marker from her mother and a B marker from her father (Figure 6-9). Thus, the mutation must have occurred on a PKU gene that had a B marker in both instances. The mother undergoes chorionic villus sampling at 10 weeks of pregnancy, and analysis of fetal DNA reveals an AB pattern. Thus, the fetus is a carrier for PKU but will not be affected.

d. Discussion. The accuracy of this prediction is close to 100% because of the very small distance between the DNA variation used to tag the gene for PKU and the actual site of the causative mutation.

IV. **DNA BANKING.** Often, when the precise mutation responsible for a disease is unknown, DNA from affected and nonaffected relatives is needed to provide DNA analysis and to determine which form of the marker is being inherited with the disease gene and with the normal gene. The most important sources of DNA in such analyses are from persons who are affected by the disease and their parents.

A. DNA banks **store DNA from crucial relatives** in an effort to ensure that no family member will be denied DNA testing due to a lack of available DNA.

B. **DNA can be extracted from any tissue.** However, for convenience, DNA usually is taken from **white blood cells.** In situations that require a large supply of DNA for analysis, white blood cells can be immortalized after exposure to the Epstein-Barr virus. This viral infection enables the cells to grow indefinitely in culture (rather than for just a few weeks) so that an unlimited supply of DNA is possible.

STUDY QUESTIONS

DIRECTIONS: Each of the numbered items or incomplete statements in this section is followed by answers or by completions of the statement. Select the ONE lettered answer or completion that is BEST in each case.

1. A woman (II-3) has a nephew (III-1) affected with Duchenne muscular dystrophy (DMD). She wishes to know if she is a carrier for this gene. The pedigree below reveals the family's DNA results using polymorphic DNA markers within the gene.

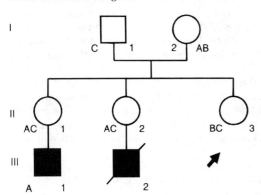

The most likely interpretation of the possibility that II-3 is a carrier for DMD is

(A) very high
(B) mildly elevated
(C) mildly reduced
(D) very low
(E) not able to be determined from this analysis

2. Two parents (I-1 and I-2) of Ashkenazi Jewish descent have had a child (II-1) with Tay-Sachs disease. They are now expecting another child (II-2) and wish to have prenatal diagnosis for this disorder. The pedigree shows the results of DNA analysis.

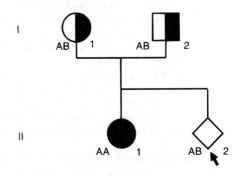

The most likely interpretation of the results for this pregnancy is that the fetus is

(A) affected
(B) completely normal
(C) a carrier
(D) unable to determine from results
(E) unlikely to be the offspring of these parents

DIRECTIONS: Each of the numbered items or incomplete statements in this section is negatively phrased, as indicated by a capitalized word such as NOT, LEAST, or EXCEPT. Select the ONE lettered answer or completion that is BEST in each case.

3. All of the following materials are necessary to perform Southern blot analysis for diagnosis of a genetic disease EXCEPT

(A) a membrane for transfer of DNA
(B) DNA from the person being tested
(C) the DNA sequence of the probe being used
(D) a specific restriction enzyme
(E) a DNA probe

4. True statements regarding the use of allele-specific oligonucleotides (ASO) for diagnosis of genetic disease include all of the following EXCEPT

(A) a precise knowledge of the mutation causing the particular disease is needed
(B) it may be helpful for the diagnosis of sickle cell anemia and α_1-antitrypsin deficiency
(C) the sequence of the whole gene, including flanking regulatory sequences, must be known prior to DNA testing
(D) DNA from only a few family members is needed for diagnosis
(E) this diagnostic method is applicable for only a small number of genetic diseases

ANSWERS AND EXPLANATIONS

1. The answer is D [II A 3 a (4)]. II-3 has a very low risk of being a carrier for Duchenne muscular dystrophy (DMD), which is an X-linked disorder. The grandfather (I-1) must have passed on a C marker to II-1, II-2, and II-3. The grandmother (I-2) has AB markers and must have passed on A markers to II-1 and II-2. The grandson, who is affected with DMD (III-1), has an A marker. Therefore, the mutation for DMD must be inherited with the A marker. Grandson III-2 died of DMD. The fact that II-3 inherited the B marker from her mother, instead of the A marker, makes the risk of II-3 being a DMD carrier very low.

2. The answer is C [II B 2 b (1)]. In this particular case, it is clear that the defect for Tay-Sachs disease is going along with the A marker. Because the fetus has inherited an A marker from one parent and a B marker from the other parent, it is most likely that the fetus is a carrier.

3. The answer is C [I A 1]. To perform Southern blot analysis, DNA is digested with a particular restriction enzyme, electrophoresed in agarose gel, transferred to a membrane, and hybridized with a labeled DNA probe. The DNA sequence of the probe being used is not necessary for the analysis.

4. The answer is C [I D]. Allele-specific oligonucleotide (ASO) hybridization is possible if the specific mutation is known, which allows synthesis of a mutant and a wild type (normal) allele. It is particularly useful when only a small number of mutations cause the disease, such as in sickle cell anemia and α_1-antitrypsin deficiency. Only the specific DNA sequence change around the mutation and the DNA sequence information of some flanking DNA are needed. DNA from numerous family relatives is not necessary to assess the presence or absence of the mutation by a particular individual.

Chapter 7

Population Genetics

J. M. Friedman

I. GENES IN POPULATIONS

A. **Population genetics** focuses on the relative distribution of genes or inherited traits within populations. The factors that change or maintain the frequency of genes or genotypes within the population are studied as well.

B. **The Hardy-Weinberg law** is used to relate the frequencies of genotypes at a single mendelian locus to the phenotype frequencies in a population.

1. **Definitions**
   a. **Selection** is the process that determines the relative share of genes that individuals of various genotypes contribute to the propagation of a population. Genotypes that are disadvantageous are selected against and contribute relatively fewer genes to the next generation. Genotypes that are advantageous are selected for and contribute a disproportionately greater number of genes to the next generation.
   b. **Migration** is the movement of individuals between populations. Migration can result in exchange of genes between populations and alteration of gene frequencies.

2. **The assumptions** upon which the Hardy-Weinberg law is based are:
   a. **There is no mutation** occurring at the locus.
   b. **There is no selection** for any of the genotypes at the locus.
   c. **Mating is completely random.**
   d. **There is no migration** into or out of the population being considered.

3. These assumptions are **never entirely correct** for any locus.
   a. If they are nearly correct, a locus is said to be in **Hardy-Weinberg equilibrium.**
   b. If the assumptions are seriously violated with respect to a given locus, the Hardy-Weinberg law may not apply.

4. **The Hardy-Weinberg law states:** In a population at equilibrium, for a locus with two alleles, D and d, having frequencies of p and q, respectively, the genotype frequencies are: $DD = p^2$, $Dd = 2pq$, and $dd = q^2$.
   a. **Note that p + q = 1** because there are only two alleles at the locus, and the sum of their frequencies (expressed as fractions of the total) must equal 1. This also means that $p = 1-q$ and that $q = 1-p$.
   b. **Note that $p^2 + 2pq + q^2 = 1$.** There are only three genotypes, and the sum of their frequencies (expressed as fractions of the total) must equal 1.

5. **For an autosomal dominant condition,** the frequency p of the mutant gene (D) is very small compared with the frequency q of the normal gene (d). The frequency of the heterozygote $[(Dd) = 2pq]$ is consequently much greater than the frequency of the abnormal homozygote $[(DD) = p^2]$. Thus, the disease frequency for an autosomal dominant condition is approximately equal to the frequency of the heterozygote (2pq).
   a. This relationship ($p^2 \ll 2pq$) explains why **homozygotes for autosomal dominant diseases are rarely observed.**
      (1) In practice, a **homozygote for an autosomal dominant disease** can usually be recognized by the fact that **both parents are affected with the disease.**
      (2) **The phenotype of the homozygote is much more severely abnormal than that of the heterozygote** for most autosomal dominant diseases in which homozygotes have actually been observed. This contrasts with the situation in

some experimental organisms in which the phenotype is usually the same in homozygotes and heterozygotes for a dominant trait.

   b. If p is very small, q is approximately equal to 1, and the frequency of the disease is approximately equal to twice the frequency of the mutant gene (2p).

6. For **autosomal recessive conditions**, the Hardy-Weinberg law permits calculation of the disease or carrier frequency from the gene frequency, and vice versa.

   a. The frequency of the disease (i.e., of the genotype *dd*) is simply the **gene frequency squared** (q^2).

   b. Conversely, the **gene frequency** (q) can be calculated as the **square root of the frequency of the disease** (q^2).

   c. The **frequency of the heterozygous carrier** (i.e., of the genotype *Dd*) is equal to **twice the product of the component gene frequencies** (2pq).

   d. For rare recessive diseases, q is very small, and p is nearly equal to 1. Under such circumstances, the **frequency of heterozygous carriers is approximately equal to 2q.**

   e. The **carrier frequency for a recessive disease is always greater than the frequency of the disease itself** because mathematically the value of 2pq must always exceed that of q^2 if p > q.

     (1) For rare recessives (where p >> q), the heterozygote frequency is far greater than the frequency of homozygotes with the disease ($2pq >> q^2$).

     (2) Thus, **almost all of the mutant genes in the population for a rare recessive disease are carried in heterozygotes.**

7. For **X-linked recessive conditions,** the Hardy-Weinberg law in its usual form refers only to females who carry two alleles for each X-linked locus. Males carry only one copy of every X-linked gene, so the genotype frequencies for *DY* and *dY* correspond directly to the gene frequencies p and q, respectively (Y represents the Y chromosome in the male).

   a. Thus, the **gene frequency** (q) for an X-linked recessive disease is **equal to the frequency of that condition among males.**

   b. The **values of p and q are the same in males and females** because a gene does not "know" whether it will end up in a male or female zygote.

   c. The **frequency of an X-linked recessive disease is much greater in males than in females,** $q >> q^2$ [the gene frequency q is expressed as a fraction, e.g., $1/100 >> (1/100)^2$].

   d. Because X-linked recessive diseases are generally uncommon, the value of q is typically very small compared with p, and $2pq >> q^2$. Thus, **heterozygous carrier females are much more common than homozygous affected females** for X-linked recessive traits.

   e. If q is very small, p is approximately equal to 1, and the frequency of female carriers (2pq) is approximately equal to twice the frequency of affected males (2q).

   f. In the population as a whole, **about two-thirds of all mutant X-linked recessive genes are found in carrier females and about one-third in affected males.**

     (1) In general, two-thirds of all X chromosomes and two-thirds of all X-linked genes are found in females; one-third are found in males.

     (2) The reason for this distribution is that males and females occur in approximately equal numbers, and females have two X chromosomes, whereas males have only one.

II. MUTATIONS IN POPULATIONS

A. Genetic load

1. Mutations are continually occurring, and most mutations are detrimental. The genetic load is the **cumulative reduction of reproductive fitness** produced by all detrimental alleles at all loci in all individuals in the population.

2. The concept of genetic load depends not only on the mutant alleles that are actually present but also upon the circumstances in which fitness is being determined. **Mutations that are deleterious in one population may be neutral or beneficial in another population** or in the same population under different circumstances. For example, the sickle cell mutation, which causes a serious disease in the homozygous state, is beneficial to populations living in regions where malaria is endemic because the more common heterozygotes are resistant to malaria.

B. **One measure of genetic load related to recessive traits** is the increase in death rate that occurs among the offspring of consanguineous parents.

1. The average number of **recessive lethal equivalents** that each person carries can be calculated from this increase. A lethal equivalent is defined as a heterozygous gene that is lethal to homozygotes or a proportionally larger number of heterozygous genes, each of which is lethal in only a portion of homozygotes. For example, each of the following is **one lethal equivalent:**
   a. **One gene** that is **lethal in 100%** of homozygotes
   b. **Two genes** that are each **lethal in half** of homozygotes
   c. **Three genes** that are each **lethal in one-third** of homozygotes

2. **Lethal equivalents are calculated from the rate of death among the children of consanguineous couples,** and the particular gene (or genes) involved is usually unknown. It is necessary to use the concept of lethal equivalents to quantitate this death rate because the number of genetic loci actually involved cannot be determined.

3. On the basis of such studies, it is estimated that **each normal person carries an average of three to five lethal equivalents**. In other words, **every person carries abnormal recessive genes.**
   a. One implication of this observation is that people who are found to be **carriers of recessive genes** for conditions such as Tay-Sachs disease, sickle cell disease, or cystic fibrosis **do not differ from others because they are carriers. They differ because they know one of the abnormal genes they carry.**
   b. Another implication is that **any strategy designed to eliminate all abnormal genes in a population can only succeed by eliminating all people in the population.**

C. **Mutations are rare in the population but common among patients with dominant or X-linked diseases that reduce fertility.** For example, consider the autosomal dominant disease **achondroplasia**, the most common kind of short-limbed dwarfism.

1. **New mutations.** About **90% of all cases** of achondroplasia arise as new mutations, but the **frequency of new mutations** of the gene for achondroplasia is only about **1/100,000.**

2. This apparent contradiction is explained by the fact that two ratios with the same numerator, but very different denominators, are being compared.
   a. The number of people with achondroplasia who have new mutant genes is the numerator in both cases. However, in the former instance, the denominator is the total number of people with achondroplasia (a small number), whereas in the latter case, the denominator is the total number of genes, normal and abnormal, at the achondroplasia locus in the population (a very large number).
   b. For example, if a population of 500,000 people included 11 people with achondroplasia and 10 of these represented new mutations, then 10/11 (91%) of the people with achondroplasia would represent new mutations, but the mutation frequency would be about 1/100,000.
      (1) Each normal person has two normal genes. Then, 500,000 − 11 = 499,989 normal people have 999,978 normal genes.
      (2) There are 11 people with achondroplasia who have 11 normal genes and 11 abnormal achondroplasia genes.
      (3) Ten of the achondroplasia genes are new mutants, so the mutation frequency is 10/(999,978 + 11 + 11) = 10/1,000,000 = 1/100,000.

D. A paternal age effect is observed with some **new dominant mutations,** in which the average age of fathers of affected children is significantly increased.

1. This observation implies that there is an increased risk of diseases owing to new dominant mutations among the children of older fathers. The exact **magnitude is unknown,** but the risk for all new dominant mutations combined is **unlikely to be more than 0.5% to 1% among the children of fathers who are older than 40 years.**

2. There appears to **be no independent association** of new dominant mutations **with the age of the mother.** Maternal age does, however, affect the rate of nondisjunction that is responsible for the occurrence of trisomy in offspring.

E. **Mutation–selection equilibrium** is the maintenance of constant gene frequencies in a population through replacement by mutation of abnormal alleles lost by death or reproductive failure. If the frequency of a monogenic disease remains constant from generation to generation, and if other causes of gene gain or loss (e.g., migration) are negligible, then **all genes lost in one generation by selection must be replaced in the next generation by mutation.**

1. **If an autosomal dominant disease is a genetic lethal** (i.e., if every carrier of the abnormal gene dies or is otherwise incapable of reproduction), **every case must arise as a new mutation.**
   a. In such circumstances, the **frequency of mutation for the abnormal gene can be calculated directly as one-half the frequency of the disease.** Every person represents two genes, and affected patients would be expected to be heterozygotes with one abnormal gene and one normal gene. If the number of people affected with the disease is A, and the total number of people in the population is N, then the disease frequency is A/N, and the mutation frequency is $A/2N$.
   b. In practice, **diseases that are complete genetic lethals are often not recognized as autosomal dominant traits** because they do not exhibit the characteristic pattern of transmission in families. This method of calculating mutation rates is therefore applied to just the subset of patients who are known to represent new mutations (i.e., those who are born to unaffected parents).
   c. **Mutation frequencies** have been calculated for several dominant diseases by this method. These frequencies have ranged from about 10^{-6} to about 10^{-4}.

2. **For an X-linked recessive disease that is genetically lethal in males, the frequency of new mutations is one-third the frequency of the disease.**
   a. If the population includes equal numbers of males and females, two-thirds of all X chromosomes occur in females and one-third in males because females have two X chromosomes and males have only one. Similarly, **two-thirds of all X-linked genes (both normal and abnormal) occur in females and one-third in males.** A gene for an X-linked recessive disease is expressed in a male, but the same gene in a female is likely not to be expressed because the female probably has a normal allele at this locus on her other X chromosome.
   b. If an X-linked disease is a genetic lethal, all males who carry the abnormal gene at that locus will die or otherwise fail to reproduce. Thus, **the one-third of all abnormal alleles that occur in males are lost in every generation.** If the disease frequency does not change, the **abnormal genes that have been lost must be replaced in the next generation by new mutations.** Because genes are distributed randomly at fertilization, one-third of the new mutant genes at the disease locus end up in affected males and two-thirds end up in carrier females.
   c. In a **sporadic case of an X-linked recessive disease that is genetically lethal in males, there is only a two-thirds chance that the mother is a carrier** because there is a one-third chance that the affected boy represents a new mutation.

III. EFFECTS OF MEDICAL INTERVENTION ON DISEASE GENE FREQUENCIES

A. **Some people have expressed concern that treatment of genetic disease would result in an increased frequency of such conditions** in the population because abnormal gene carriers who would otherwise die would be permitted to survive and reproduce. In general, **this concern is unfounded.**

1. **Treatment of autosomal recessive diseases** has almost no effect on gene frequencies because most abnormal alleles are carried in unaffected heterozygotes.

2. **Treatment of a dominant or X-linked disease** could increase the disease frequency, but the change would probably be quite small.
   a. **Many dominant diseases do not affect reproduction** because they have late onset or are relatively mild. Thus, carriers may reproduce normally even without treatment.
   b. **Genetic counseling** in families of patients with serious autosomal dominant or X-linked diseases tends to discourage having children and thus decreases the likelihood that such traits will be transmitted to the next generation.

3. Conversely, **genetic counseling has very little effect on reducing the frequency of abnormal genes** in a population.

4. **Prevention and treatment of genetic disease benefits individual patients and families.** The effect on disease frequencies in the population is, in general, negligible.

B. **Eugenics** can be defined as improvement of the human species by selective breeding. For centuries, selective breeding has been used successfully in plants and domesticated animals. The best specimens were crossed to improve the quality of the stocks. Eugenics attempts to apply the same principles to humans.

1. **Positive eugenics** seeks to increase the propagation of "more desirable" types of people.

2. **Negative eugenics** seeks to decrease the propagation of "less desirable" types.

3. **Eugenic policies** became quite popular and were implemented in Europe and North America during the early decades of the twentieth century.
   a. Some of the proponents of eugenics were **eminent scientists,** but their advocacy was often based on unconvincing data or on interpretations or extrapolations that went far beyond the facts.
   b. The popularity of eugenics was partly due to its **resonance with the contemporary social and cultural milieu,** which included broad acceptance of racism, imperialism, and social darwinism.

4. Eugenics was used to provide "scientific" support for restrictive **immigration policies, laws prohibiting marriage on the basis of race and certain handicaps, and laws requiring sterilization** of people considered to have serious genetic defects. A perversion of eugenic doctrine was used as a "scientific" basis for the extermination of Jews and other ethnic minorities by the Nazis during World War II.

5. Current understanding of genetics provides **little scientific support** for eugenic programs, all of which must entail subjugation of the interests of the individual to the interests of future society, and thus loss of personal freedom.

STUDY QUESTIONS

DIRECTIONS: Each of the numbered items or incomplete statements in this section is followed by answers or by completions of the statement. Select the ONE lettered answer or completion that is BEST in each case.

1. Cystic fibrosis is the most common autosomal recessive disease among white Americans, occurring with a frequency of 1/2500 births. What is the approximate frequency of heterozygous carriers for cystic fibrosis in this population?

(A) 1/25
(B) 2/25
(C) 1/50
(D) 1/2500
(E) 2/2500

2. Sickle cell disease, an autosomal recessive condition that occurs with a frequency of 1/625 among African-Americans, produces anemia, pain crises, and an increased risk of certain infections. What is the approximate chance that the clinically normal sister of a person with sickle cell disease will have an affected child if she marries an unrelated African-American man?

(A) 1/4
(B) 1/25
(C) 1/50
(D) 1/75
(E) 1/625

3. Albinism is an autosomal recessive disease that produces a lack of skin and hair pigmentation. The frequency of the gene for albinism in a population is known to be 1/190. What is the approximate risk for albinism in the child of an albino woman who marries an unrelated and unaffected man with no family history of albinism?

(A) 1/95
(B) 1/190
(C) 1/380
(D) 1/570
(E) 1/760

4. Duchenne muscular dystrophy is an X-linked recessive disease that produces progressive loss of muscle function. Affected boys usually die by early adulthood; they are unable to reproduce. The frequency of Duchenne muscular dystrophy is about 1/25,000 males. What is the approximate frequency of carrier females for this disease?

(A) $2/\sqrt{25{,}000}$
(B) 1/25,000
(C) 1/25,000
(D) 2/75,000

5. Which one of the following is a correct statement regarding genetic load?

(A) Effective treatment of autosomal recessive diseases is likely to increase the frequency of such diseases in a few generations
(B) Genetic counseling is likely to reduce the frequency of autosomal dominant diseases substantially
(C) Mutations that are deleterious in one population may be beneficial in others
(D) Lethal equivalents are largely confined to populations with a high rate of consanguinity
(E) Eugenic policies, if conscientiously applied, could eliminate almost all abnormal genes from the population

DIRECTIONS: The item in this section is negatively phrased, as indicated by the capitalized word EXCEPT. Select the ONE lettered answer or completion that is BEST in each case.

6. All of the following observations can be explained by mutation–selection equilibrium EXCEPT

(A) new dominant mutations occur more often among the children of fathers who are over age 40 than among the children of younger fathers

(B) the frequency of mutation for an autosomal dominant disease that is genetically lethal is equal to one half the frequency of the disease

(C) new mutations are often observed among patients with autosomal dominant diseases that substantially impair reproduction

(D) the chance of a new mutation is 1/3 in a boy who is the first in his family to be af-

fected by an X-linked recessive disease that is genetically lethal in males

(E) the mothers of some heterozygous female carriers of X-linked recessive diseases that are lethal in males are not carriers themselves

---

DIRECTIONS: The set of matching questions in this section consists of a list of four to twenty-six lettered options (some of which may be in figures) followed by several numbered items. For each numbered item, select the ONE lettered option that is most closely associated with it. To avoid spending too much time on matching sets with large numbers of options, it is generally advisable to begin each set by reading the list of options. Then, for each item in the set, try to generate the correct answer and locate it in the option list, rather than evaluating each option individually. Each lettered option may be selected once, more than once, or not at all.

Questions 7–10

Stenosis of the aqueduct of Sylvius is sometimes inherited as an X-linked recessive trait. Affected individuals have severe hydrocephalus and do not reproduce. In each of the following pedigrees, the affected boys have X-linked aqueductal stenosis. Match the recur-

rence risk for a future son of the woman indicated by the asterisk in each pedigree with the appropriate value.

(A) Essentially 0 (risk of mutation)
(B) 1/6
(C) 1/4
(D) 1/3
(E) 1/2

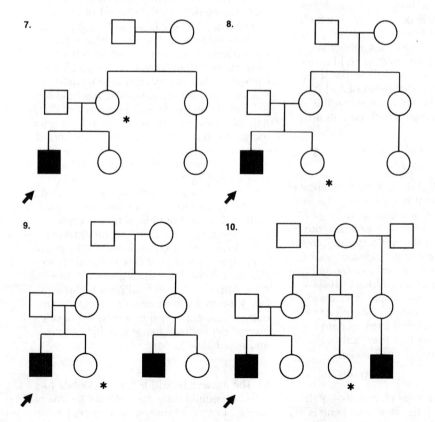

ANSWERS AND EXPLANATIONS

1. The answer is A [I B 6]. According to the Hardy-Weinberg law, the frequency of affected homozygotes for an autosomal recessive disease is q^2. In this case, $q^2 = 1/2500$, and

$$q = \sqrt{1/25,000} = 1/50$$

The heterozygote frequency is represented by $2pq$, where $p = 1-q$. Since this is an uncommon disease, the heterozygote frequency is approximately equal to $2q$, or $2/50 = 1/25$.

2. The answer is D [I B 6]. An unaffected woman whose brother has sickle cell disease has a 2/3 chance of being a carrier of the abnormal gene. The disease occurs among homozygotes with a frequency of $1/625 = q^2$. The frequency of the abnormal gene (q) is

$$\sqrt{1/625} = 1/25$$

According to the Hardy-Weinberg law, the frequency of carriers in the general population is $2pq = 2(24/25)(1/25)$ or about 2/25, which is the chance that the woman's husband carries the sickle cell gene. The chance that the woman would have an affected child is determined by multiplying the chance that she is a carrier by the chance that her husband is a carrier, multiplied by the chance that the child would be affected if both parents are carriers:

$$2/3 \times 2/25 \times 1/4 = 4/300 = 1/75$$

3. The answer is B [I B 6]. If the frequency of the abnormal gene (q) is 1/190, then the frequency of carriers is approximately $2q = 2/190 = 1/95$. The woman is homozygous for the disease gene, so she will transmit it to her offspring. If her husband is a heterozygous carrier, he will have a 1/2 chance of transmitting the abnormal gene to his children. The chance that this woman would have an affected child is the product of her risk of carrying the gene, her husband's risk of carrying the gene, and the risk that they both would transmit it to a child. This is:

$$1 \times 1/95 \times 1/2 = 1/190$$

Note that in this case the chance that both parents will transmit the abnormal gene is 1/2 and not the usual 1/4 because the mother MUST transmit the abnormal gene, and the father has a 1/2 chance of transmitting it.

4. The answer is C [I B 7 e]. For an X-linked recessive disease, the gene frequency (in both males and females) is the same as the frequency of the disease in males. In this case, $q = 1/25,000$. The frequency of female heterozygotes is indicated by the term $2pq$ in the Hardy-Weinberg law. If the disease is rare (i.e., if q is very small), the frequency of carrier females is approximately equal to $2q$ or $2/25,000$ in this case.

5. The answer is C [II A 2, B; III A]. Whether or not a gene exerts a deleterious effect depends on many factors, such as environmental conditions, population density, and the "genetic background" (i.e., the types of genes that are common in the population). A gene that is deleterious under one set of circumstances may be beneficial under others. Treatment of autosomal recessive diseases has almost no effect on gene frequencies because most abnormal autosomal recessive alleles are carried in clinically normal heterozygotes. Conversely, genetic counseling has little beneficial effect on the overall frequency of dominant diseases because many are due to new mutations, have onset after the usual period of reproduction, exhibit incomplete penetrance, or have variable and often mild expression. Lethal equivalents (genes that, when homozygous, cause death in some affected individuals) are measured in consanguineous matings but are found in almost everyone. Each normal person carries approximately three to five lethal equivalents in a heterozygous state. Eugenic policies are unlikely to eliminate most deleterious genes for three reasons: Almost every normal person carries a few abnormal genes; new mutations continually occur; and whether a gene is considered normal depends on many variable genetic and nongenetic factors.

6. The answer is A [II E 1 a, 2]. Mutation–selection equilibrium accounts for the maintenance of constant disease (and gene) frequencies in a population by replacement of all genes lost to selection in one generation by new mutations in the next generation. New mutations occur more often among the children of older fathers, but this appears to be related to the continuing cell division that occurs among spermatogonia throughout life. Selection and gene loss are not factors in the paternal age effect. Because every person represents two genes at each locus, there are twice as many genes at each locus as there are people in a population. The frequency of individuals with a disease due to a mutant gene is thus twice the frequency of new mutant genes among all genes at that locus. For a genetic lethal, all cases of the disease must represent new mutations. A dominant disease that substantially impairs fertility would disappear in a few generations if new mutations did not occur. Among people affected by such diseases, new mutations are common. According to mutation–selection equilibrium, one-third of boys who have sporadic cases of an X-linked recessive disease that is lethal in males represent new mutations. In the other two-thirds of cases, the mothers are carriers. These women represent new mutations themselves in half of the cases because new mutant genes may first appear in either males or females.

7–10. The answers are: 7-D, 8-B, 9-C, 10-A [II E 2]. X-linked aqueductal stenosis is an X-linked recessive disease that is genetically lethal in males. In the pedigree in question 7, there is just one affected boy. According to mutation–selection equilibrium, there is a 1/3 chance that this case arose as a new mutation and a 2/3 chance that the mother carries the abnormal gene. If she is a carrier, the risk that her son would inherit the abnormal gene and be affected is 1/2. Thus, the overall risk that her son would have X-linked aqueductal stenosis is:

$$2/3 \times 1/2 = 2/6 = 1/3$$

In the pedigree in question 8, the son of the sister of the proband is at risk. Again, the mother's risk of being a carrier of the gene for X-linked aqueductal stenosis is 2/3 because of mutation–selection equilibrium. Her daughter has a 1/2 chance of inheriting the abnormal gene if the mother is a carrier. If the daughter is a carrier, her son has a 1/2 risk of inheriting the abnormal gene from her and being affected with the disease. The overall risk that the daughter's son would have X-linked aqueductal stenosis is thus:

$$2/3 \times 1/2 \times 1/2 = 2/12 = 1/6$$

The pedigree in question 9 differs from the previous pedigrees because two boys are affected with X-linked aqueductal stenosis, and they are related to each other through their mothers. It is therefore very likely that the proband's mother and her sister both carry the abnormal gene. Two separate new mutations are an extremely unlikely explanation for this pedigree. If the proband's mother is a carrier, the proband's sister has a 1/2 chance of being a carrier as well. If the proband's sister is a carrier, her son has a 1/2 chance of inheriting the abnormal gene and being affected with the disease. The overall risk that the proband's sister's son would have X-linked aqueductal stenosis is:

$$1/2 \times 1/2 = 1/4$$

In the pedigree in question 10, the mother of the proband is almost certainly a carrier of the abnormal gene because her maternal half-sister also has a boy with X-linked hydrocephalus. In this family, however, the risk to the sons of the mother's brother's daughter is the concern. This woman (the one with the asterisk) cannot have inherited the abnormal gene because her father did not inherit it from his mother; if he did, he would have been affected with the disease. If a woman does not carry the abnormal gene, she cannot transmit it to her son, so the risk of the proband's cousin's son being affected is extremely small.

Chapter 8

Biochemical Basis of Disease

Barbara McGillivray

I. **INTRODUCTION.** There are few instances in which either normal development or a disease state occurs without interaction of both genetic ("intrinsic") and nongenetic ("extrinsic") factors. Even if only genetic factors are considered, it is important to remember that mutant genes do not act in isolation; they are influenced by the action of many other genes.

A. **Inborn errors of metabolism** are largely determined by genetic mutations, which may be caused by a single gene with mendelian inheritance (e.g., Tay-Sachs disease) or a more complex process (e.g., coronary artery disease).

B. **Treatment.** Some diseases can be treated or ameliorated by dietary or other nongenetic manipulations, but the development of such strategies requires that the pathophysiology or the underlying process be understood.

II. **RELATIONSHIP OF GENES AND PROTEINS.** Genes either specify the ultimate amino acid sequence of a protein or control the rate or timing of synthesis of a specific protein. The immediate consequence of a gene mutation is a change in the quality or quantity of a specific protein. Currently, more than 500 single-gene biochemical abnormalities are partly or completely understood. Rather than attempting to remember each individually, **physicians should be familiar with how various types of mutations influence the final protein and determine the clinical pathology.**

A. **Underlying principle.** The concept of **"one gene–one enzyme"** is now called **the "one cistron–one polypeptide" principle** because the gene product may not be an enzyme and because there may be subunits both within and among enzymes. The principles that comprise this concept include the following.

1. **All biochemical processes are genetically controlled.**

2. **Each biochemical pathway is made up of steps, each of which is under the control of a different enzyme.**

3. **Each enzyme is encoded by one or more genes.**

4. **A single gene mutation can result in an alteration in a biochemical reaction.** All single-gene disorders are the result of an abnormal protein molecule or the abnormal control of such molecules.

B. **Protein functions and disorders.** Proteins function as enzymes, and they are involved in metabolism and structure. For each function of a protein, mutation can cause specific genetic disorders.

1. **Direct biologic effects.** Some mutations directly act in a way to cause disease.
   a. **Osteogenesis imperfecta** describes a group of disorders that involves defects in the production of type I collagen.
      (1) **Type I collagen** is the major structural protein of bone. It is a helical structure composed of two procollagen proα1(I) chains and one procollagen proα2(I) chain.
      (2) Infants with a particularly severe type of osteogenesis imperfecta have been found to have a **point mutation** involving a substitution of a glycine, which results in instability of the collagen, interference with its secretion, or difficulty in the assembly of collagen fibrils in the extracellular matrix.

(3) **Affected infants** are heterozygous for the mutation and usually die of severe fracturing and bone crumpling.

b. **β-Thalassemia.** As a consequence of a number of different mutations affecting the β-globin gene, there is decreased synthesis of β chains. The normal function of the hemoglobin molecule is to transport oxygen from the lungs to the peripheral tissues. The mutation leads to **altered oxygen transport and increased red cell destruction with anemia.** Homozygotes have severe anemia, and they require repeated blood transfusions.

c. **Kartagener syndrome (immotile cilia syndrome).** This autosomal recessive syndrome combines bronchiectasis, dextrocardia, and male infertility. On electron microscopy, sperm tails are absent, which causes immotile sperm. Also on electron microscopy, the dynein arms of cilia are absent, which leads to an inability to clear the lung of secretions. Because cilia are made up of many structural proteins, it is likely that the mutations are heterogeneous.

2. **Proteins affecting the metabolism of other molecules.** Many biochemical defects are manifested through secondary effects. If synthesis or transport is impaired, there could be either a deficiency of the product or a harmful accumulation of precursor. If membrane transport is involved, there may be malabsorption or increased renal loss. Often, the exact mechanism of the production of disease symptoms is still unclear.

a. **Phenylketonuria (PKU).** Hepatic phenylalanine hydroxylase converts the essential amino acid phenylalanine to tyrosine. Deficiency of phenylalanine hydroxylase leads to increased levels of both phenylalanine and its metabolites, which results in mental retardation and pale coloring in affected children. Treatment involves severe restriction of oral phenylalanine.

b. **Galactosemia.** The most common enzyme deficiency involves galactose-1-phosphate uridyl transferase. Infants present with hepatomegaly, jaundice, and hypotonia. Death may occur from sepsis. The enzyme deficiency results in accumulation of galactose, which cannot be converted to glucose. Treatment involves elimination of lactose from the diet.

c. **Tay-Sachs disease.** Hexosaminidase A is involved in complex lipid metabolism. It removes sugars from a particular branched long-chain lipid (ceramide), which acts as a surface membrane receptor in the brain. In patients affected with Tay-Sachs disease, the enzyme abnormality leads to massive accumulation of the lipid in brain cells (i.e., it is a storage disorder). Affected children gradually lose skills (e.g., sitting) and sight. Death occurs at a young age. There is no treatment.

d. **Mucopolysaccharidosis type I (MPS I)**
   (1) Deficient levels of α-l-iduronidase result in **three overlapping clinical phenotypes,** which are all part of MPS I.
      (a) **Hurler syndrome (MPS IH)** is the most severe phenotype. Affected children have stiff joints, hepatosplenomegaly, corneal clouding, and progressive mental retardation. The children die of respiratory infection or cardiac failure.
      (b) **Scheie syndrome (MPS IS)** has some similar features (e.g., joint stiffness, corneal clouding) to MPS IH, but the effects are milder, and the children do not develop mental retardation. The diagnosis may not be made until early adulthood.
      (c) **Hurler-Scheie syndrome (MPS IHS)** is an intermediate phenotype with joint involvement and corneal clouding but little mental retardation.
   (2) All three clinical conditions are associated with abnormal mucopolysaccharide excretion, and low α-l-iduronidase levels. Hurler and Scheie syndromes result from different mutant alleles of the α-l-iduronidase gene, while the Hurler-Scheie syndrome is a compound.

e. **Cystic fibrosis (CF).** The gene involved in CF has been found to encode for a transmembrane conductance regulator protein that is involved in the transport of chloride across the membranes of cells in the pancreas, lungs, and sweat glands. It is postulated that the defect involves chloride permeability and leads to chronic obstructive lung disease and pancreatic insufficiency. Treatment is still only symptomatic.

    f. **Thyroid hormone deficiencies.** A number of thyroid hormonogenesis defects exist (e.g., thyroid peroxidase deficiency, abnormal carrier substance, abnormal iodine receptor), all of which are inherited as autosomal recessive traits.

      (1) Some thyroid hormone deficiencies, such as **thyroid peroxidase deficiency,** involve an inability to convert accumulated iodide to organically bound iodine. A number of abnormal alleles are now defined that can determine the clinical severity.

      (2) The end result is **congenital hypothyroidism,** which presents as an infant with coarse features, delayed growth, and eventual mental retardation.

      (3) Treatment involves administering exogenous thyroid hormone.

C. **Types of protein alterations.** Protein synthesis is the result of transcription of DNA into mRNA in the nucleus of the cell and translation of mRNA into protein on the ribosomes. Transcription is, therefore, nucleotide to nucleotide, while translation is a nucleotide-to-amino acid sequence. The regulation of transcription and translation determines the normal process of development. The **process of protein synthesis** can be broken down into the following steps.

    1. Transcription and RNA splicing (see Chapter 1 II B 1). Alterations in the amount of transcribed RNA are seen when deletions or mutations involve regulation or splice sites, or introduce a stop codon. This results in an inability for the complete DNA sequence to be read and converted to mRNA. The **thalassemias** result from a decreased or absent amount of the globin product (see II B 1 b).

    2. Translation (see Chapter 1 II B 3). If a mutation results in a frameshift, transcription may occur, but there may not be translation into a polypeptide if the sequence was shifted in such a way that a stop codon exists near its beginning.

    3. Secondary and tertiary structure of the polypeptide. Mutations affecting a protein's secondary and tertiary structure result in production of a protein. However, abnormal folding may occur, which results in an unstable molecule.

      a. Mutations in the collagens may produce abnormal cross-linking, which results in a weak structural protein.

      b. An **example of weak structural proteins due to collagen mutations** is seen with the highly elastic skin and hyperextensibility in certain types of **Ehlers-Danlos syndrome.**

    4. Three-dimensional localization. A completed protein may be destined to occupy a specific position in the cell structure. Alterations in key amino acid sequences may interfere with the ability of a protein to be localized appropriately. Many proteins require normal localization for normal function.

      a. In some patients with **methylmalonicacidemia,** the enzyme lacks a leader sequence, which prevents entry of the enzyme into the mitochondrion. The enzyme does not function normally except within the mitochondria.

      b. Infants present with **vomiting** and **failure to thrive.**

III. **DIAGNOSIS OF A BIOCHEMICAL DISEASE** involves the identification of accumulated or missing metabolites, the measurement of specific enzyme levels, or the identification of protein variants. See Chapter 6 for discussions of techniques used in DNA diagnosis of biochemical diseases and other genetic disorders.

A. **Suspecting a biochemical disease.** Although many of the mutations responsible for metabolic disease have been characterized, the clinician and the biochemist first note certain features in the patient or in the patient's biochemistry profile. Until the basic defect is clarified, what the clinician sees is the consequence of a variety of mutation types.

1. **Initial suspicions.** Some biochemical disorders are diagnosed as a result of **newborn screening tests** performed before the infant develops any clinical symptoms. **Clinical findings** also may suggest a disorder of a particular system. For example, excessive bleeding may be the initial presentation for hemophilia; muscle weakness may signal Duchenne muscular dystrophy (DMD); ambiguous genitalia may indicate androgen insensitivity.

2. **Direct analysis of enzymes or proteins.** When the biochemical pathway is known, a direct assay for an enzyme or enzyme product is available. Blood, cultured skin fibroblasts, or urine may be used. For example, a child may be suspected of having Tay-Sachs disease because she shows progressive physical and mental deterioration after appearing normal in the first few months of life. Measurement of hexosaminidase A activity in the child's blood can be used to establish or rule out the diagnosis.

3. **Cell culture studies.** Either skin fibroblasts or transformed lymphoblasts have been used to examine complex biochemical pathways. The incorporation of radioactive precursors in growing cells, the ability to perform repeated studies, and the comparison of results from a number of individuals with the same condition are all advantages of a long-term culture.

4. **Molecular techniques.** Both linkage analysis and direct mutation analysis are available for an increasing number of biochemical conditions. These enable early diagnosis as well as identification of heterozygotes.

B. **Genotype–phenotype correlations.** An important question to answer is whether the clinical presentation can be predicted from knowledge of the gene involved. Present knowledge of specific mutations suggests the following.

1. **Allelic mutations may result in different clinical phenotypes.** The mutations in the dystrophin gene may lead to DMD or Becker muscular dystrophy (BMD), depending on the amount of functioning dystrophin in the patient. In patients with the thalassemias, there may be enormous variation, depending on the type and location of allelic mutations.

2. **The clinical presentation may not be predictable from knowledge of the specific mutation.** Although the basic defect may be known, the actual development of a disease may not be clear. For example, the changes seen in the fragile X gene (i.e., the increased size of a repeat segment) do not yet explain the speech delay and other predictable findings of fragile X syndrome.

3. **Inheritance patterns are not always recessive.** The majority of enzyme deficiency conditions (e.g., PKU) are manifested only in the homozygote, although the normal heterozygote may have intermediate levels of the involved enzyme. However, many biochemical diseases [e.g., familial hypercholesterolemia (FH), type I osteogenesis imperfecta] that involve structural or transport proteins are manifested in the heterozygote. An affected homozygote with such conditions may be rare.

C. **Clinical considerations after diagnosis.** Once a metabolic disorder has been precisely diagnosed, at least four issues must be considered clinically.

1. Genetic counseling of the affected individual or the family

2. Identification of heterozygotes either in the extended family or, in some biochemical disorders, in the general population

3. Prenatal diagnosis

4. Early and appropriate treatment for the affected individual

STUDY QUESTIONS

DIRECTIONS: The numbered item or incomplete statement in this section is followed by answers or by completions of the statement. Select the ONE lettered answer or completion that is BEST.

1. Hurler and Scheie syndromes are both mucopolysaccharide disorders. Hurler syndrome presents in early childhood with severe bony changes and coarse facies. Scheie syndrome is much milder and later in onset. If the two disorders are allelic, which one of the following results would be expected?

(A) Both syndromes should show similar levels of enzyme activity

(B) If cells from each patient are cultured together, the increased mucopolysaccharide excretion characterizing both should normalize

(C) Sibships should occasionally demonstrate some children with Hurler syndrome and some with Scheie syndrome

(D) Offspring of one Hurler heterozygote parent and one Scheie heterozygote parent should have an intermediate disorder, not one or the other

(E) Molecular analysis will not demonstrate any differences with the genetic sequence

DIRECTIONS: The numbered item or incomplete statement in this section is negatively phrased, as indicated by a capitalized word such as NOT, LEAST, or EXCEPT. Select the ONE lettered answer or completion that is BEST.

2. All of the following clinical features may indicate an inborn error of metabolism EXCEPT

(A) a child who is the second pregnancy to parents who are known to be inbred through generations

(B) the parents of a child with mental retardation, who have also had two early miscarriages, as did the maternal grandmother

(C) an infant who was initially bright and alert and is now losing skills and paying little attention to the external environment

(D) a previously well infant with no dysmorphic features who suffers vascular collapse at 2 days of age

DIRECTIONS: The set of matching questions in this section consists of a list of four to twenty-six lettered options (some of which may be in figures) followed by several numbered items. For each numbered item, select the ONE lettered option that is most closely associated with it. To avoid spending too much time on matching sets with large numbers of options, it is generally advisable to begin each set by reading the list of options. Then, for each item in the set, try to generate the correct answer and locate it in the option list, rather than evaluating each option individually. Each lettered option may be selected once, more than once, or not at all.

Questions 3–7

Match the following clinical findings with the most likely type of alteration in protein function.

(A) Enzyme deficiency
(B) Abnormality of membrane transport protein
(C) Structural protein abnormality
(D) Altered cellular receptor
(E) Abnormal control of growth and differentiation

3. Affected males with Menkes syndrome, an X-linked disorder, have a progressive loss of skills and are found to have increased intracellular levels of copper with decreased serum levels

4. A female infant has multiple episodes of pneumonia, skin infections, and encephalitis; she has a combined immune deficiency; carriers in the family may be identified

5. A young woman presents with joint dislocations, hyperextensible skin, and easy bruising; electron microscopy demonstrates abnormal-appearing collagen fibrils; both her father and sister have had similar problems

6. Hereditary spherocytosis causes anemia in a woman because of an increased destruction of red blood cells with increased fragility

7. A phenotypically normal female infant presents with inguinal hernia and at surgery has a testicular structure identified in the hernia; her chromosomes are 46,XY; she is diagnosed as having androgen insensitivity

ANSWERS AND EXPLANATIONS

1. The answer is D [II B 2 d]. Hurler-Scheie offspring show the effect of two allelic mutations. Children with both Hurler and Scheie syndromes have been described. Both syndromes are the result of an abnormality in the enzyme α-l-iduronidase. In patients with Hurler syndrome, the enzyme is severely deficient; in patients with Scheie syndrome, the enzyme has better residual levels. In classic coculturing experiments, mixing the two cells did not correct the defect because the same enzyme was involved (in contrast to experiments using Hunter and Hurler syndrome cell lines, in which separate enzymes are involved). Both Hurler syndrome and Scheie syndrome are inherited as autosomal recessive traits. Offspring of Hurler heterozygous parents produce children with Hurler syndrome, whereas offspring of Scheie heterozygote parents produce children with Scheie syndrome.

2. The answer is B [II A–C]. Inborn errors of metabolism, whether enzyme or cofactor problems, are usually inherited as autosomal recessive traits. A clue may be the history of consanguinity. Some enzyme deficiencies lead to a buildup of substrate, which may be toxic or may be stored in various organelles. The process is ongoing, leading to progressive involvement. The initial presentation of some children with metabolic abnormalities is at the onset of feeding immediately after birth. Until that time, the placenta and maternal enzyme function protect the fetus. The history of both a developmentally delayed child and miscarriages is more suggestive of an inherited chromosome rearrangement (e.g., translocation; see Chapter 2 III E–F).

3–7. The answers are: 3-B, 4-A, 5-C, 6-C, 7-D [II C 3 b, III]. Menkes syndrome involves an abnormal copper transport protein, such that a differential is seen with copper both intra- and extracellularly. The condition leads to severe cerebral degeneration and death in infancy. One type of severe combined immune deficiency is secondary to adenosine deaminase deficiency (an enzyme involved in white blood cell function). In many enzyme deficiencies, heterozygotes are identified by intermediate enzyme levels. The inheritance is often autosomal recessive. Both the woman with the connective tissue problem (a subtype of Ehlers-Danlos syndrome) and the woman with hereditary spherocytosis have an abnormal structural protein (with spherocytosis, the spectrin forming the red cell membrane skeleton is abnormal). Structural protein abnormalities are often autosomal dominant in inheritance. The child with androgen insensitivity (see Chapter 12 II C 4) has an abnormal androgen receptor, such that androgen is not presented to the nucleus. The XY child consequently develops as a phenotypic female.

Chapter 9

Genetic and Environmental Interaction

J. M. Friedman
Michael R. Hayden
Barbara McGillivray

I. **INTRODUCTION.** Arguments are sometimes heard about the relative importance of "nature" and "nurture" in determining human traits, but there are few instances in which either normal development or a disease state occurs without interaction of both genetic and nongenetic factors. Even if only genetic factors are considered, it is important to remember that mutant genes do not act in isolation; they are influenced by the action of many other genes. Pharmacogenetics provides a vivid demonstration of the interaction of genotype and environmental agents. Most normal traits (e.g., behavior) and most common diseases of middle life (e.g., diabetes mellitus, hypertension, or manic-depressive illness) exhibit **multifactorial inheritance** (i.e., they are due to a combination of genetic and nongenetic factors). Most common isolated congenital anomalies also are multifactorial.

II. **PHARMACOGENETICS** refers to the **influence of genes on the response to drug therapy.** These responses may take the form of an exaggerated physiologic response to a drug, resistance to drug effects, or an increased frequency of side effects. Pharmacologic agents can also trigger the effects of certain genetic diseases.

A. Genes affecting drug metabolism. Polymorphisms of certain genes can have important effects on the activities of enzymes that are crucial in the metabolism of some drugs.

1. **Acetylation** is involved in the metabolism of many drugs. Polymorphisms in the rate of acetylation can result in differing effects of drugs administered to different patients.
    a. For example, patients who have a phenotype of **slow acetylation** for drugs such as **isoniazid,** which is used for treating tuberculosis, are **more likely to develop the side effects** of isoniazid therapy even with conventional doses.
    b. On the other hand, patients who have **rapid acetylation** of drugs like isoniazid may be inadequately treated because isoniazid levels in the blood will be decreased. Therefore, a patient who is a rapid acetylator and is taking isoniazid for tuberculosis may be **more prone to recurrence of the disease.**
    c. **Genetic polymorphisms of acetylation** have been described for many drugs that are commonly used in medicine.

2. The **cytochrome P_{450}-dependent enzyme system** is also involved in metabolism of many different drugs. Variation in genes for this enzyme system can result in an increased frequency of side effects in certain persons.
    a. Approximately 8%–10% of the American Caucasian population and less than 1% of the Chinese population are **poor metabolizers** of drugs that utilize this system.
    b. Drugs that fall into this category include **propranolol,** which is a β-blocker commonly used in the treatment of hypertension and angina.
    c. **Poor metabolizers** have **increased sensitivity** to propranolol and an **increased frequency of side effects** at conventional doses.

3. Individuals vary markedly in their responses to **ethanol.** There are significant ethnic differences in the pharmacologic effects of ethanol because of differing rates of metabolism.
    a. **Persons of Asian descent,** including most Chinese and Japanese individuals, **metabolize ethanol at a higher rate than Europeans,** with more rapid production of by-products of ethanol and increased clinical effects.

  b. The variation in metabolism of ethanol in different population groups is due to **polymorphism in the enzyme alcohol dehydrogenase.**

B. Pharmacologic effects of drugs on certain genetic diseases

  1. Glucose-6-phosphate dehydrogenase (G6PD) deficiency. Patients who are deficient in this enzyme may develop **rapid hemolysis** as an adverse reaction to treatment with certain commonly used drugs, including **antimalarial agents and sulfonamides.** This is seen in **people of Mediterranean and African descent.**
    a. People with G6PD deficiency do *not* have hemolysis unless their red cells are subjected to chemical or pharmacologic stresses.
    b. The locus controlling G6PD is situated on the X chromosome; therefore, this condition is inherited as an **X-linked recessive trait.**

  2. Malignant hyperthermia is usually triggered by anesthetic agents, such as halothane. Affected people present with muscle spasm, hyperthermia, and subsequent acidosis. If untreated, death may occur.
    a. Malignant hyperthermia is a **genetically heterogeneous** condition.
    b. It may be seen in patients with a variety of myopathies that are inherited as autosomal dominant or autosomal recessive traits.
    c. Some patients who are otherwise normal exhibit malignant hyperthermia, which is inherited as an **autosomal dominant trait.**
      (1) The genetic defect in some such families is in a **skeletal muscle calcium release channel** gene on chromosome 19.
      (2) In other families, the genetic defect is caused by a gene on the long arm of chromosome 17.
      (3) In still other families with dominantly inherited malignant hyperthermia, other genes appear to be involved.

  3. Human leukocyte antigen (HLA) and adverse reactions. Some adverse reactions to drugs are influenced by HLA genes involved in the immune response. For example, patients receiving gold therapy who have the HLA antigen DRW3 are more likely to have side effects than individuals who do not have this HLA antigen.

  4. Succinylcholine sensitivity. The enzyme **butyrylcholinesterase** (also called "pseudocholinesterase") hydrolyzes **choline esters,** including acetylcholine and succinylcholine, which is widely used in anesthesia as a muscle relaxant. Approximately 1/3000 Caucasian individuals is homozygous for an atypical butyrylcholinesterase allele, which results in an inability to break down succinylcholine. Such people have **prolonged muscle relaxation and apnea** after anesthesia with succinylcholine. The abnormal butyrylcholinesterase activity can be detected through a laboratory test.

C. Clinical concerns in pharmacogenetics

  1. Genes can significantly alter the therapeutic responsiveness to drugs, and in some instances these drugs may precipitate clinical manifestations of genetic diseases. A key to detecting these susceptibilities is a **thorough family history.**
    a. The family history may reveal an adverse drug reaction that is known to be inherited. For example, if a patient's parent is found to have suffered malignant hyperthermia, the patient is probably at risk for the same condition.
    b. In such cases, the physician should either **undertake appropriate investigations before subjecting the patient to a drug** that might precipitate a similar adverse reaction or **avoid the use of such drugs** altogether.
    c. The challenge is to identify patients and their families who are susceptible to adverse drug reactions by virtue of their genetic constitution.
    d. Remember that **drug metabolism,** including absorption, distribution, binding to receptors, and degradation, is **determined in large part by genetic factors.**

  2. The presence of unusual adverse reactions to pharmacologic agents may reflect the presence of **a genetic allele** in that particular individual, which predisposes the person to the adverse event.

3. **Certain drugs may be teratogenic** in some individuals because of variations in genes of the mother or the fetus (see Chapter 10 II). In other instances, genetic traits may protect a fetus from the harmful effects of certain drugs.

III. **MULTIFACTORIAL INHERITANCE** is responsible for most normal phenotypic differences among individuals as well as for many congenital anomalies and common diseases of adulthood.

A. **Definitions and terminology**

1. The term **multifactorial** is used in medicine to describe traits that are caused by a **combination of many genetic and nongenetic factors.** If only the genetic factors are considered, the inheritance is called **polygenic.**
   a. This definition of a multifactorial trait implies **both a familial nature and an environmental dependence.** A child of tall parents is more likely to be tall than is a child of short parents, but poor nutrition (an environmental factor) may compromise the growth of either child.
   b. The **genetic predisposition** to multifactorial traits is usually **inherited from both parents.**
   c. The **genes and environmental factors** affecting a given multifactorial trait may **vary among different individuals.** Black hair may be the result of genes inherited from an Asian genetic background in one individual, of genes inherited from an African genetic background in another person, and of hair dye in a third individual whose genetic background would ordinarily produce brown hair.

2. **Quantitative traits** are those that **can be measured.** Examples include height, weight, and serum cholesterol level.
   a. In general, quantitative traits exhibit **continuous variability.** This means that they can assume an unlimited number of intermediate values between extremes. This **contrasts with discrete or qualitative traits,** which are all-or-none phenotypes like achondroplasia or Huntington disease.
   b. **Quantitative phenotypes are typically inherited as multifactorial traits in normal individuals.**

B. **Normal variation**

1. **Most phenotypic variations among normal individuals are due to multifactorial traits.** Examples include the range of skin pigmentation, height, and intelligence seen among normal people.

2. **Extreme values** may occur as a result of normal variation. A man is unlikely to be 4'10" tall just on the basis of normal variation, but it is possible.

3. **Children tend to resemble their parents** with respect to normal traits because of the underlying genetic components. Tall parents tend to have tall children. **For normal quantitative traits, a child's phenotypic value tends to resemble the average of his or her parents' values.** This average is called the midparent value.

4. **Each parent contributes half of the genetic factors** for any multifactorial trait in his or her child, on the average. This means that the **children of a parent who exhibits an extreme value for a multifactorial trait tend to have less extreme values themselves,** a phenomenon known as "regression to the mean."

5. Although quantitative traits are continuously variable, only a **limited range of values** may occur. For example, human adults with heights of 5 inches or 40 feet do not exist.

6. **Quantitative characteristics that exhibit continuous variation among normal individuals may also exhibit a major alteration as a result of genetic or environmental factors of large effect.** Thus, achondroplasia or thyroid ablation by radiation may

greatly reduce the height of a child in whom average stature would otherwise have been expected.

C. **Multifactorial diseases.** Many diseases are inherited as multifactorial traits.

1. **Some multifactorial diseases are defined clinically in terms of quantitative traits.** For example, hypertension is diagnosed on the basis of a patient's blood pressure being higher than a certain number.
   a. **The difference between "normal" and "disease" in such cases is arbitrary.** Blood pressure is a continuous variable, and the pathologic effect of having "high" blood pressures of 140/110, 120/85, or 125/81 compared with "normal" blood pressures of 120/80 or 110/75 is only one of degree.
   b. Inheritance of diseases such as essential hypertension can be thought of in terms of **extreme manifestations of a multifactorial quantitative trait.**

2. **Other multifactorial diseases differ qualitatively from the normal state.** Cleft palate is one example. In such cases, a multifactorial predisposition to the disease is inherited, and the disease either occurs or does not occur, depending on the aggregate strength of the predisposing factors.
   a. The **multifactorial-threshold model** (Figure 9–1) is a formal explanation of how a multifactorial predisposition can produce a trait that is qualitatively distinct from normal.
      (1) According to this model, **all of an individual's genetic and environmental disease-predisposing factors when considered together constitute liability.** Liability follows a **normal distribution** in the population.
      (2) **If an individual's liability exceeds a certain threshold value, he or she will have the disease.** If the liability does not exceed that threshold, the disease will not occur.
   b. **Other models** can also be used to explain genetic predispositions to disease and often fit available data as well as or better than the multifactorial-threshold model.
      (1) **Mixed models** postulate a major gene of large effect (i.e., a mendelian factor with relatively high penetrance) operating on a multifactorial background.
      (2) **Oligogenic (i.e., few gene) models** postulate the presence of a small number of genes operating in combination.
      (3) **Genetic heterogeneity** may occur, in which some cases have a mendelian cause and others have a nongenetic or multifactorial cause.
   c. **Linkage studies** and the isolation of contributory genes by **molecular methods** should help to clarify the underlying basis of most multifactorial diseases.

3. **Diseases transmitted as multifactorial traits**
   a. **Most isolated congenital anomalies** appear to be multifactorial traits. Examples include cleft lip with or without cleft palate, congenital heart disease, and anencephaly.

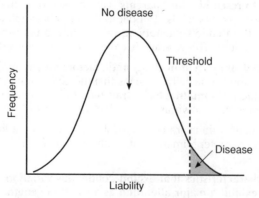

FIGURE 9–1. The multifactorial-threshold model.

    b. Many common diseases of adulthood also seem to be multifactorial traits. Noninsulin-dependent diabetes mellitus, arteriosclerotic heart disease, and schizophrenia are examples.

4. **Clinical characteristics of multifactorial diseases** include the following:
   a. The disease tends to be **familial but does not follow any monogenic pattern of inheritance.**
   b. Multifactorial disorders tend to **occur more frequently in one sex than in the other.** Examples include:
      (1) Pyloric stenosis, which is much more common in males
      (2) Systemic lupus erythematosus (SLE), which is more common in females
   c. **The recurrence risk is the same for all relatives who share the same proportion of genes.**
      (1) For example, each sibling, child, and parent shares half of his or her genes with a proband, on the average.
      (2) The recurrence risk in all such first-degree relatives is expected to be about the same.
   d. **The recurrence risk in a family drops off quickly as the relationship to an affected individual becomes more remote.** For example, the recurrence risk for cleft lip with or without cleft palate is about 4% for the sibling but only about 0.5% for the first cousin of an affected child.
   e. **The recurrence risk in first-degree relatives of an affected individual is approximately equal to the square root of the frequency of the condition in the population.**
      (1) This means that the recurrence risk is lower in populations exhibiting a lower incidence of a condition.
      (2) For **multifactorial congenital anomalies** that have population incidences of about 1/1000, the **recurrence risk in siblings or children of an affected individual is usually 2%–4%.**
      (3) For **multifactorial diseases of adulthood** that have population prevalences in the range of 1%, the **recurrence risk in siblings and children is usually in the range of 5%–10%.**
   f. Multifactorial diseases are **more common among the children of consanguineous parents.** This is because parents who are related are more likely to share similar disease-predisposing genes.

5. **Factors that influence the recurrence risk** for multifactorial disorders in a family include the following:
   a. **The recurrence risk is higher if more than one close relative is affected.**
      (1) For example, the risk for cleft lip with or without cleft palate in a child who has one affected sibling is approximately 4%. If the child has two affected siblings, the risk is approximately 10%.
      (2) This reflects the fact that a couple who have already had more than one affected child are more likely to have more predisposing factors (i.e., more liability) than a couple with just one affected child.
      (3) Note that this is quite **different from monogenic inheritance,** in which the risk of recurrence depends on the parental genotypes and is independent of the number of previously affected children.
   b. **The recurrence risk is higher in the relatives of an affected individual of the *less* frequently involved sex.**
      (1) Individuals of the less frequently involved sex must have more predisposing factors to manifest the disease so their relatives are at greater risk of being similarly affected.
      (2) For example, pyloric stenosis occurs five times as often in males as in females. The recurrence risk in the brother of an affected child is 3.8% if the affected child is male, but 9.2% if the affected child is female.
   c. **The recurrence risk is higher in relatives of more severely affected probands.**
      (1) Such individuals must have more predisposing factors to manifest the disease severely; therefore, their relatives are at greater risk.

(2) For example, the risk of recurrence of cleft lip with or without cleft palate is 2.5% in the sibling of a child with unilateral cleft lip but almost 6% in the sibling of a child with bilateral cleft lip and palate.

(3) Note that this is very **different from** the situation with **monogenic and chromosome disorders,** in which the severity of disease in the proband does not influence the recurrence risk.

6. Multifactorial inheritance is a **diagnosis of exclusion.**
   a. **The clinical features of a multifactorial disorder rarely distinguish it from similar lesions that have another cause.**
      (1) For example, cleft lip and cleft palate, alone or in combination, usually exhibit multifactorial inheritance.
      (2) There are, however, about 200 other conditions that have cleft lip or cleft palate as a feature.
      (3) Some of these conditions are due to chromosome abnormalities, others to monogenic disorders, and still others to teratogenic environmental effects.
   b. **Multifactorial congenital anomalies typically occur in patients who do not have embryologically unrelated birth defects.**
      (1) Cleft lip and clubfeet are examples of abnormalities that are embryologically unrelated to each other.
      (2) Cleft lip and cleft palate are embryologically related because morphologic alterations that produce one can also produce the other.
      (3) A common congenital anomaly, such as spina bifida, in a child who is otherwise completely normal is likely to be multifactorial. Spina bifida in a child who also has congenital heart disease, kidney malformations, and cleft lip is not likely to be multifactorial.
   c. **The recurrence risks used for multifactorial conditions do _not_ apply to situations in which the condition is not multifactorial.**
      (1) The recurrence risk for the sibling of a child with congenital heart disease, omphalocele, and clubfeet cannot be calculated from the recurrence risks estimated for these conditions when they occur as isolated anomalies.
      (2) The recurrence risk for the sibling of such a child is determined by the underlying cause of the child's anomalies, and this is unlikely to be multifactorial when multiple congenital anomalies are present.

7. Because multifactorial diseases are caused by combinations of genetic and environmental predispositions, **environmental triggers have the greatest chance of causing disease in individuals with existing genetic predispositions.**
   a. This means that **identification of environmental factors** that predispose to a given disease should be easiest among genetically predisposed individuals.
   b. **Manipulation of these environmental triggers to prevent disease may be most effective among genetically predisposed individuals.**
   c. Identification of individuals with genetic predispositions to multifactorial disease may lead to **disease prevention through manipulation of nongenetic factors.**

D. **Twin studies** are often used to distinguish multifactorial traits from those caused by nongenetic factors or by mendelian single genes.

1. **Because monozygotic (MZ) twins have all of their genes in common, MZ twins should be 100% concordant for fully penetrant monogenic diseases.** Dizygotic (DZ) twins should be concordant 50% of the time for monogenic dominant conditions and 25% of the time for monogenic recessive conditions.

2. **Familial traits are not necessarily genetic.** For example, chickenpox very often runs in families but it is not genetic. If MZ and DZ twins are assumed to share similar common environments, **concordance should be the same in MZ and DZ twins for diseases caused entirely by environmental factors.**
   a. Differences in concordance rates between MZ and DZ twins are attributed to genetic differences between DZ twins that do not occur between MZ twins.
   b. The environment of two DZ twins is probably not quite as much alike as the environment of two MZ twins, especially if the DZ twins are of different sexes.

TABLE 9–1. Twin Concordance for Some Common Multifactorial Diseases

	Percent Concordance	
Disease	MZ Twins	DZ Twins
Manic depressive psychosis	67	5
Rheumatoid arthritis	34	7
Bronchial asthma	47	24
Hypertension	25	7
Cancer, same site	7	3
Congenital hip dislocation	40	3
Clubfoot	33	3
Cleft lip (with or without cleft palate)	38	8

DZ = dizygotic; MZ = monozygotic.
(Data from Nora JJ, et al: *Nora and Fraser Medical Genetics,* 4th ed., 1994, p 401.)

3. **If one of a pair of MZ twins has a multifactorial disease, the chance that the second twin is also affected** (i.e., is concordant) **is less than 100%** and usually less than 50%.

4. The **concordance** for multifactorial conditions **in DZ twins is much less than the concordance in MZ twins** and usually is similar to the recurrence risk in ordinary siblings. Table 9–1 lists the concordances for several common multifactorial diseases in MZ and DZ twins.

5. The main **advantage** of twin studies is that they provide a powerful method of distinguishing diseases caused purely by genetic factors and those caused purely by nongenetic factors from diseases caused by a combination of genetic and nongenetic factors.

6. Twin studies are subject to several **limitations.** These include the following:
    a. The frequency of concordance in MZ twins does not reveal anything about the mode of transmission of the predisposing genes.
    b. Assignment of pairs as MZ or DZ is inaccurate in some studies. The value of a twin study is greatly compromised by incorrect or uncertain determination of zygosity.
    c. Biased sampling
        (1) **Small samples.** Twins account for about 1% of all births. If the disorder being studied is also uncommon, small sample size may limit the power of a study. To obtain adequate numbers of twins with a specific disorder, twin registries or clubs are sometimes useful.
        (2) **Biased selection.** Concordant pairs, especially concordant MZ pairs, may be more likely to be identified or to participate in studies of a particular disease.
        (3) **Varied sources of twins.** Twins may be drawn from different sources in different studies. This may result in mildly affected patients being compared with those who are more seriously ill.

7. **Variations of twin studies** may be used to overcome some of these limitations. Such variations include:
    a. Comparison of MZ twins reared together with MZ twins separated by adoption and reared apart
    b. Studies of the children of MZ twins

IV. **GENETICS OF COMMON ADULT DISORDERS.** By 25 years of age, approximately 5% of individuals will suffer from a genetic disease. However, if disorders that have a genetic component in their causation (e.g., heart disease, cancer) are included, approximately 60% of the population will suffer from a disorder with a major or minor genetic contribution during their lifetime. Many of these diseases are caused by the interaction of genetic and environmental factors. By identifying susceptible individuals, it may be possible to modify known environmental factors and prevent the illness in genetically susceptible persons.

A. **Diabetes** affects approximately 5% of the population. There are different genetic contributions to insulin-dependent (type 1) and noninsulin-dependent (type 2) adult-onset diabetes.

1. **Type 1 (juvenile-onset, insulin-dependent) diabetes mellitus**
   a. **Genetic background.** An association with HLA-DR3 and HLA-DR4 is documented, and 95% of insulin-dependent diabetics have one or both of these antigens compared with 50% of the general population. The risk to a first-degree relative of a person with insulin-dependent diabetes mellitus is approximately 10%.
      (1) Because the subgroups HLA-DR3 and HLA-DR4 can be rapidly identified by molecular analysis, refinement of prediction has now become possible.
         (a) The hypothesis is that genes closely linked to these HLA antigens control immune responses, making a person susceptible to environmental factors such as viruses, which can result in pancreatic damage and subsequent diabetes.
         (b) These patients develop antibodies to insulin and islet cells of the pancreas and require insulin therapy.
      (2) It is now possible to identify persons at risk for juvenile-onset diabetes by using a combination of molecular, serologic, and immunologic markers.
   b. **Environmental aspects.** Approximately 50% of monozygous twins are concordant for this disease, indicating that environmental factors—probably viral infections (e.g., rubella)—play a major role in addition to genetic factors. The greatest risk is to subjects who have antigens HLA-DR3 and HLA-DR4 and a family history of insulin-dependent diabetes mellitus.

2. **Type 2 (adult-onset, noninsulin-dependent) diabetes mellitus**
   a. **Genetic aspects.** Type 2 diabetes mellitus has a very strong genetic predisposition, and concordance in monozygous twins is close to 100%. The risk to siblings for developing diabetes increases with age. The risk to first-degree relatives of a person with noninsulin-dependent diabetes mellitus is approximately 5%. Recently, different genes in different regions of the genome have been shown to play a role in determining the genetic susceptibility to diabetes.
   b. **Environmental aspects.** The major factor that unmasks the presentation of diabetes is obesity. One way to prevent the onset of type 2 diabetes mellitus is for those individuals who have a first-degree relative with this disorder to maintain optimal body weight. In other words, knowledge of a family history of diabetes can have a significant influence on modification of lifestyle in an effort to prevent the expected outcome.

B. **Hemochromatosis**

1. **Clinical aspects.** Hemochromatosis is caused by the accumulation of toxic quantities of iron in different organs. The disease has a frequency of approximately 1/3000.
   a. **Iron concentration,** which is highest in the liver and pancreas, sometimes reaches 50 to 100 times the normal range.
   b. Iron concentration can also increase in the joints, skin, spleen, kidney, stomach, and in the thyroid, adrenal, and pituitary glands.
   c. As a result, patients present with pain in their joints, increased skin pigmentation, and feelings of weakness and malaise.
   d. With time, the iron accumulation affects liver and pancreatic function, causing cirrhosis and diabetes.
   e. Hypogonadism, which is caused by involvement of the pituitary gland with testicular atrophy, and loss of libido also occur.

2. **Diagnosis of hemochromatosis** is made by a significantly increased transferrin saturation level to between 80% and 100%, which is associated with increased serum ferritin and serum iron.

3. **Treatment.** The clinical manifestations of this disease are completely preventable if recognized early and treated with regular phlebotomy. If untreated, hemochromatosis results in premature death due to diabetes, cirrhosis, or cardiac failure.

4. **Genetic aspects.** Approximately 1/10 Caucasian individuals is a carrier of hemochromatosis, which is an autosomal recessive trait. The disease is associated with HLA antigen A3, and it has been shown that the gene causing this disorder is closely linked to the HLA region. In some instances, there may be a family history of hemochromatosis in first-degree relatives. The presence of hemochromatosis in a parent and child reflects the high frequency of the carrier state for this disease and indicates that someone who is affected with hemochromatosis has mated with a carrier with subsequent transmission of two affected alleles to their offspring.

C. **Cancer**

1. **Genetic contribution to common malignant tumors of adulthood.** Genes play a major role in the development of cancer; there are some genetic syndromes predisposing to malignancy and some tumors that follow a strict mendelian inheritance (see Chapter 11 II B).

2. **Recent advances.** Recently, tumor suppressor genes (in particular, the p53 gene) have been shown to play a key role in the development of human cancer in different tissues (see Chapter 11 III).

3. **Genetic implications of some common cancers.** The common cancers of adult life include those of the breast, colon, lung, prostate gland, and stomach, as well as cancers affecting the central nervous system (CNS).

   a. **Breast cancer.** Genetic studies have convincingly shown a significant increase in the frequency of breast cancer in close relatives of a person with the disease.
      (1) **Risks for breast cancer**
         (a) In the general population, the risk of breast cancer in women is approximately 9%.
         (b) If a first-degree relative is affected, a woman has two to three times the population risk.
         (c) If there are two first-degree relatives with bilateral premenopausal onset, a woman's risk might be as high as 50%.
      (2) The presence of breast cancer in a first-degree relative should increase the early detection screening for a woman. Breast self-examination should begin earlier, and in some instances, examinations would include more frequent mammograms.
      (3) Many of the hereditary forms of breast cancer have early onset, bilateral occurrence, and are multicentric (see Chapter 11 II B 1).
      (4) Recently, a gene underlying some forms of familial breast and ovarian cancers has been identified (the BRCA-1 gene). Many different mutations have been found underlying breast cancer in different families. Familial breast cancer in some patients is caused by mutations in another gene (BRCA-2) [see Chapter 11 II B 1].

   b. **Gastrointestinal cancer.** The genetic contribution is low for esophageal cancer, slightly higher for gastric cancer, and highest for colon cancer. The presence of colon cancer in a first-degree relative, especially occurring at an early age, should prompt more frequent testing for occult blood in the stool and sigmoidoscopy examinations in first-degree relatives. Recently, mutations in genes underlying a common form of colon cancer have been determined. These mutations impair the function of a DNA repair gene, which renders these cells in the colon susceptible to malignant transformation.

   c. **Lung cancers,** especially bronchial carcinomas, were rare before the twentieth century. Most epidemiologic studies have focused on environmental factors, such as smoking. Whereas the major cause for lung cancer is tobacco smoking, genetic factors also have an important, although smaller, role in conferring predisposition to this malignancy. Recently, the first-degree relatives of lung cancer patients have been shown to have a risk that is two to three times higher than the risk for lung cancer in the general population.

D. **Coronary artery disease** remains the most frequent cause of morbidity and mortality in Western industrialized countries, accounting for more deaths than all forms of cancer combined.

1. The **role of genes** in the causation of atherosclerosis is supported by family studies and concordance rates of 65% for coronary artery disease in monozygous twins.

2. **Patients with genetic hyperlipidemia** present with cholesterol levels that are markedly elevated and, in some instances, may have been elevated since childhood.
   a. The **importance of the recognition** of a genetic hyperlipidemia is that it influences therapy and management.
   b. In general, genetic hyperlipidemias **do not respond adequately to environmental modulation by diet;** drug therapy is often needed to bring down the cholesterol levels.
   c. Genetic hyperlipidemia should be suspected when there is a positive family history, as defined by the presence of angina, heart attack, or stroke in a first-degree relative before 60 years of age.

3. **Genes are particularly implicated in premature atherosclerosis** when a first-degree relative has a history of either angina or heart attack before 60 years of age.
   a. In this group, the **family history** is the most important indicator that the individual is at increased risk for coronary disease.
   b. In addition, **clinical examination** may reveal particular findings, including tendon xanthomas and an arcus cornealis, which is indicative of a genetic hyperlipidemia. Genetic hyperlipidemia should also be considered if a patient has a very elevated low-density lipoprotein (LDL) cholesterol level.

4. **Important genetic disorders causing premature atherosclerosis**
   a. **Familial hyperlipidemia** (FH) [see Chapter 3 II A 1 c; Chapter 6 II A 3 c] is inherited as an autosomal dominant trait and is penetrant early in life. The molecular basis for this disorder is different mutations in the LDL receptor gene.
   b. **Familial combined hyperlipidemia (FCH)** occurs with a frequency of approximately 1%–2% in the general population. The diagnosis of FCH can be made in the presence of an elevated LDL cholesterol or triglyceride level in the patient and siblings or other first-degree relatives. The pathogenesis of the disorder is unknown.

E. **Predictive testing.** As a result of significant advances in the molecular genetics of different illnesses, it is now possible to assess an asymptomatic individual who has a family history of a genetic illness to determine whether that person has inherited the mutation for a particular disease. If the patient has inherited a particular mutation that is present in other symptomatic persons of the family, then the finding of the DNA change is predictive of the person developing signs and symptoms of the illness in the future.

1. **Advantages.** Predictive testing has been offered for a few late-onset illnesses, including Huntington disease and a genetic form of colon cancer. In the absence of any treatment known to modify the course of the illness, an individual who chooses to participate in predictive testing may receive test results that remove uncertainty and allow that person to plan for the future. Furthermore, for illnesses for which there is treatment, such as familial forms of colon cancer, the demonstration that a person has inherited DNA changes associated with the disease allows the implementation of treatment for the disorder. In some instances, predictive testing may result in preventive removal of part of the colon.

2. **Concerns.** Predictive testing that provides clues about genetic susceptibility of predisposition for genetic disorders is likely to be more common in the future. Numerous concerns about predictive testing have been raised, including the possibilities of discrimination and the potential for harm caused by inappropriate preventive or therapeutic measures. The importance of quality control in the laboratory, as well as counseling before and after the test result is received, is imperative for helping the patient use the information advantageously.

TABLE 9-2. Study Methods in Behavioral Genetics

Method	Features
Family studies	
Pedigree analysis	Fast, inexpensive; underestimates morbidity
Interviews	Direct contact best; "blind" interview required
Twin studies	Allow heritability studies; need accurate zygosity data; may have biased selection
Adoption studies	Separate genetic from environmental factors; allow long-term prospective studies

V. **BEHAVIORAL DISORDERS.** Recent advances in the area of genetics and behavior suggest a significant link between genetic factors and major psychiatric illnesses such as schizophrenia and mood disorders. The genetic influence was suggested in the early 1900s by family studies that demonstrated an increased incidence of schizophrenia among close relatives of affected patients. Historically, genetic research relevant to psychiatric illness has been limited by the reliance on behavioral or phenotypic traits. Until recently, the genotype could only be inferred.

A. **Study methods in behavioral genetics.** Three basic methods (Table 9-2)—family, twin, and adoption studies—are used to assess the genetic component of psychiatric conditions and to derive risk figures (empiric figures), both for use in counseling and for determining the possible mode of inheritance of the disorders.

1. **Family studies** compare the prevalence of a certain psychiatric disorder among relatives of an affected individual with the prevalence in a normal or control population. These studies involve either taking a family history from an affected or unaffected family relative or interviewing individual family members. The pedigree obtained can then be analyzed to compare single gene and multigene models of inheritance.

  a. **Advantages.** This method requires direct contact with the family and should allow maximum information to be gathered regarding the family. Specifically, the following information should be gathered from family studies.

    (1) **Precise diagnosis.** The investigator is able to confirm a diagnosis and is more likely to discover less severely affected family members with careful history taking and individual examination.

    (2) **Separation of multiple factors.** If two psychiatric conditions are coexisting, pedigree analysis may allow separation of the conditions into two family branches. Families may be excluded to allow cleaner analysis.

    (3) **Availability of family members for other studies.** Direct interaction with a family facilitates the discussions necessary to elicit the family's participation in other research studies (e.g., linkage analysis, mutation identification).

  b. **Limitations.** The most significant drawback of family studies is their inability to differentiate genetic from environmental influences. Also, unless a specific biologic or genetic marker is available, the genotype usually cannot be identified with certainty. Other problems encountered in family studies include the following.

    (1) **Imprecise or incorrect diagnosis.** Although strict diagnostic criteria exist for common psychiatric disorders [i.e., in the *Diagnostic and Statistical Manual of Mental Disorders,* 4th ed. (DSM-IV) of the American Psychiatric Association], an inexperienced interviewer may interpret findings incorrectly. A highly structured interview setting is best for less-experienced interviewers.

    (2) **Biased data**

      (a) **A family history (pedigree) obtained by telephone or from only one individual** may exclude mildly affected relatives, thus underestimating psychiatric morbidity. Ideally, formal family interviews are conducted in person.

      (b) **The diagnosis of the proband should not be known to the interviewer.**

Blind interviews are especially important when several diagnostic categories are being considered.

2. **Twin studies** (see III D)

3. **Adoption studies** compare the prevalence of a psychiatric disorder among the biologic relatives of affected individuals with the prevalence among the adopted relatives. These studies provide a unique opportunity to separate genetic from long-term environmental influences on the development of an individual.

4. **Prospective studies** of at-risk individuals involve long-term comparison of disease prevalence in persons at increased risk and in low-risk controls. These studies allow identification of predisposing environmental factors.

B. **Schizophrenia**

1. **Definition.** Schizophrenia is a psychosis involving loss of contact with the environment, disintegration of the personality, and disordered or inappropriate thought. The DSM-IV criteria for the diagnosis include two or more of the following characteristic symptoms, each of which is present for much of a 1-month period, with some signs persisting for at least 6 months:
   a. Delusions
   b. Hallucinations
   c. Disorganized speech
   d. Grossly disorganized or catatonic behavior
   e. Affective flattening, poverty of speech, or an inability to participate in goal-directed activities

2. **Prevalence.** Published prevalence studies are difficult to compare because of differences among diagnostic standards, life expectancies, and courses of illness. The lifetime prevalence of schizophrenia ranges from 0.03% in the Amish to 2.3% in the Swedish. In the United States, prevalence studies average 0.5% among the general population.

3. **Evidence for genetic contribution**
   a. **Family studies.** Recent studies using strict diagnostic criteria and control groups indicate that the risk for schizophrenia among first-degree relatives of probands is increased about 4% over controls.
   b. **Twin studies.** Concordance rates for schizophrenia generally are higher among MZ twins (15%–85%) than DZ twins (2%–10%). The discordance among MZ twins may suggest that environmental factors contribute to schizophrenia.
   c. **Adoption studies.** A large ongoing study among Danish adoptees has identified schizophrenia in 8.7% of close biologic relatives of schizophrenic probands compared with 1.9% of adoptive relatives.

4. **Inheritance of schizophrenia.** Although evidence indicates a genetic role in the development of schizophrenia, the exact mode of transmission is unknown. Autosomal inheritance with decreased penetrance has been explored in a number of linkage studies. Because direct genotype studies usually are not available, other methods of studying the genetics of schizophrenia are used to define inherited factors segregating with schizophrenia and to delineate subtypes concordant in sibling pairs.
   a. **Physical and laboratory markers**
      (1) **Monoamine oxidase (MAO) activity.** Platelet MAO activity is inherited and tends to be decreased in schizophrenic patients. It is not clear whether catechol or indoleamine metabolism is important.
      (2) **Brain morphology.** Lateral ventricular enlargement is seen in some schizophrenics, but the significance of this finding is unclear.
   b. **Linkage data**
      (1) A family with mental retardation, dysmorphic features, and schizophrenia segregating with a partial trisomy of the long arm of chromosome 5 (5q) has been described, and linkage to this cytogenetic region has been established

in some large families in which schizophrenia appears to segregate as a dominant trait.

   (2) Most families do not show linkage to this chromosome region.

   (3) Linkage to the genes for dopamine receptors D2, D3, and D5 has been excluded.

   (4) Anticipation (earlier and more severe disease with vertical transmission) is seen in schizophrenia. Dynamic mutations involving triplet repeats are now being considered.

   (5) The results of linkage studies demonstrate genetic heterogeneity even in families with an apparently dominant mode of transmission.

C. **Mood disorders**

1. **Definition.** Mood disorders are conditions characterized by two forms of pervasive pathologic changes in mood.

   a. **Bipolar disorder** (formerly referred to as **manic-depressive illness**) is marked by the presence of one or more manic or hypomanic episodes, usually with a history of depressive episodes. Manic episodes may be severe enough to impair functioning.

   b. **Unipolar disorder** (also referred to as **depressive disorder**) is marked by the presence of one or more major depressive episodes without a history of manic or hypomanic episodes. The DSM-IV defines the major depressive episodes as periods of depression with a variety of symptoms lasting at least 2 weeks.

2. **Prevalence.** An estimated 0.4% to 1.2% of adults have bipolar disorder. Prevalence figures for unipolar disorder vary widely; recent reports indicate that 4.5% to 9.3% of women and 2.3% to 3.2% of men have the disorder.

3. **Evidence for genetic contribution**

   a. **Family studies.** Hereditary factors have been suspected in the causation of mood disorders since the early part of the twentieth century and are now known to play a major role.

   (1) Generally, family studies show the risk for bipolar disorder among first-degree relatives of affected patients to be higher (19.2%) than the risk for unipolar disorder (9.7%).

   (2) If age of onset is considered in bipolar disorder, the risk is 20% for first-degree relatives of a patient affected before 40 years of age and 11% with onset after 40 years of age.

   b. **Twin studies** show a striking difference in concordance rates for mood disorders in MZ twins (70%) versus DZ twins (13%). Concordance rates in MZ twins are high regardless of whether the twins are reared apart.

   c. **Adoption studies** confirm the importance of genetic factors in bipolar disorder, with a more modest component seen in unipolar disorder.

4. **Inheritance of mood disorders.** Evidence strongly suggests that genetic factors participate in the etiology of mood disorders. A single mode of inheritance has not been documented.

   a. **Possible physical and laboratory markers**

   (1) **Response to drug therapy.** Bipolar disorder shows a better response to lithium, whereas unipolar disorder shows a better response to the tricyclic antidepressants. These findings suggest involvement with different neurotransmitters.

   (2) **Catecholamine levels** have been shown to be increased with mania and decreased with depression. Other brain peptides have similar associations. Because tyrosine hydroxylase is the rate-limiting enzyme in catecholamine synthesis, the tyrosine hydroxylase gene is an obvious candidate for further study.

   b. **Linkage data.** Genetic marker studies have examined the relationship between mood disorders and red blood cell types, HLA types, and chromosome variants, to name a few.

   (1) Linkage studies have involved X-linked and autosomal markers. Linkage of manic-depressive illness and the X-linked genes for deuteranopia (color blindness) and the Xg blood group has been suggested in some families.

(2) A large Old Order Amish pedigree has shown a dominant transmission pattern, with strong evidence of linkage with an area on the short arm of chromosome 11 (11p). The tyrosine hydroxylase gene is also on 11p, but current results suggest linkage to neither tyrosine hydroxylase nor the dopamine D4 receptor, both of which are in the area of 11p15.5. Linkage to distal 5q has been found in a subgroup of families. These results probably reflect heterogeneous causes of the mood disorders and indicate the need for further study.

D. Other disorders

1. **Anxiety disorders**
   a. **Definition.** Anxiety disorders are characterized by anxiety and avoidance behavior; these illnesses do allow perception of reality. Included in this group are panic disorders, generalized anxiety disorders, phobias, and obsessive-compulsive disorders. Of these, panic disorders appear to be the most familial in nature.
   b. **Prevalence.** Recent studies show anxiety disorders to be the most frequent psychiatric disorder, with phobias the most common of the anxiety disorders. Patients who actually seek treatment are most likely to have panic disorders.
   c. **Evidence for genetic contribution** comes from both family and twin studies. Twin studies of those with depression secondary to anxiety disorders show a concordance rate of 50% in MZ twins, but only 15% concordance in DZ twins.

2. **Personality disorders**
   a. **Definition.** Personality disorders are chronic patterns of maladaptive and inflexible behavior that significantly impair function or cause subjective distress. Specific disorders that show genetic influence include schizotypal, antisocial, histrionic, and compulsive personality disorders.
   b. **Evidence for genetic contribution**
      (1) Family studies indicate an increased risk for schizotypal personality disorder among close relatives of schizophrenics. The risk for antisocial personality disorder is greatly increased (5–10 times) in first-degree relatives of affected persons; a lesser risk exists for histrionic and compulsive personality disorders.
      (2) **Twin studies** show that concordance rates for personality disorders are generally much higher in MZ twins than in DZ twins.
      (3) A subset of families with compulsive personality disorder also has **Tourette syndrome,** which is a dominant condition with tics and coprolalia. The affected individuals do not respond well to serotonin-uptake blockers, as do the main group with obsessive-compulsive disorders. This suggests genetic heterogeneity.

3. **Chromosome disorders associated with behavioral disorders.** Combined psychiatric and chromosome disorders are rare. However, some generalizations can be made about sex chromosome aneuploidies.
   a. **Klinefelter syndrome** (see Chapter 2 II A 2 d). As children, XXY males may be immature, with poor judgment and learning problems. The incidence of XXY among schizophrenic males is 0.55%, compared with the expected 0.1% in the general population.
   b. **Trisomy X** (see Chapter 2 II A 2 f). The incidence of XXX females also is higher among schizophrenics than in the general population.
   c. **XYY syndrome** (see Chapter 2 II A 2 e). Early reports that XYY males were more likely to be aggressive and to commit violent crimes have been dismissed, but affected males do tend to be more immature and impulsive.
   d. **X monosomy and other Turner variants** (see Chapter 2 II B, C 2 b; III C 1 c). Affected individuals have space-form perceptual defects and are immature, although overall intelligence is normal. No increase in psychiatric disorders, such as schizophrenia, has been found.

4. **Single gene defects associated with behavioral disorders**
   a. **Fragile X syndrome** (see Chapter 3 I D 3 b)
      (1) Affected **males** not only have overall developmental delay but also have a disproportionate delay in speech and later abnormal speech patterns. As young

children, they exhibit autistic features; true autism is less frequent. As adults, their behavior often is described as friendly and cooperative.

  (2) Females are less severely affected, on average, and may have learning disabilities.
  b. **Phenylketonuria** (see Chapter 8 II B 2 a). As well as being mentally retarded, untreated children are irritable and unhappy. These traits disappear with treatment.
  c. **Homocystinuria.** Affected adults are more likely to have unusual personalities with psychoses associated with a schizophrenia-like picture.
  d. **Adult metachromatic leukodystrophy** presents as schizophrenia.
  e. **Lesch-Nyhan syndrome** produces a compulsion to self-mutilation.

VI. CONGENITAL ANOMALIES

A. Perspective

1. An **anomaly** is any abnormal deviation from the expected type in structure, form, or function. **Congenital** means present at birth.

2. Congenital anomalies are **common causes of morbidity and mortality,** especially in childhood.

3. **Many congenital anomalies are not apparent at birth,** although, by definition, all are present at birth. External malformations, such as polydactyly or cleft lip and cleft palate, are generally noted in the immediate newborn period, but internal or functional anomalies (involving, for example, the heart, kidneys, or brain) may not become apparent until later in life.

4. **Similar congenital anomalies in different individuals may have different causes.** This phenomenon is called **etiologic heterogeneity.**
  a. The **cause** of a congenital anomaly **cannot usually be determined by its appearance alone.**
  b. To determine the cause, one must consider any **other congenital anomalies** that may be present in the child, as well as the **pregnancy history** and **family history.**
  c. It is particularly **important to determine if a congenital anomaly is isolated** (i.e., the only anomaly in a child who is otherwise completely normal) or part of a more generalized pattern of anomalies.
    (1) Isolated congenital anomalies usually (but not always) **are of multifactorial etiology** (see III C 6 b).
    (2) Multiple congenital anomalies in a child **are usually** *not* **of multifactorial etiology.**

B. Types of congenital anomalies

1. **Malformations** are morphologic defects resulting from **intrinsically abnormal developmental processes.**
  a. Malformations may have a variety of causes.
  b. A malformed structure exhibits abnormal development **early in embryogenesis.**
  c. Examples include polydactyly (too many fingers or toes), oligodactyly (too few fingers or toes), most spina bifida, most cleft palates, and most kinds of congenital heart disease.

2. **Disruptions** are morphologic defects resulting from **breakdown of, or interference with, an originally normal developmental process.**
  a. Disruptions may result from the effects of a teratogenic agent or may have an unknown cause; they are **usually not caused by single gene or chromosome abnormalities.**
  b. Disruptions may occur at **any time during gestation.** The manifestations tend to differ with gestational timing, however.

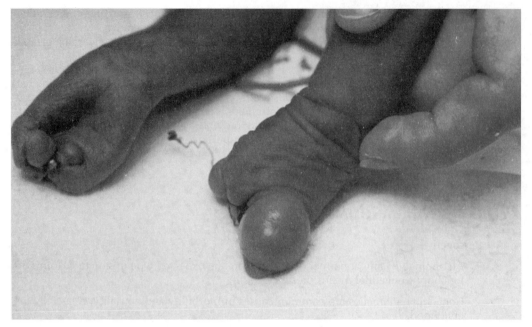

FIGURE 9–2. Amniotic band disruptions in the limbs of an infant.

    c. Examples include amniotic band disruptions (see Figure 9–2) and most cases of porencephaly (cystic lesions within the brain).

3. Deformations are abnormalities of form or position of a part of the body **caused by nondisruptive mechanical forces.**
    a. Deformations result from mechanical interference with the normal growth, function, or positioning of the fetus in utero. **Constraining factors** that may predispose to deformations include:
      (1) First pregnancy (uterus more resistant to stretch)
      (2) Small maternal size
      (3) Small uterus
      (4) Uterine malformation
      (5) Large uterine fibroids
      (6) Small maternal pelvis
      (7) Early engagement of the fetal head into the mother's pelvis
      (8) Unusual fetal position (e.g., transverse lie)
      (9) Oligohydramnios
     (10) Large fetus
     (11) Multifetal gestation
    b. Deformations are **usually *not* caused by chromosome or single gene abnormalities** unless the deformations are associated with malformations in the same infant.
    c. Deformations usually develop in the **second half of pregnancy** when the size of the fetus is large compared with the size of the uterus.
    d. Because deformations are caused by mechanical factors, they can often be **treated by mechanical means.** For example, positional deformations of the feet can usually be treated successfully by physical therapy or casting.
    e. Examples of deformations include positional abnormalities of the feet and molding of the head.

4. Dysplasias are morphologic defects caused by **abnormal organization of cells into tissue.**
    a. Dysplasias are **often due to single abnormal genes.**
    b. Dysplasias **develop during embryogenesis.**

    c. Examples include hemangiomas and thanatophoric dysplasia (a form of lethal short-limbed dwarfism).

C. **Patterns of anomalies** should be sought in individuals with two or more congenital defects. Such patterns may be of **four types:**

1. **Sequences** are patterns of anomalies **derived from a single known or presumed structural defect or mechanical factor.**
   a. A sequence can be thought of as a **cascade of anomalies, all of which derive directly or indirectly from a single primary defect.**
   b. A sequence may have **several different causes,** just as a malformation may have several different etiologies.
   c. One example is the **Robin sequence,** which consists of a broad, U-shaped cleft palate, small mandible, and a tendency for the tongue to obstruct the airway.
      (1) The **primary error of morphogenesis** in this instance is a small jaw (micrognathia). This, in turn, causes the oropharynx to be too small to contain the tongue normally while the palate is forming. As a consequence, the tongue remains partially in the nasopharynx and prevents the palatal shelves from approximating so that they can fuse.
      (2) The broad cleft palate is a more serious problem in a child than the small jaw, but the cleft palate is a secondary consequence of the micrognathia.
      (3) There are many causes of Robin sequence (e.g., Stickler syndrome, which is an autosomal dominant condition, and trisomy 18) since many different factors can cause an embryo to have a small jaw.
   d. Another example is the **oligohydramnios sequence.**
      (1) Features of this sequence include pulmonary hypoplasia (which is often fatal), positional deformities of the hands and feet, and Potter facies (a compressed appearance of the face and body).
      (2) Causes. The oligohydramnios sequence can occur as a consequence of decreased amniotic fluid or other cause. Commonly encountered causes include amniotic fluid leakage and decreased amniotic fluid production due to placental hypoperfusion or fetal anuria.

2. **Developmental field defects** are patterns of anomalies resulting from the **disturbed development of a morphogenic field or a part thereof.**
   a. Developmental (or morphogenic) fields can be thought of as **regions of the embryo that develop in a related fashion.** The derivative structures are not necessarily close spatially.
   b. Similar developmental field defects in different children **may have different causes.**
      An **example** is holoprosencephaly, a serious abnormality of midline brain development that is often associated with eyes that are set too closely together, hypoplasia of the nose, and midline cleft lip and palate. All of these abnormalities can be traced to a single localized defect of the prechordal mesoderm in the third to fourth week of embryonic development.

3. **Syndromes** are patterns in which **all of the component anomalies are pathogenically related.**
   a. In clinical genetics, the term "syndrome" implies a **similar etiology in all affected individuals.**
   b. The implication of causal specificity does *not* apply to "syndromes" in other medical contexts.
   c. **Examples** of genetic syndromes include Down syndrome (caused by trisomy of chromosome 21), fetal alcohol syndrome (caused by maternal alcohol abuse during pregnancy), and Marfan syndrome (caused by a dominantly inherited mutation of the fibrillin gene).
   d. **Syndrome identification** is one goal of genetic evaluation because it permits precise genetic counselling.

4. **Associations** are patterns of **anomalies that occur together more frequently than expected by chance** but are not identified as sequences, syndromes, or developmental

field defects. In other words, an association is simply a nonrandom grouping of congenital anomalies in an individual.

    a. The same group of anomalies may also occur in a sequence, a syndrome, or a developmental field defect.

    b. A similar association may have **different causes in different children.**

    c. **Examples** of associations include abnormal external ears and renal anomalies; single umbilical artery and cardiac defects; or vertebral, cardiac, and renal anomalies.

    d. As more is learned about the pathogenesis of congenital anomalies, some children with certain associations are likely to be reclassified as having a syndrome, a sequence, or a developmental field defect.

D. **Minor anomalies are unusual morphologic features that are of no serious medical or cosmetic consequence.**

    1. **Examples** include dermatoglyphic alterations, abnormal scalp hair whorls, alterations in the shape of the auricles, and bifid ribs.

    2. Minor anomalies are important because they **may be characteristic of certain patterns of anomalies** and permit their classification as specific syndromes. Down syndrome, fetal alcohol syndrome, and many other syndromes are recognized clinically on the basis of characteristic patterns of minor anomalies rather than on the presence of specific major anomalies.

    3. Recognition of minor anomalies is also important because the presence of multiple minor anomalies in a child suggests a generalized disorder of early embryogenesis. **The more minor anomalies a child has, the more likely he or she is to have an associated major congenital anomaly.**

    4. **Certain minor anomalies tend to be associated with certain malformations.** For example, absence of the occipital hair whorl and wide-spaced eyes tend to be associated with brain malformations, such as microencephaly and holoprosencephaly, respectively.

STUDY QUESTIONS

DIRECTIONS: Each of the numbered items or incomplete statements in this section is followed by answers or by completions of the statement. Select the ONE lettered answer or completion that is BEST in each case.

1. Quantitative traits are best described by which one of the following statements?

(A) They are the number of structures of a given type that occur in a person's body, such as the number of fingers, ribs, or kidneys

(B) They usually exhibit multifactorial inheritance

(C) They are more frequent in monozygotic twins than in dizygotic twins

(D) They are continuously variable and may assume any value

(E) They usually exhibit more extreme values in children than in either parent

2. A 21-year-old black man on vacation in Greece developed acute hemolytic anemia after treatment of malaria with primaquine. Which one of the following statements regarding this man is true?

(A) His reaction to primaquine is likely to be caused by sickle cell disease

(B) His sisters should not be treated with primaquine

(C) His father is likely to have hemolytic anemia if he is treated with primaquine

(D) He may also develop hemolytic anemia if he is treated with other drugs such as sulfonamides

(E) He is at risk for malignant hyperthermia if he undergoes general anesthesia

3. A young woman whose sister developed a bipolar disorder at 23 years of age asks her physician if she is at risk for the disorder. No other family members are known to be affected. This woman's risk for developing bipolar disorder is which one of the following percentages?

(A) 1%
(B) 5%
(C) 10%
(D) 15%
(E) 20%

DIRECTIONS: Each of the numbered items or incomplete statements in this section is negatively phrased, as indicated by a capitalized word such as NOT, LEAST, or EXCEPT. Select the ONE lettered answer or completion that is BEST in each case.

4. All of the following characteristics suggest that a disease under consideration is inherited as a multifactorial trait EXCEPT

(A) the disease occurs more frequently in women than in men

(B) the disease occurs more often among the children of an affected patient than among the grandchildren

(C) the risk of recurrence of the disease in a child is greater if both parents are affected than if only one parent is affected

(D) the incidence of the disease is 4% in the population and 50% among the children of an affected parent

5. Mr. K, who is 40 years old, has previously had difficulty breathing after anesthesia. A blood test performed on him after this episode showed that he was completely deficient for serum butyrylcholinesterase activity. All of the following statements regarding his case are correct EXCEPT

(A) Mr. K is likely to have breathing difficulties after future anesthetics if succinylcholine is administered

(B) Mr. K should be given intravenous anticholinesterase antibodies before surgery

(C) halothane and similar general anesthetics can be safely administered to Mr. K during surgery

(D) regional anesthetics can be safely administered to Mr. K during surgery

(E) members of Mr. K's family should be
aware of this problem

6. All of the following statements about schizophrenia are true EXCEPT

(A) linkage to an autosomal locus has been
proposed

(B) nearly 2% of the population is affected

(C) it is a psychosis characterized by disordered or inappropriate thought

(D) increased concordance rates in monozygous (MZ) twins indicate that genetic factors are important

(E) abnormal smooth pursuit eye movements
are positively correlated

7. A 49-year-old woman is being assessed
preoperatively. She informs the anesthesiolo-
gist that her mother died during an anesthetic
procedure and that her mother's brother also
had significant medical problems, including
high fever, during an operation. All of the following statements are correct EXCEPT

(A) this woman should be considered at increased risk for the autosomal dominant
condition, malignant hyperthermia

(B) she should be encouraged to wear a
Medic Alert bracelet stating she is at risk
for malignant hyperthermia

(C) the medical records of her relatives
should be obtained to learn more about
the reason for problems during anesthesia

(D) she should only have emergency surgery

(E) problems in surgery can be reduced by
medications or by use of different anesthetics

8. An 18-year-old man has a strong family
history of premature atherosclerosis; his father
and grandfather died of a heart attack in their
mid-30s. The young man's father was known
to have high cholesterol. All of the following
statements are true EXCEPT

(A) he has up to a 50% chance of having
high cholesterol levels

(B) dietary therapy is unlikely to lower his
cholesterol levels to normal if they are
elevated

(C) his siblings should have their cholesterol
measured

(D) treatment for hypercholesterolemia
should begin when he is in his 30s

(E) modification or elimination of other risk
factors, such as smoking, is especially important for this young man

9. All of the following statements regarding
the genetics of cancer are true EXCEPT

(A) all types of cancer involve changes of
DNA, but these may not be inherited

(B) cloning of the gene causing familial polyposis has now allowed development of
predictive testing for people at risk for
this disorder

(C) specific changes in the p53 gene have
been shown to be associated with Li-
Fraumeni syndrome

(D) changes in the tumor suppressor gene
p53 are only seen in patients with inherited forms of cancer

(E) a family history of breast cancer significantly alters the risk for first-degree relatives

DIRECTIONS: The set of matching questions in this section consists of a list of four to twenty-six lettered options (some of which may be in figures) followed by several numbered items. For each numbered item, select the ONE lettered option that is most closely associated with it. To avoid spending too much time on matching sets with large numbers of options, it is generally advisable to begin each set by reading the list of options. Then, for each item in the set, try to generate the correct answer and locate it in the option list, rather than evaluating each option individually. Each lettered option may be selected once, more than once, or not at all.

Questions 10–13

Match each of the following congenital anomalies with the category it is most likely to represent.

(A) Deformation
(B) Disruption
(C) Dysplasia
(D) Malformation
(E) Sequence

10. Polydactyly inherited as an autosomal dominant trait

11. Clubfoot occurring in an otherwise normal baby born of a triplet pregnancy at 37 weeks

12. A brain cyst resulting from an intrauterine stroke in the infant of a woman who abused cocaine during pregnancy

13. Congenital heart disease in an infant with trisomy 18

ANSWERS AND EXPLANATIONS

1. The answer is B [III A 2, B 3–5]. Quantitative traits are those that can be measured on a continuous scale. They usually exhibit multifactorial inheritance and have a normal population distribution, with average values being most common. Monozygotic (MZ) twins tend to resemble each other closely with respect to quantitative phenotypes, but such traits occur in everyone. Although quantitative traits are continuously variable, the range of values that occurs is limited by physiologic and anatomic constraints. Because children inherit only half of the genes that determine a quantitative multifactorial trait from each parent, a parent who manifests an extreme value for a trait tends to have children who exhibit less extreme values.

2. The answer is D [II B 1]. Glucose-6-phosphate dehydrogenase (G6PD) deficiency is an X-linked enzyme disorder that affects approximately 5% of males of African ancestry in the United States. Affected males may develop an acute hemolytic anemia when treated with a variety of drugs, including primaquine and sulfonamides. Because G6PD deficiency is an X-linked recessive disorder, an affected man's sisters may be carriers but are unlikely to have G6PD deficiency unless their father also has this condition. The chance that the father is affected is approximately 5%. It is usually safe to treat females with primaquine and other drugs that may unmask G6PD deficiency in males, but it is possible to test people for this deficiency before treatment. Malignant hyperthermia is a completely separate pharmacogenetic condition that has nothing to do with primaquine sensitivity.

3. The answer is E [V C 2, 3 a]. Although bipolar disorder affects roughly 0.4%–1.2% of the general adult population, the recurrence risk for first-degree relatives is much higher. The risk is highest (20%) when the onset of illness in the proband occurs before 40 years of age. This may reflect the severity of the disorder.

4. The answer is D [III C 4]. Isolated congenital anomalies and common diseases of adulthood often are inherited as multifactorial traits. Such conditions characteristically occur in one sex more frequently than in the other. The incidence of multifactorial diseases is higher among individuals who are more closely related to an affected person than in those who are less closely related. Individuals who are more closely related are likely to share with the proband more genetic and nongenetic factors that predispose to the disease. Multifactorial diseases typically exhibit a higher recurrence risk in families with more affected members because such families are likely to possess, and thus transmit, more factors that contribute to the disease. The incidence of multifactorial diseases in the first-degree relatives of an affected patient typically equals approximately the square root of the population frequency.

5. The answer is B [II B 4]. Serum butyrylcholinesterase is an enzyme that breaks down succinylcholine. In some populations, particularly those of Caucasian descent, about 1/3000 individuals has an abnormal enzyme that is unable to degrade succinylcholine, which often results in prolonged apnea after anesthesia. Because the problem is inactivity of this enzyme, a treatment such as administration of antibody against cholinesterase would not be helpful. Both general and regional anesthesia can safely be administered to patients with serum butyrylcholinesterase deficiency if succinylcholine (or similar drugs) are avoided. Family members should certainly be aware of this problem and should inform their anesthesiologists of it prior to surgery.

6. The answer is B [V B 2]. Schizophrenia is seen in approximately 0.5% of the general population and has an increased recurrence risk in first-degree relatives. Schizophrenia is defined as a psychosis characterized by disordered thought that lasts longer than 6 months. In some families, the disorder is linked with altered smooth pursuit eye movements, suggesting that these families have a dominant disorder. Twin studies indicate a higher concordance rate for schizophrenia in monozygotic (MZ) twins than in dizygotic (DZ) twins. However, even MZ twins do not show 100% concordance, which suggests that genetic factors alone do not cause schizophrenia.

7. The answer is D [II B 2]. Clearly, the woman should be considered at increased risk for malignant hyperthermia, and wearing a Medic Alert bracelet might prevent a catastrophic outcome. If surgery is needed for this particular woman, it can be undertaken; however, appropriate medications (e.g., dantrolene sodium) should be available during the operation to prevent or reduce the severity of the hyperthermic response.

8. The answer is D [IV D 1–4]. Treatment of high serum cholesterol should strongly take into account the family history. In this instance, with the father having a high cholesterol level and a history of a heart attack in his mid-30s, it is most likely that there is a genetic hyperlipidemia. In this instance, dietary therapy alone is usually insufficient to lower the levels. In view of the significant family history of very marked premature atherosclerosis, treatment should begin before the age of 30 years in an effort to reduce the likelihood of this particular outcome. Of course, in this young man, as in other patients with hyperlipidemia, modification of other risk factors is essential to try to reduce the risk for later atherosclerotic events.

9. The answer is D [IV C 2]. All cancer involves changes in DNA of somatic cells. However, in most instances, these genetic changes do not involve the germ line and therefore are not inherited. Familial polyposis is a disorder that is inherited as an autosomal dominant trait and is characterized by the presence of multiple polyps in the colon, which eventually become cancerous. The cloning of the gene for this disorder now allows predictive testing using DNA markers close to or within this particular gene. Changes in the p53 gene, which is a tumor suppressor gene, have now been shown to be associated with familial cancer syndrome. Patients with this syndrome may present with cancers in many different tissues, including the breast and the brain. The p53 gene is also changed in sporadic forms of many different cancers. In all of these, inactivation of this gene results in loss of tumor suppression, which results in cancer. This was initially seen in sporadic forms of cancer and later recognized as the defective gene in Li-Fraumeni syndrome. Breast cancer has a strong genetic component and a woman's risk of developing breast cancer is significantly increased if a first-degree relative is affected. The risk increases if more than one relative is affected.

10–13. The answers are: 10-D, 11-A, 12-B, 13-D [VI B]. Polydactyly and congenital heart disease, especially when they occur in the context of a genetic condition, are likely to represent malformations. They are the consequences of intrinsically abnormal developmental processes during embryogenesis. The movement of fetuses in a triplet pregnancy is likely to be constrained near term. An otherwise normal baby with a clubfoot born of a triplet pregnancy is likely to have a deformation.

A cyst resulting from an intrauterine stroke is an example of a disruptive process. The brain probably developed normally during embryogenesis but has subsequently been damaged.

Chapter 10

Teratogenesis and Mutagenesis

J. M. Friedman

I. INTRODUCTION. Both teratogens and mutagens can cause alterations in the structure and function of the body, but the mechanisms by which they cause alterations differ. Epidemiologic studies are an important means of evaluating potential teratogens and mutagens in human populations.

A. Teratogens cause damage by altering embryonic or fetal development either directly or indirectly.

B. Mutagens cause changes within the genetic material that may lead to inherited disease if the germ cells are affected or to cancer if somatic cells are involved.

C. Epidemiology is the study of the frequency and distribution of diseases within groups of people and of factors that affect this frequency and distribution.

II. TERATOGENESIS

A. A teratogen is an agent that can produce a permanent alteration of structure or function in an organism after exposure during embryonic or fetal life. Teratogens include environmental factors, medications, drugs of abuse, and occupational chemicals.

B. Clinical teratology is concerned with the following:

1. The relationship between the anomalies in a child and teratogenic exposure

2. The risk of anomalies for a child of a woman who has been exposed to a teratogen

3. The risks to a pregnant woman for whom treatment with or exposure to a potential teratogen is being considered

C. Principles of clinical teratology

1. **There are no absolute teratogens,** but many agents can exhibit a teratogenic effect under some circumstances. The **timing and conditions of exposure** are as important as the nature of the agent itself in determining teratogenic risk. For example:
   a. Thalidomide is not teratogenic if the exposure is just holding a pill in one's hand.
   b. However, **any agent** that is administered in a manner and dose that is **toxic to a pregnant woman** may present a **danger to her fetus.** This is even true of "nonteratogenic" agents, such as table salt.

2. **An embryo is not a little adult.**
   a. The likelihood that an agent will produce a teratogenic effect in an embryo or fetus usually cannot be predicted on the basis of its pharmacologic action in an adult.
   b. The biochemical processes involved in the development of an organ or structure may have no relationship to the processes involved in maintaining the function of that organ or structure once formation is complete.

3. **Teratogens act at vulnerable periods of embryogenesis and fetal development.**
   a. In general, the embryo is **most sensitive** to damage **between 2 and 10 weeks after conception** (4 to 12 weeks after the beginning of the last menstrual period).

During this time, most structures and organs are differentiating and forming. Each structure has its own period of greatest sensitivity within this time.

(1) The period of **embryonic development** that is most sensitive to teratogenic effects has **already passed** by the time many women know that they are pregnant.

(2) Therefore, the **teratogenic potential** of any drug given to a woman who is capable of having children **should be discussed** with her **when the drug is prescribed**.

b. The **first 2 weeks after conception** is generally considered to be a period during which the conceptus is **resistant to the induction of malformations** by teratogens. During this time, the conceptus consists of few cells, and damage is usually repaired completely or results in the death of the embryo.

c. **By 10 weeks** after conception, most structures in the embryo have been formed, so **malformations are unlikely** to be produced by subsequent exposures.

(1) However, disruptions, disturbances of growth, or altered tissue maturation may be caused by teratogenic exposures throughout pregnancy.

(2) Such effects are most likely to manifest as fetal growth retardation and abnormal central nervous system (CNS) function.

4. **Individual differences in susceptibility to teratogens exist.**

a. In experimental animals, genetic differences can greatly alter the susceptibility to teratogenic damage.

b. In humans, **both maternal and fetal susceptibility** are probably important in determining the likelihood of teratogenic effects.

5. **Combinations of exposures to teratogenic agents may have effects different from those resulting when exposures occur individually.**

a. In some cases, the risk inherent in exposure to combinations of teratogens may be substantially **greater than the sum of risks** of individual exposures.

b. In other cases, exposure to certain agents may **decrease the risk** usually associated with exposure to another agent.

6. **Teratogenic exposures tend to produce characteristic patterns of multiple anomalies** rather than single defects.

a. The **recognition** of most human teratogens has resulted from clinical identification of an unusual pattern of congenital anomalies among children of women who had similar exposures during pregnancy.

b. **Examples** include the embryopathies caused by rubella, alcohol, and isotretinoin.

D. Teratogenic factors are thought to be responsible for about **10% of all congenital anomalies**. These factors fall into several groups.

1. **Maternal metabolic imbalance** includes factors intrinsic to the mother that cause alterations of the intrauterine environment of the embryo or fetus.

a. The children of women with **insulin-dependent diabetes mellitus** have a risk of congenital anomalies that is two to three times greater than that of the general population.

(1) The **most common malformations** among infants of diabetic mothers are **congenital heart disease** (occurring in 2%–3%) and **neural tube defects** (occurring in 1%–2%). Some other congenital anomalies, such as caudal dysplasia and proximal femoral hypoplasia, are rare, but they occur much more often in the infants of diabetic mothers than in other infants.

(2) **Many of these congenital anomalies can be detected prenatally** by high-resolution ultrasound examination, fetal echocardiography, or measurement of the α-fetoprotein concentration in maternal blood or amniotic fluid. **Prenatal diagnosis should be offered to all pregnant women with insulin-dependent diabetes mellitus.**

(3) **Malformations develop early in gestation.** Improved control of maternal diabetes established later in pregnancy cannot influence the frequency of malformations in infants of diabetic mothers. Thus, **pregnancies in women with insulin-dependent diabetes should be planned so that excellent control can be maintained from the moment of conception.**

b. **The children of women with phenylketonuria (PKU),** particularly if untreated during pregnancy, are almost certain to be born with mental retardation, microcephaly, and other anomalies. Such children usually do not have PKU themselves, but they are damaged by developing in a uterine environment of hyperphenylalaninemia.

c. **Children of women with certain endocrinopathies** (e.g., androgen-secreting tumors) are at high risk of being born with abnormalities resulting from such pathologic hormone exposure.

d. **Pregnant women with systemic lupus erythematosus (SLE)** have an increased risk for fetal cardiac conduction defects, which may be transient or permanent and which may cause fetal death.

2. **Infectious agents** can involve the embryo or fetus transplacentally.

   a. **Syphilis** can cause congenital infections that present at birth or in early infancy. Features may include stillbirth, various cutaneous lesions, rhinitis, hepatosplenomegaly, meningoencephalitis, and osteochondritis.

   b. **Congenital toxoplasmosis** (*Toxoplasma gondii*) may be asymptomatic or present with a variety of abnormalities. Severely affected infants may exhibit chorioretinitis, hydrocephaly or microcephaly, intracranial calcification, and mental retardation.

   c. **Rubella (German measles)** embryopathy produces fetal growth retardation, hepatosplenomegaly, purpura, jaundice, microcephaly, cataracts, deafness, congenital heart disease, and mental retardation.

   d. **Congenital cytomegalovirus (CMV)** infection may produce fetal growth retardation, hepatosplenomegaly, hemolytic anemia, purpura, jaundice, intracranial calcification, and microcephaly.

   e. **Varicella (chickenpox)** infection in utero is rare but may be devastating. Manifestations include cutaneous lesions or scarring and disruptions (e.g., limb reduction defects, cortical atrophy).

   f. **Congenital human immunodeficiency virus (HIV)** results in the development of AIDS and death in early childhood. Microcephaly and failure to thrive may also occur.

   g. **Parvovirus** infection of the fetus may produce severe anemia, hydrops, and death.

3. **Ionizing radiation** causes DNA damage and can injure the developing embryo.

   a. In utero exposure to **large doses of ionizing radiation** (e.g., those that are used for cancer radiotherapy) can produce microcephaly and mental retardation. Diagnostic radiographs during pregnancy are rarely associated with radiation doses that pose a substantial risk to the embryo or fetus, but they should be avoided if possible.

   b. **Radioactive iodine** is concentrated in the fetal thyroid gland after the thirteenth week of pregnancy and may produce cretinism.

4. **Environmental agents and occupational chemicals** are often of concern to pregnant women.

   a. Exposure to only two chemicals has been **proved to be teratogenic in humans.**

      (1) Maternal poisoning during pregnancy by food contaminated with **methyl mercury** has resulted in damage to the fetal CNS. Ataxia, weakness, and features of cerebral palsy may be produced.

      (2) Maternal ingestion of large amounts of **polychlorinated biphenyls (PCBs)** during pregnancy produces fetal growth retardation, diffuse hyperpigmentation, and natal teeth.

   b. **Suspected environmental teratogens.** The following agents are suspected of being teratogenic in humans.

      (1) Hyperthermia, regardless of cause, that produces sustained elevation of maternal body temperature to levels substantially above normal (e.g., 40°C). This is usually due to fever but may occur with extreme use of saunas or hot tubs.

      (2) Maternal exposure to large amounts of **lead** during pregnancy has been associated with CNS damage in the offspring. However, available studies do not permit clear separation of the effects of prenatal and postnatal exposures.

    c. Unlikely teratogens. It is unlikely that maternal use of a video display terminal (VDT) during pregnancy poses any measurable risk to the fetus.

  5. Drugs of abuse not only may damage the health of the mother but also may interfere with the development of the embryo or fetus.

    a. Established human teratogens

      (1) Alcohol

        (a) Classic **fetal alcohol syndrome** occurs among the children of women with chronic, severe alcoholism during pregnancy.

          (i) Mothers of infants with fetal alcohol syndrome usually drink **more, and often much more, than 3 ounces of absolute alcohol daily** (i.e., the equivalent of about six beers, six glasses of wine, or six mixed drinks every day.

          (ii) Features of fetal alcohol syndrome include growth deficiency, mental retardation, behavioral disturbances, and typical facial appearance (Figure 10-1). The facies are characterized by short palpebral fissures, hypoplastic midface, long and flat philtrum, and narrow upper lip vermilion. Congenital heart disease and structural brain anomalies are common.

        (b) The risks of maternal **binge drinking** during pregnancy have not been clearly defined but may be substantial.

        (c) Smaller amounts of maternal alcohol drinking during pregnancy have been associated with less severe disturbances of growth, intellectual performance, and behavior among offspring. **No safe level of maternal drinking during pregnancy has been established.**

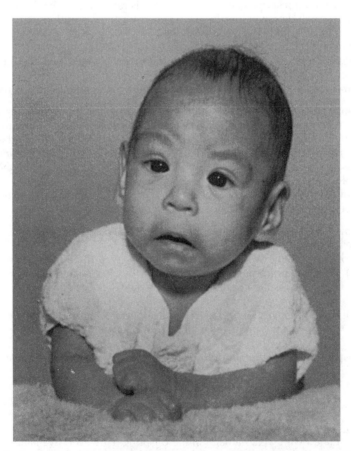

FIGURE 10-1. Infant with fetal alcohol syndrome–typical facies. (Photograph courtesy of T. Kellerman.)

(2) Cocaine. Maternal use of cocaine during pregnancy has been associated with abruptio placentae and the occurrence of vascular disruptions (e.g., encephaloclastic lesions) in the fetus.

(3) Maternal **abuse of organic solvents** such as toluene by inhalation can cause fetal brain damage.

b. Recreational drugs **not proven to be teratogenic** in humans with usual exposures include:

(1) Marijuana

(2) Heroin

(3) LSD

(4) Caffeine (as small or moderate amounts of coffee, tea, or soft drinks)

6. Medications

a. Maternal treatment with some medications in usual therapeutic doses **early in pregnancy** is known to cause congenital anomalies in humans.

(1) Thalidomide exposure in the first trimester of gestation may produce limb reduction defects, facial malformations, and other congenital anomalies.

(2) Aminopterin and other **cytotoxic drugs** kill rapidly growing cells in the fetus and cause growth deficiency and a variety of other anomalies.

(3) An increased rate of congenital anomalies is observed among the children of epileptic women treated with **anticonvulsant medications** during pregnancy.

(a) Whether this increased risk of congenital abnormalities is caused by the mother's epilepsy, by a teratogenic effect of the medications, or by some combination thereof is uncertain. In general, **therapy with multiple anticonvulsant drugs is associated with a higher risk than therapy with a single anticonvulsant medication.**

(b) Drugs that have been implicated as having teratogenic effects when used as anticonvulsants include **phenytoin, trimethadione, paramethadione, carbamazepine, phenobarbital, and valproic acid.**

(i) Maternal treatment with **valproic acid** during pregnancy has also been associated with approximately a 2% risk of **neural tube defects** in the offspring. The risk of neural tube defects may also be somewhat increased among the children of women treated with **carbamazepine** during pregnancy.

(ii) The **risk** of having a child with a neural tube defect may be **decreased** in women taking valproic acid or carbamazepine if they also take **folic acid supplements** prior to conception and through the first 2 months of pregnancy.

(iii) Prenatal diagnosis of neural tube defects should be offered to women who have been treated with valproic acid or carbamazepine during early pregnancy.

(4) Maternal use of **androgenic hormones** during pregnancy can produce virilization of the external genitalia of female infants.

(5) Daughters of women treated with **diethylstilbestrol (DES)** during early pregnancy often exhibit abnormalities of the vaginal epithelium and cervix and have a greatly increased risk of clear cell adenocarcinoma of the vagina or cervix.

(6) Maternal treatment with **lithium** during early pregnancy has been associated with an increased frequency of Ebstein anomaly of the heart (a malformation of the tricuspid valve) in offspring.

(7) CNS anomalies, ocular malformations, midface hypoplasia, and radiographic evidence of epiphyseal stippling may occur among the children of women treated with **warfarin** during pregnancy.

(8) Isotretinoin and **etretinate** are vitamin A congeners that can cause craniofacial, brain, cardiac, and other serious fetal malformations.

b. Maternal treatment with the following medications is **suspected but not proved to be teratogenic.**

(1) Penicillamine

(2) Quinine

(3) Retinol (vitamin A) in very large doses (> 25,000 IU/day)

    c. Maternal treatment with other medications **later in pregnancy** does not cause malformations but can have serious adverse effects in the offspring.

      (1) Oligohydramnios, fetal renal failure, and fetal or neonatal death occur with greatly increased frequency among women treated with **angiotensin-converting enzyme (ACE) inhibitors** (e.g., **captopril, enalapril**) late in pregnancy. The ACE inhibitors are not known to pose a substantial teratogenic risk in early pregnancy.

      (2) Maternal treatment with **tetracycline** during the second or third trimester of pregnancy often causes discoloration of the teeth in offspring.

      (3) A greatly increased frequency of intestinal atresia occurs in twin pregnancies in which **methylene blue** was **instilled into the amniotic fluid** during amniocentesis.

      (4) Maternal treatment with **indomethacin** late in pregnancy may be associated with the development of fetal anuria, oligohydramnios, premature closure of the ductus arteriosus, and consequent problems in perinatal adaptation.

    d. Some medications that are commonly used in pregnancy have been shown **not** to be **teratogenic** in conventional human doses.

      (1) Metronidazole

      (2) Aspirin

      (3) Contraceptives

        (a) Oral contraceptives

        (b) Vaginal spermicides

      (4) Bendectin

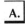

III. MUTAGENESIS

A. **Definition and overview.** A **mutagen** is an agent that can alter the DNA or chromosomes.

1. Whereas teratogens act only during embryonic or fetal development (see II A), **mutagens may act at any time of life.** Thus, mutations may occur in the gamete, zygote, embryo, fetus, child, or adult.

2. Teratogens affect the development of a tissue, organ, or structure. In contrast, **a mutation always affects a single cell.**

    a. If this single cell is a germ cell, the mutation may be transmitted to subsequent generations.

    b. If a single cell in a very early embryo sustains a mutation, many tissues of the embryo (including the germ cells) may be affected as embryogenesis progresses.

    c. If a single cell in an embryo, fetus, child, or adult sustains a mutation, only cells derived from the mutated cell will carry the mutation. Most cells in the individual will not contain the mutation.

B. **Clinical importance of environmental mutagens**

1. **Radiation and thousands of chemicals can produce mutations** in bacteria, fruit flies, mice, rats, and cultured human or animal cells. Examples of such experimental mutagens include urethane, cyclophosphamide, and dioxin.

2. **Somatic cell mutations** play an important part in the development of human **neoplasia** (see Chapter 11 III), but it is usually not possible to attribute these mutations to exposure to a specific mutagenic agent.

3. **No chemical agent has been proved to produce transmissible gametic mutations in humans.** It is likely, however, that mutagens do affect human germ cells but that available studies have just been unable to show this effect. There are several explanations for this.

    a. **Most potential mutations are repaired to the normal state** by efficient DNA correction mechanisms that exist within human cells.

    b. Most mutations are recessive and will be expressed only when they occur in homozygotes.

    c. The rate of disease caused by new gametic mutations in the general population is probably substantially less than 1%, and many different conditions can be produced by such changes. It is, therefore, very difficult to carry out human studies that are large enough to show a measurably increased rate of disease caused by new gametic mutations.

4. From a practical point of view, concerned patients can be told that there is **no evidence that remote preconceptional exposure of either parent to any mutagenic environmental agent substantially increases the risk of congenital anomalies among offspring**.

    a. Even though the risk of inducing birth defects in future children by exposure of the parents to mutagens is small in any individual case, **the risk for the population as a whole may be substantial.**

    b. There may be no completely safe level of exposure to radiation or to a mutagenic chemical. Thus, **absolute safety is usually not possible.**

IV. EPIDEMIOLOGY OF CONGENITAL ANOMALIES

A. Definitions and overview

1. Epidemiology is the study of factors that determine the frequency and distribution of disease within or between populations.

2. Birth defects epidemiology seeks to demonstrate associations among a particular congenital anomaly (or congenital anomalies) and various potential etiologic factors.

3. Etiologic heterogeneity

    a. Clinically indistinguishable **congenital anomalies in different patients may have different causes**. For example, cleft palate may be caused by a chromosome abnormality in one patient, by a teratogenic exposure in another, and by a single-gene mutation in a third patient. In most patients, however, cleft palate results from a multifactorial predisposition. It is sometimes possible to determine the cause of the congenital anomalies in an individual patient by dysmorphic evaluation (see Chapter 13 I B).

    b. In epidemiologic studies, **it is important to consider etiologic heterogeneity when trying to determine whether a particular exposure is likely to be associated causally with a given congenital anomaly.**

B. Types of studies.
Studies of associations between possible causative factors and congenital anomalies may be of several types. Most often, such investigations deal with exposure of the mother to putative teratogens early in pregnancy.

1. Case reports are simply descriptions of patients with a given congenital anomaly or pattern of anomalies whose mothers were exposed to certain agents during gestation.

    a. Case reports are valuable in **raising suspicion** regarding the possible teratogenic effect of an agent but **cannot be used to prove that the association is causal.**

    b. Most associations observed in individual case reports are spurious (i.e., the associations are due to chance or some noncausal relationship).

2. A **clinical series** consists of cases that are similar with respect to exposures or that have similar anomalies.

    a. If a **recurrent pattern of congenital anomalies** is observed among infants born to women with similar exposures during pregnancy, a causal relationship may be suggested, particularly if the pattern of anomalies, the exposure, or both are rare.

    b. Almost all human teratogens have been recognized initially in clinical series. Thus, the **most effective means of recognizing human teratogens is the alert clinician** who notices a similar unusual pattern of congenital anomalies among the children of women who have had a similar unusual exposure during pregnancy.

    c. Because of the biases inherent in collecting cases for a clinical series, this approach **usually cannot be used to estimate the magnitude of risk** associated with exposure to an agent.

3. Cohort studies compare the frequency of congenital anomalies among the children of women exposed to an agent during pregnancy to the frequency among children of women who were not exposed.

    a. Cohort studies **can be used to estimate the risk and statistical significance** of an observed association.

    b. Cohort studies are often subject to serious **biases of ascertainment** and may be difficult to interpret because of **confounding factors.** Appropriate experimental design and analysis are essential to proper interpretation of cohort studies.

    c. Cohort studies of congenital anomalies are usually **difficult** and quite **expensive** to perform.

4. Case-control studies compare the frequency of maternal exposure during pregnancy to a given agent among children with and without congenital anomalies.

    a. Case-control studies **can be used to estimate the risk and statistical significance** of an observed association.

    b. Case-control studies are often subject to serious **biases of ascertainment and recall,** and they may be difficult to interpret because of **confounding factors.** Appropriate experimental design and analysis are essential to proper interpretation of case-control studies.

5. Animal experiments are essential to elucidating the mechanisms by which teratogenic effects occur. Such studies may also be useful in identifying agents that should be suspected of having teratogenic potential in humans, but **animal studies alone cannot prove that an exposure is teratogenic in humans**.

    a. Experimental animals **differ from humans in physiology, metabolism, and embryonic development**.

    b. **Exposures** used experimentally **often differ** in dose and route from those encountered in humans.

    c. Humans may exhibit a wide range of **individual susceptibilities** to teratogenic effects, but this variability is often controlled in experimental animals by employing genetically inbred strains.

    d. Animal experiments deal with **populations**. In humans, the physician is generally concerned about the risks for an **individual patient**.

C. Interpretation of studies

1. Types of associations

    a. An association between the occurrence of a congenital anomaly in a child and a prenatal exposure in the mother may be due to **chance.** This is most likely if the exposure or the anomaly or both are relatively common or poorly defined. Even rare coincidences are expected to occur occasionally in a country as large as the United States.

    b. An association between a congenital anomaly in a child and a prenatal exposure may occur because **both the anomaly and the exposure are related to another variable.** For example, maternal cigarette smoking during pregnancy might be associated with small head size in infants. However, women who smoke are more likely to drink alcohol, and maternal drinking is associated with small head size in infants.

    c. An association is said to be **causal** if the exposure produced the congenital anomaly. The following factors support the interpretation that an association is causal:

        (1) Consistency of the association in studies of different design and in different populations

        (2) Dependence of the effect **on dose and time of exposure**

        (3) Existence of a similar effect in an **experimental animal model**

        (4) Biologic plausibility

2. Cohort studies and case–control studies can be evaluated statistically. Four parameters are often used to assess the outcome of such studies.

a. **Statistical significance** is an expression of how likely the association is to have occurred due to chance alone. For example, if an observed association is statistically significant at a level of $P < 0.05$, the probability is less than 0.05 (or 1/20) that the observation would have occurred by chance alone.

b. **Absolute risk** is the rate of occurrence of a condition among the children of individuals who have had a given exposure. If 20% of infants born to women who took isotretinoin in the first trimester of pregnancy are found to have congenital anomalies in a study, then the absolute risk is 20%.

c. **Relative risk** is the ratio of the rate of a condition among those exposed to the rate among those not exposed. A relative risk of 3.0, for example, implies that an anomaly occurs three times more often among the children of women with a particular exposure than among the children of women without that exposure.

   (1) A very high relative risk may be associated with a small absolute risk if the defect under consideration is rare.

   (2) For example, an exposure that produces a relative risk of 10 would increase the frequency of a congenital anomaly that normally occurs with a rate of 1/100,000 to 1/10,000.

d. **Attributable risk** is the proportion of cases of a condition in exposed individuals that can be attributed to the exposure. **Population attributable risk** is the proportion of cases of the condition in the population as a whole that results from the exposure.

   (1) The population attributable risk provides an estimate of the **amount by which the rate of a condition might be reduced by prevention of an exposure.**

   (2) For example, in a study of childhood deafness, the population attributable risk for maternal rubella is found to be 10%. One could, therefore, estimate that the overall frequency of childhood deafness would be reduced by 10% if rubella infection of pregnant women could be entirely eliminated.

STUDY QUESTIONS

DIRECTIONS: Each of the numbered items or incomplete statements in this section is followed by answers or by completions of the statement. Select the ONE lettered answer or completion that is BEST in each case.

1. Maternal abuse of which one of the following substances is known to be teratogenic in humans?

(A) Marijuana
(B) LSD
(C) Heroin
(D) Alcohol
(E) Coffee

2. Mutagens are correctly described as

(A) agents that can produce a permanent alteration of structure or function in an organism after exposure during embryonic or fetal life
(B) common causes of congenital anomalies in humans

(C) responsible for causing most autosomal recessive diseases
(D) responsible for causing most autosomal dominant diseases
(E) capable of affecting both somatic cells and germ cells in humans

Questions 3–5

A study is done on low–birth-weight among infants born during a 12-month period. The mothers of some of these infants drank soft drinks containing a new artificial sweetener called Nomoflab during pregnancy. The mothers of the remaining infants did not drink such beverages. The findings of the study are as follows:

| Mothers | Birth Weight of Infant | |
	> 2500 g	< 2500 g
Did not consume Nomoflab	2609	123 (4.5%)
Consumed Nomoflab	1915	192 (9.1%)

Statistical significance: $P < 0.001$
Relative risk = 2.0
Population attributable risk = 31%

3. If none of the women had used beverages containing Nomoflab during pregnancy, which one of the following statements would be true, according to the data in the table?

(A) The frequency of low–birth-weight infants would have been more than 1000 times lower
(B) 2.0% of infants would have had low birth weights
(C) 9.1% of infants would have had low birth weights
(D) The overall frequency of low–birth-weight infants would have been 31% lower

(E) Only half as many infants would have had low birth weights

4. The observed association between maternal use of Nomoflab during pregnancy and low–birth-weight infants is best described by which one of the following statements?

(A) It is likely to be due to chance alone
(B) It is two times more likely to be causal than due to chance alone
(C) It is about nine times stronger than expected by chance alone

(C) It is about nine times stronger than expected by chance alone
(D) It has about a 2% probability of being due to chance alone
(E) It has a probability of less than 0.1% of being due to chance alone

5. The risk of birth weight below 2500 g among infants of women who used Nomoflab during pregnancy in this study is how many times as great as the risk among infants of women who did not consume soft drinks containing this sweetener during pregnancy?

(A) More than 1000 times as great
(B) Approximately 31 times as great
(C) Approximately 9 times as great
(D) Approximately twice as great
(E) Approximately 1/3 as great

6. Which one of the following patients, all of whom are 10 weeks' pregnant, has had an exposure that is most likely to have harmed her fetus? A woman who

(A) attempted suicide by taking 500 aspirin tablets 8 weeks into her pregnancy, who was in a coma with salicylate toxicity for 2 days and required treatment with hemodialysis, and who has now fully recovered

(B) continued taking oral contraceptive pills for 2 months after having become pregnant
(C) works in the office of a nuclear power plant that has operated normally for the past 12 years while maintaining ambient radiation levels within government safety levels
(D) injects cell cultures with isotretinoin two to three times a week in a research laboratory
(E) was hospitalized repeatedly for chronic alcoholism but has not had a drink for the past 10 months

7. None of the following women is currently pregnant, but they all wish to become pregnant within the next year or so. Which one of these women is at increased risk for having an infant with congenital anomalies? A woman who

(A) is an airline flight attendant and is concerned about cosmic ray exposure during flight
(B) works for an insurance company entering data into a video display terminal for 8 hours every day
(C) currently has rubella
(D) is just completing a course of treatment with isotretinoin
(E) has insulin-dependent diabetes mellitus, which has been well controlled for the past 5 years

DIRECTIONS: Each of the numbered items or incomplete statements in this section is negatively phrased, as indicated by a capitalized word such as NOT, LEAST, or EXCEPT. Select the ONE lettered answer or completion that is BEST in each case.

8. A substantial teratogenic risk is associated with treatment of a woman in the first trimester of pregnancy with each of the following drugs EXCEPT

(A) lithium
(B) captopril
(C) etretinate
(D) carbamazepine
(E) warfarin

9. Each of the following statements regarding the action of mutagens is true EXCEPT

(A) they may affect somatic cells
(B) they are most likely to produce a mutation between the second week and the tenth week of embryonic development
(C) they act at the level of single cells
(D) they produce genetic alterations in cells from humans as well as in cells from experimental animals
(E) they often produce cellular damage that is subsequently repaired

DIRECTIONS: The set of matching questions in this section consists of a list of four to twenty-six lettered options (some of which may be in figures) followed by several numbered items. For each numbered item, select the ONE lettered option that is most closely associated with it. To avoid spending too much time on matching sets with large numbers of options, it is generally advisable to begin each set by reading the list of options. Then, for each item in the set, try to generate the correct answer and locate it in the option list, rather than evaluating each option individually. Each lettered option may be selected once, more than once, or not at all.

Questions 10–12

Match each statement with the kind of teratology study it most closely describes.

(A) Case report
(B) Clinical series
(C) Double-blind controlled trial
(D) Cohort study
(E) Case-control study

10. Compares the frequency of maternal exposure to an agent during pregnancy between two groups of children, one of which has congenital anomalies

11. Is particularly valuable in establishing a characteristic pattern of congenital anomalies produced by maternal exposure to a particular teratogenic agent during pregnancy

12. May be useful in raising suspicion of a teratogenic effect, but associations observed are usually not causal

ANSWERS AND EXPLANATIONS

1. The answer is D [II D 5 a (1)]. Alcohol abuse is the most frequently encountered human teratogenic exposure. Chronic maternal alcohol abuse during pregnancy can cause fetal alcohol syndrome. Maternal use of marijuana, heroin, lysergic acid diethylamide (LSD), or coffee during pregnancy is not thought to increase the risk of malformations among offspring.

2. The answer is E [II A; III A, B 1–3]. Ionizing radiation and various chemicals have been shown to cause mutations in human somatic cells, and it is likely that such mutagens affect human germ cells as well, although this has not yet been formally proven. Germ line mutations have been induced in various experimental animals with mutagenic agents. Teratogens, not mutagens, produce permanent alterations of structure or function after exposure during embryonic or fetal life. New mutations, whether spontaneous or caused by environmental agents, are uncommon causes of congenital anomalies in humans. Most induced mutations are recessive, but most dominant and recessive diseases result from altered genes inherited as such from heterozygous carrier parents.

3–5. The answers are: 3-D, 4-E, 5-D [IV C 2]. In a cohort study such as this one, the population attributable risk provides an estimate of the amount by which the rate of a condition would be reduced if the exposure did not occur. In this instance, the population attributable risk is 31%, so the data are consistent with a 31% reduction in the frequency of low birth weight if none of the women drank beverages containing Nomoflab during pregnancy.

The statistical significance of an association is an expression of how likely the association is to have occurred by chance alone. In this study, the association is statistically significant at a value of $P < 0.001$, indicating that the probability is less than 1/1000 (0.1%) for the association to have occurred just by chance.

The relative risk is an expression of how much more frequently an anomaly occurs among the exposed group than among those not exposed. The observed relative risk of 2.0 indicates that low birth weight is about twice as common among the infants of women who drank Nomoflab-containing soft drinks during pregnancy as among the infants of women who did not.

The occurrence of low birth weight in 9.1% of infants of women who drank beverages containing Nomoflab during pregnancy is called the absolute risk. This figure includes infants (4.5% overall) who would have been of low birth weight even if their mothers had not consumed beverages containing the sweetener.

6. The answer is A [II C 1 6, D 3, 5 a (1), 6 a (8), d (3) (a)]. Although maternal use of aspirin in usual therapeutic doses during pregnancy is not thought to be associated with a measurable teratogenic risk, the situation is much different in the woman who attempted suicide. Because the mother suffered serious toxic effects of her aspirin overdose, there is a danger that the fetus may also have suffered toxic (or teratogenic) effects as well. As a rule, any agent that is taken by a pregnant woman in a manner and dose that is toxic to her may present a danger to her fetus.

Oral contraceptives in usual doses do not appear to present a serious teratogenic risk, even if the exposure occurred during the critical period of embryogenesis. It is unlikely that the woman who works in a nuclear power plant or the woman who works in the laboratory was exposed to a sufficient amount of the agent to raise concern, despite the fact that both radiation and isotretinoin are well-recognized human teratogens and the "exposures" occurred during the critical period of embryogenesis.

Fetal alcohol syndrome is due to maternal ingestion of large amounts of alcohol during pregnancy. The woman with chronic alcoholism did not drink during the current pregnancy so her fetus is not at risk for alcohol embryopathy.

7. The answer is E [II C 1, 3, D 1 a, 2 c, 3, 4 c, 6 a (8)]. Children of women with insulin-dependent diabetes mellitus have a twofold to threefold increased risk of congenital anomalies. Good control of diabetes in pregnancy from the time of conception is important, but it does not reduce the teratogenic risk. Although ionizing radiation is a well-recognized human teratogen, it is unlikely that either the flight attendant or the woman who works with the video display unit will encounter enough radiation in her job to be of concern. The woman who now has rubella should have recovered completely from her infection and be immune to the disease when she becomes pregnant. Similarly, the woman who is completing her course of treatment with isotretinoin now should not be at risk for teratogenic effects related to this drug in a few months, assuming that she does not take the medication again at that time.

8. The answer is B [II D 6]. Maternal treatment with captopril and other angiotensin-converting enzyme (ACE) inhibitors late in pregnancy has been associated with fetal anuria, oligohydramnios, or death. Maternal treatment with captopril in the first trimester is not thought to pose a substantial risk of damage to the embryo or fetus. Lithium, etretinate, valproic acid, and warfarin are all considered to be potentially teratogenic in humans. Maternal treatment with any of these agents in usual therapeutic doses during the first trimester of pregnancy poses a teratogenic risk to the embryo or fetus.

9. The answer is B [III A 1, 2, B 1, 3]. Mutagens are agents that can alter the DNA or chromosomes in either germ cells or somatic cells. Mutations can occur in any nucleated cell, regardless of whether the cell is contained in a conceptus, embryo, fetus, child, or adult. However, cells have efficient DNA repair mechanisms, and most mutations that occur are repaired to normal. Human cells, like experimental animal cells, are subject to the effects of mutagens in vitro. It is likely that some human congenital anomalies are a result of the action of mutagens despite the fact that this has never been clearly demonstrated in humans. Because each cell usually has its own nucleus (and thus its own set of chromosomes and genes), a mutation that occurs in one cell only affects that one cell and its descendants. Other cells in the same tissue or organ are not affected.

10–12. The answers are: 10-E, 11-B, 12-A [IV B]. Case–control studies compare the frequency of exposure to a putative teratogen during pregnancy in two groups of mothers—those whose children have a congenital anomaly and those whose children do not. Case–control studies can be used to calculate the statistical significance and to estimate the relative risk of an observed association.

Such calculations can also be made from cohort studies, in which the frequency of congenital anomalies is determined among the children of women who were exposed to a given agent during pregnancy and among the children of women who were not so exposed.

Most human teratogens have been identified by recognizing a recurrent and characteristic pattern of congenital anomalies among a series of children whose mothers were exposed to the same agent during pregnancy. Clinical series are thus an extremely important method of detecting teratogenic effects in humans, although such studies usually do not permit calculation of statistical significance or estimation of risks.

Case reports are sometimes valuable in raising suspicion of a teratogenic effect. However, the observation of a congenital anomaly in an infant whose mother was exposed to a particular agent during pregnancy is more often just coincidental. This is especially likely if the exposure or congenital anomaly or both are relatively common.

Chapter 11

Cancer and Genetics

J. M. Friedman

I. GENERAL NATURE OF NEOPLASIA

A. A **neoplasm** is abnormal tissue that grows beyond normal cellular control mechanisms. Neoplasms may involve almost any tissue in the body and may be either **benign** or **malignant,** depending on whether they possess the potential to spread to other parts of the body (i.e., to **metastasize**).

B. **Neoplasia** is the pathologic process that results in the development of neoplasms. It appears to be a **multistep process** that varies for patients with histologically similar tumors, as well as for patients with different kinds of tumors.

II. MALIGNANCY AS A PHENOTYPE

A. **Most neoplasms are of multifactorial etiology** in the sense that both inherited and noninherited factors are involved in their pathogenesis. Many of the noninherited factors are genetic, however; **somatic mutation** is a key component of the neoplastic process. In some instances, strong **environmental predispositions** to neoplasia exist; often, these act through somatic genetic mechanisms.

B. **A small percentage (5% or less) of patients with malignant neoplasms have a strong predisposition that is inherited as a simple mendelian trait.**

1. The **tumors in these patients do not differ in type or histology** from tumors that occur in most patients with neoplasms, but, in general, patients with monogenic predispositions to neoplasia are characterized by the following features.
   a. The neoplasms have an **earlier age of onset.**
   b. The neoplasms tend to be **bilateral and/or multifocal.**
   c. **Only one or a few specific types of neoplasms** occur in each mendelian condition. There are many such conditions, however, and as a group they involve many different types of tumors.
   d. In some conditions, there are **associated phenotypic abnormalities** that are characteristic of the specific mendelian trait.

2. In individuals with mendelian conditions, the **risk of developing a malignancy may be very high** (75%–100%), **but most cells of the affected types do not develop into tumors.** Thus, the **predisposition to develop neoplasia,** not the neoplasia itself, is inherited. Even in patients with strong genetic predispositions, **other events are necessary** to cause the cells to become neoplastic.

3. **Mendelian conditions that produce strong predispositions to neoplasia** are of several types:
   a. **Syndromes of multiple benign or malignant neoplasms**
      (1) Affected individuals develop increasing numbers of characteristic kinds of tumors throughout life.
      (2) These conditions are inherited as **autosomal dominant** traits.
      (3) **Examples** include:
         (a) Neurofibromatosis
         (b) Multiple endocrine neoplasia
         (c) Familial adenomatous polyposis of the colon
         (d) Li-Fraumeni syndrome

  b. Abnormalities of DNA or chromosome repair
    (1) Affected individuals exhibit abnormal DNA repair or increased frequencies of chromosome breakage.
    (2) Most of these syndromes are associated with other phenotypic abnormalities and are inherited as **autosomal recessive traits. Examples** include:
      (a) Xeroderma pigmentosum
      (b) Fanconi pancytopenia syndrome
      (c) Ataxia-telangiectasia
    (3) Hereditary nonpolyposis colon cancer (HNPCC), an autosomal dominant condition, is not associated with any other phenotypic abnormalities.
      (a) Patients with HNPCC have an **inherited defect in correction of nucleotide mismatches in DNA.**
      (b) Inherited mutations in any one of **at least four different genes** involved in the DNA mismatch repair pathway can cause HNPCC.
      (c) The risk of colon cancer in a person with an inherited mutation in one of the HNPCC genes is greatly increased. In at least some of these families, the risk of developing certain other kinds of cancer also seems to be increased.
      (d) Approximately 10% of people with colon cancer may have an inherited defect of DNA mismatch repair.
  c. Immunodeficiency syndromes
    (1) Affected patients have congenital abnormalities of immunologic function.
    (2) These syndromes are inherited as **recessive traits,** either autosomal or X-linked.
    (3) Examples include:
      (a) X-linked agammaglobulinemia
      (b) Wiskott-Aldrich syndrome
  d. Some monogenic predispositions to neoplasia do not fall into these categories. Examples include **tylosis** (keratosis palmaris et plantaris), which is associated with esophageal cancer, and α_1-**antitrypsin deficiency,** in which hepatocellular carcinoma may occur.

C. **Chromosome abnormalities and neoplasia**

  1. Some **constitutional chromosome abnormalities** are associated with an increased frequency of certain kinds of malignancy.
    a. Leukemia occurs in about 1% of patients with **Down syndrome.**
    b. Retinoblastoma develops regularly in children with **constitutional deletions of band q14.1 of chromosome 13.**
    c. Wilms tumor of the kidney often occurs in children with **constitutional deletions of band p13 of chromosome 11.**

  2. Acquired chromosome abnormalities arise in most malignant neoplasms. In these instances, the patient does not usually have a constitutional chromosome abnormality, but karyotypic changes develop during the formation of the neoplasm.
    a. Often, a neoplasm exhibits **cytogenetic changes that are characteristic of a specific tumor type.** For example, a t(8;14)(q24;q32) occurs in most cases of Burkitt's lymphoma, and a t(9;22)(q34;q11) is found in most cases of chronic myelogenous leukemia (CML). The der(22)t(9;22) of CML is sometimes called the **Philadelphia (Ph) chromosome.**
    b. Some chromosome abnormalities are associated with differences in the malignant behavior of a neoplasm. In acute myelocytic leukemia (AML), for example, the presence of t(8;21) is a good prognostic sign, whereas the presence of t(9;22) is a poor prognostic sign.
    c. Frequently, neoplasms exhibit multiple chromosome abnormalities. Some of these cytogenetic alterations are characteristic of a specific tumor type, others may be changes that occur in many different kinds of neoplasms, and still others are more or less unique to an individual patient.

    d. Cell lines exhibiting different karyotype abnormalities are often seen within a single neoplasm. Sometimes, almost every cell has a karyotype that varies from other cells studied from the same tumor.

    e. In general, however, **all of the cell lines are clonally related,** which means it is possible to trace the cytogenetic evolution of the lines back to a single abnormal progenitor.

    f. As the neoplasm progresses (i.e., becomes more malignant), **the karyotype tends to become more abnormal.** For example, AML associated with t(8;21) usually has a relatively benign course until other cytogenetic changes, such as trisomy 8, appear. Once the additional chromosome alterations are present, the disease usually behaves in a more malignant fashion.

    g. Karyotypic abnormalities may precede clinical evidence of relapse or worsening of the disease. For example, the appearance of additional changes such as trisomy 8, trisomy 19, or an isochromosome 17q in Ph chromosome-positive CML may precede the development of a blast crisis by weeks or months.

D. **Most malignant neoplasms have a clonal origin.** This means that all of the neoplastic cells derive from a **single abnormal progenitor.** In contrast, normal tissues develop from cells that are not clonally related after the first few postzygotic divisions.

    1. Cells that do not exhibit neoplastic behavior but are developmentally related to a neoplasm may share in the neoplasm's clonal origin. This indicates that an initial somatic mutation led to clonal proliferation of a cell line, but additional events were necessary to produce neoplasia.

    2. The clonal origin of malignancies is consistent with a multistep neoplastic process because multiple independent events are much more likely to occur sequentially in a single cell lineage than simultaneously in many different cells.

III. **MALIGNANCY AS A GENOTYPE.** Two main classes of genes involved in the neoplastic process are **oncogenes** and **tumor suppressor genes.**

A. **Oncogenes** are normal genes that when altered, inappropriately expressed, or overexpressed can lead to neoplasia.

    1. Oncogenes are widely **conserved in evolution.**

    2. More than 100 oncogenes have been identified as **part of the normal genome** of human cells. These normal cellular genes are called **proto-oncogenes** or *c-oncogenes* to indicate that in their normal state and under normal physiological controls, these genes do not cause tumors.

    3. Proto-oncogenes are generally thought to have **important functions in cell growth and differentiation.** Examples include the following:

        a. The *c-src* proto-oncogene codes for a cytoplasmic **protein kinase** that affects phosphorylation of certain amino acids in target proteins and thereby influences their activity.

        b. Some proto-oncogene products appear to be **growth factors and growth factor receptors** expressed in certain cell types.

            (1) The *c-erbB* proto-oncogene codes for the **epidermal growth factor receptor,** which has protein tyrosine kinase activity. Therefore, *c-erbB* can also be considered as one of the proto-oncogenes that codes for a protein kinase.

            (2) *nt-2* is a proto-oncogene related to the **fibroblast growth factor** gene.

        c. The product of the *c-jun* proto-oncogene is a **transcription factor** that regulates gene expression.

        d. The product of the *c-ras* proto-oncogene is a guanosine triphosphate (GTP)-binding protein that plays a key role in a **signal cascade** that transmits messages from cell surface receptors to the nucleus.

4. Proto-oncogenes must be **activated** to express their oncogenic potential. **Activation of a proto-oncogene can occur in a variety of ways:**
   a. **Point mutation**
      (1) The **c-ras** proto-oncogene provides the best-studied example of activation by point mutation. Transfection of some cell lines with DNA from certain mutated c-ras oncogenes transforms these lines to a neoplastic phenotype.
      (2) The **mutations** that activate ras are **highly specific,** usually involving one of only two amino acids within the ras protein.
   b. **Other structural alterations of oncogenes** can also activate their products. An example is the **t(9;22) chromosome rearrangement characteristically associated with CML** (see II C 2 a).
      (1) This translocation moves the **c-abl** proto-oncogene from chromosome 9 into a region called **bcr** on chromosome 22.
      (2) The oncogene becomes included in the bcr transcription unit, producing a **fusion protein** that has a structure substantially different from that of the normal c-abl protein.
   c. **Gene amplification**
      (1) Gene amplification **increases the number of copies of a normal proto-oncogene** within a cell.
      (2) Unique chromosome structures called **double minutes** and **homogeneously staining regions (HSRs)** may be formed in neoplastic cells that contain many copies of an oncogene.
   d. **Control of a proto-oncogene by a more active promoter** (e.g., when a retrovirus promoter is inserted near or within a proto-oncogene sequence)
   e. **Control of a proto-oncogene by an enhancer sequence**
      (1) This appears to be a mechanism associated with **chromosome translocations** characteristic of some malignancies.
      (2) An example is **Burkitt's lymphoma,** in which the **c-myc** proto-oncogene on chromosome 8 is translocated into proximity with an **immunoglobulin locus,** most often locus IgH on chromosome 14, which codes for the heavy chain of immunoglobulin.

5. **Activation of more than one oncogene is usually necessary** to change a normal cell line into one that exhibits fully neoplastic properties. This observation is in accord with the **multistep nature of the neoplasia.**

6. **An activated oncogene exhibits a dominant phenotype at the cellular level.** One copy of an activated oncogene is sufficient to produce its oncogenic effect, even in the presence of a normal, nonactivated proto-oncogene of the same type elsewhere in the cell. Tumorigenesis results from a **gain of function.**

7. **Mutated oncogenes may occur in the germ line and be transmitted from generation to generation.** When this happens, a **dominantly inherited tumor predisposition** may be produced. For example, **multiple endocrine neoplasia (MEN) type II (MEN II)** is due to germ-line transmission of an activated **c-ret** oncogene.

8. In experimental animals, the **oncogenic potential of most tumorigenic retroviruses** has been shown to be **caused by their inclusion of an activated oncogene.**
   a. Such oncogenes appear to have originated in the genome of a vertebrate host and to have been picked up by the virus during a transducing event.
   b. The structure of the viral version of the oncogene, called a **v-oncogene,** is altered from that of the host, reflecting the mechanism of origin and activation of the v-oncogene.

B. **Tumor suppressor genes** are normal genes that function to **prevent the development of neoplasia.**

1. Tumor suppressor genes are **widely conserved in evolution.**

2. **Tumor suppressor genes are defined by the effect of their absence.** Tumors tend to develop in cells in which **both normal alleles** of a tumor suppressor gene have been lost or inactivated.

    a. Tumor suppressor genes usually have a **recessive effect at the cell level.** One normal allele is sufficient to prevent the neoplastic effect, even if the second allele has been inactivated or lost. The development of neoplasia results from a **loss of function.**

    b. Loss or inactivation of a normal tumor suppressor gene may be **constitutional** (i.e., affecting every cell of the body, including the germ line) or **acquired somatically** in a single clone of cells.

3. The **Rb gene** is a good example of a tumor suppressor gene. The Rb gene product is a phosphoprotein involved in control of the cell cycle. Normal activity of the Rb gene helps prevent the development of **retinoblastoma** and other neoplasms.

    a. Retinoblastoma, which is a **malignant tumor of the retina,** develops in early childhood and is usually fatal if not treated.

        (1) The incidence of retinoblastoma is about 1/20,000 infants.

        (2) Most retinoblastomas occur sporadically, but **approximately 10%** of affected children have a parent who also had retinoblastoma. The inherited form of the disease, called **hereditary retinoblastoma,** is transmitted as an **autosomal dominant trait.**

        (3) Tumors in hereditary retinoblastoma are often **bilateral or multifocal** and exhibit an **earlier age of onset** than sporadic retinoblastomas.

    b. Retinoblastoma develops when *both* **alleles of the Rb tumor suppressor gene are lost or inactivated** in a retinoblast. Loss or inactivation of the Rb gene may be **constitutional** or acquired as a **somatic mutation.**

        (1) In **hereditary retinoblastoma,** a chromosome containing an **allele** of the Rb gene that has been **deleted or inactivated by mutation** is transmitted in typical autosomal dominant fashion. **All of the cells of the body** of a person who has inherited this abnormality begin with **only one normal copy** of the Rb gene.

            (a) Retinoblastoma develops in a person who has inherited this mutation **only if the second Rb allele is also inactivated or lost somatically in a retinoblast.**

            (b) Although the abnormal Rb phenotype (i.e., loss of tumor suppression) is **recessive at the cellular level,** the predisposition to hereditary retinoblastoma is **transmitted dominantly at the level of the whole organism.**

        (2) The Rb gene lies in band q14.1 of chromosome 13. Children with multiple congenital anomalies due to cytogenetically apparent **constitutional deletions of chromosome 13q14.1** have only one normal Rb allele in every cell of their bodies. Development of retinoblastoma occurs in these children if their remaining Rb allele is inactivated or lost somatically in a retinoblast.

        (3) In most people with **sporadic unilateral retinoblastoma, loss or inactivation of both Rb alleles occurs somatically** in the clone of cells that give rise to the tumor.

    c. Loss or inactivation of a normal Rb allele may occur by a variety of mechanisms.

        (1) Mutation producing absent or altered transcripts is a common mechanism of inactivation of the Rb allele transmitted in hereditary retinoblastoma. This is a less common mechanism of Rb allele inactivation in somatic cells.

        (2) Deletions of the Rb locus account for most other cases of hereditary retinoblastoma. Most of these deletions are submicroscopic; that is, they are not apparent on conventional cytogenetic studies.

        (3) Loss of a whole chromosome 13 is a common somatic event associated with loss of a normal Rb allele from a cell. In some cases, duplication of the other chromosome 13, which carries a deleted or inactivated Rb allele, is seen with loss of the normal chromosome 13.

        (4) Mitotic crossing over between a chromosome with a normal Rb allele and one with an inactive Rb allele can result in homozygosity for the inactivated state in one of the daughter cells, which may then go on to produce a malignant cell clone.

4. Knudson's "two-hit" hypothesis states that the development of tumors, such as retinoblastoma, requires two separate mutations: **In hereditary retinoblastoma, the first**

mutation is inherited and the second mutation is acquired somatically. In most **sporadic retinoblastomas, both mutations occur somatically.**

   a. This explains why hereditary retinoblastomas usually exhibit an earlier age of onset and bilateral or multifocal occurrence more often than sporadic retinoblastomas. The occurrence of a second mutation in a cell that already carries a first (inherited) mutation is much more likely than two independent somatic mutations in a single cell lineage.

   b. Molecular studies have proven that Knudson's hypothesis is correct for the *Rb* gene in retinoblastoma.

5. In general, **each tumor suppressor gene locus is involved in controlling the development of several different kinds of tumors.** For example, the *Rb* locus is involved in the development of at least some cases of osteosarcoma and small cell carcinoma of the lung.

6. A general method of identifying chromosome regions containing tumor suppressor genes is by observing **reduction to homozygosity** of markers in these regions within tumor cells. Reduction to homozygosity implies **loss of one chromosome or a part thereof** with elimination of one allele of a tumor suppressor gene.

   a. For example, if a patient is heterozygous for a series of markers on chromosome 17p in his normal tissues but is found to show only one allele at each of these loci in tissue from a neoplasm, reduction to homozygosity is said to have occurred.

   b. Reduction to homozygosity may result from a variety of mechanisms [see II B 3 c].

   c. This phenomenon accounts for some of the **characteristic chromosome abnormalities** associated with specific neoplasms.

   d. Observing reduction to homozygosity implies that the **retained homologous chromosome carries a tumor suppressor gene** that has been lost or inactivated either somatically or by an inherited mutation.

C. **Other genes** are also involved in the development of neoplasia.

1. The various **monogenic conditions that predispose to tumor development** suggest the nature of some of these additional genes (see II B 3), including those that control repair of DNA damage and those involved in immunologic function.

2. The *p53* gene produces a DNA binding protein that affects a variety of functions including the cell cycle, DNA synthesis, and programmed cell death. The p53 protein induces the activity of some genes and represses the activity of many others.

   a. **The *p53* gene functions as a tumor suppressor gene in normal cells.** It is lost or inactivated during the development of many different neoplasms.

   b. In some tumors, especially colon cancers, **increased amounts of p53 protein occur,** indicating that the action of this gene sometimes promotes tumor development. This is thought to represent a **dominant negative effect** (see Chapter 3 II G 2).

   c. **Constitutional mutations of *p53* occur in Li-Fraumeni syndrome,** a dominantly inherited condition that strongly predisposes to several kinds of malignancy.

   d. **Mutation or loss of the *p53* gene is the most common genetic change** that occurs in neoplasia and is seen in a wide variety of cancers, including those of the colon, breast, lung, and brain.

      (1) Similar tumors often have similar *p53* mutations, and **different tumors usually have different *p53* mutations.**

      (2) **Certain specific *p53* mutations occur in tumors associated with particular environmental exposures.** For example, a G→T point mutation at nucleotide 249 of the *p53* gene is seen in most cases of hepatocellular carcinoma associated with exposure to aflatoxin, a mutagen that is common in the diet in some parts of the world.

D. **Genes involved in the development of neoplasms in rare mendelian tumor-predisposition syndromes often are also involved in common tumors in the general population.**

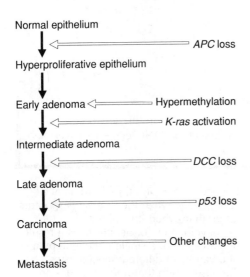

Normal epithelium

Hyperproliferative epithelium

Early adenoma

Intermediate adenoma

Late adenoma

Carcinoma

Metastasis

APC loss

Hypermethylation

K-ras activation

DCC loss

p53 loss

Other changes

FIGURE 11-1. Steps that commonly occur in the pathogenesis of carcinoma of the colon. The transition from normal colon epithelium to metastatic carcinoma is a multistep process. *K-ras* is a c-oncogene; *APC, DCC,* and *p53* are tumor suppressor genes.

1. Examples include the **Rb gene** and the **p53 gene,** as discussed previously.

2. **Mutation is a critical component of the neoplastic process.** Mendelian tumor predisposition syndromes often involve constitutional mutations of genes that more frequently affect neoplastic development through somatic mutation or acquired chromosomal abnormalities.

3. **Development of neoplasia is a multistep process.**
   a. The best example is **carcinoma of the colon,** in which several of the specific events, and the order in which they usually occur, have been determined (Figure 11-1).
   b. Although the specific steps may differ among patients with similar tumors as well as among those with different tumors, there is often **considerable overlap of the genes involved.**
   c. **Environmental factors** that predispose to the development of neoplasia may act by promoting mutation or alteration of expression of cellular genes, thereby disrupting their normal control over division and differentiation.
   d. **Environmental factors, inherited genetic factors, acquired somatic mutations, and acquired chromosome alterations all may interact** in the development of neoplasia.
   e. **Prevention** may involve intervention at any one or more of these steps.

STUDY QUESTIONS

DIRECTIONS: Each of the numbered items or incomplete statements in this section is followed by answers or by completions of the statement. Select the ONE lettered answer or completion that is BEST in each case.

1. Which one of the following features is usually exhibited by tumors occurring in patients with mendelian conditions that predispose to neoplasia?

(A) The tissues affected are rarely involved by neoplasia in patients without the mendelian disease

(B) The age of onset is later than similar tumors in other patients

(C) The tumors are of different types in various affected relatives

(D) The tumors are bilateral, multifocal, or both

2. The most common genetic change that occurs in the development of tumors is

(A) inherited activation of the *c-myc* gene

(B) activation of the *c-myc* gene by somatic mutation

(C) activation of the *c-myc* gene by chromosome rearrangement

(D) inherited inactivation or loss of the *p53* gene

(E) inactivation or loss of the *p53* gene by somatic mutation

3. Evidence that the development of malignancy is a multistep process includes

(A) the observation that certain tumor suppressor genes and oncogenes are involved in a sequential manner in the development of colon cancer

(B) the fact that *c*-oncogenes are widely conserved through evolution

(C) the occurrence of retinoblastoma at a younger age when the disease is sporadic rather than when it is inherited

(D) the development of neoplasia as a result of activation of a single oncogene by any of a variety of different mechanisms

(E) the observation that normal tissues are usually of clonal origin, whereas adjacent tumor tissue develops from multiple progenitor cells

4. Chromosome abnormalities that occur in association with cancer can best be described by which one of the following statements?

(A) They are often characteristic of a specific tumor type

(B) They usually disappear as the neoplasm becomes more malignant

(C) They usually are present in all cells of the body

(D) They often vary from cell to cell in a random fashion

(E) They usually result from clonal evolution of constitutional chromosome abnormalities

5. Hereditary nonpolyposis colon cancer (HNPCC) is an autosomal dominant condition that produces a greatly increased risk of developing malignancy. Patients with HNPCC have an inherited

(A) activated *c*-oncogene

(B) immune deficiency

(C) abnormality in metabolism of dietary carcinogens

(D) chromosome aberration

(E) defect in the correction of DNA nucleotide mismatches

DIRECTIONS: The set of matching questions in this section consists of a list of four to twenty-six lettered options (some of which may be in figures) followed by several numbered items. For each numbered item, select the ONE lettered option that is most closely associated with it. To avoid spending too much time on matching sets with large numbers of options, it is generally advisable to begin each set by reading the list of options. Then, for each item in the set, try to generate the correct answer and locate it in the option list, rather than evaluating each option individually. Each lettered option may be selected once, more than once, or not at all.

Questions 6–9

Match each of the following statements with the class of gene that it describes.

(A) Oncogenes or proto-oncogenes
(B) Tumor suppressor genes
(C) Both
(D) Neither

6. May be activated by gene amplification, translocation, or mutation

7. Loss of function promotes tumor development

8. Present in normal cells of normal people

9. Exhibits a dominant effect at the cellular level

ANSWERS AND EXPLANATIONS

1. The answer is D [II B 1]. Tumors in patients with mendelian syndromes that predispose to neoplasia are characterized by an earlier-than-usual age of onset, by multifocal or bilateral occurrence, and by involvement of only one or a few specific tissues. There are many different mendelian disorders that predispose to neoplasia, and among them are syndromes associated with the occurrence of many different kinds of tumors, including those that are most common in the general population.

2. The answer is E [III C 2 d]. Inactivation of the *p53* tumor suppressor gene by somatic mutation or loss occurs in a wide variety of malignancies, including those of the colon, breast, lung, and brain. The *p53* gene is the gene most frequently involved in the pathogenesis of cancer. Germ-line mutation of *p53* occurs in Li-Fraumeni syndrome, which is a rare dominantly inherited tumor predisposition syndrome. *C-myc* is an oncogene that is often activated by a chromosome translocation in Burkitt's lymphoma. Germ-line mutation of *c-myc* has not been recognized in association with any cancer-predisposing syndrome.

3. The answer is A [II D 2; III A 5, D 3]. The sequence of changes in the behavior of normal colonic epithelium as it progressively becomes more malignant is often accompanied by a parallel series of somatic changes in tumor suppressor genes and oncogenes (see Figure 11-1). This provides direct evidence for the multistep nature of neoplasia. Both *c-onco*genes and tumor suppressor genes are widely conserved in evolution, but this does not indicate how they are involved in the neoplastic process. Retinoblastoma occurs at a younger age in the hereditary form of the disease than in the sporadic form. This is consistent with the Knudson hypothesis that retinoblastoma is a "two-hit" phenomenon, with the first mutation being inherited in hereditary retinoblastoma but both changes being somatic in the sporadic form of the disease. Experimental studies indicate that activation of a single oncogene in normal cells is not usually sufficient to produce a fully neoplastic phenotype. The development of a fully malignant state requires more than one genetic alteration. Normal tissues are usually derived from multiple precursors, whereas neoplasms usually show clonal origin. This is compatible with the multistep nature of neoplasia, because multiple changes are more likely to occur sequentially in the descendants of a single abnormal cell than simultaneously in many cells.

4. The answer is A [II C 2]. Acquired chromosome abnormalities occur during the neoplastic process in most malignancies. Although the cytogenetic changes vary somewhat from tumor to tumor, they are often characteristic of the tumor type. In general, the karyotype of a neoplasm becomes more abnormal as its behavior becomes more malignant. Chromosome abnormalities usually arise by somatic mutation in a cell line of an individual whose constitutional karyotype is normal; cells not involved in the neoplastic clone usually have a normal karyotype. Although different cells in a tumor may exhibit different chromosome abnormalities, the changes are not random but clonally related.

5. The answer is E [II B 3 b (3)]. Hereditary nonpolyposis colon cancer (HNPCC) is caused by an inherited abnormality of DNA mismatch repair. Affected individuals do not have other phenotypic abnormalities but are at a greatly increased risk of developing colorectal cancer, and sometimes other malignancies as well. HNPCC is a relatively common disorder that may account for as many as 10%–15% of all colon cancers.

6–9. The answers are: 6-A, 7-B, 8-C, 9-A [III A, B]. Proto-oncogenes (*c*-oncogenes) can be activated by gene amplification, translocation, mutation, or other means. Once a *c*-oncogene is activated, it promotes neoplastic development even in the presence of a normal allele of the same *c*-oncogene in the same cell. Thus, oncogenes function dominantly at the cellular level.

Tumor suppressor genes must be lost, not activated, to predispose to neoplasia. This loss may occur by mutation that results in failure of transcription, translation, or function of the product; deletion; mitotic crossover; or by loss of the entire chromosome that carries the tumor suppressor gene. Both alleles of a tumor suppressor gene must be lost to promote tumor development; the presence of just one normal allele prevents this effect. Thus, tumor suppressor genes act as recessives at the cellular level.

Both proto-oncogenes and tumor suppressor genes are present in normal cells in normal individuals. Both classes of genes are thought to be important in physiological control of cell differentiation and proliferation.

Chapter 12

Developmental Genetics

J. M. Friedman
Barbara McGillivray

I. **EMBRYONIC DEVELOPMENT** is controlled by the genome. The zygote contains all of the information necessary to produce an entire organism from a single cell.

A. Although the structural changes involved in embryogenesis have been well described for many years, **little is known about the molecular processes that control human embryonic development.**

1. Considerable insight has been gained recently regarding molecular and genetic control of embryogenesis in other organisms, especially ***Drosophila melanogaster*** and ***Caenorhabditis elegans.*** Although these organisms differ greatly from humans, many fundamental genetic mechanisms underlying their embryonic development are similar.

2. Molecular and genetic understanding of embryogenesis in the **mouse,** the mammal that has been studied most extensively, is less advanced but is progressing rapidly.

3. **Current understanding of the genetic and molecular nature of human embryogenesis is largely based on analogy** to the mouse and lower organisms.

B. The **major events of early mammalian embryogenesis** include:

1. **Cell lineage specification,** which is the allocation of cells into lineages that have more restricted developmental potential

2. **Segmentation,** which is the establishment of periodic structures along the length of the embryo

3. **Regional specialization** in both segmental structures (e.g., vertebrae) and nonsegmental structures (e.g., the gastrointestinal tract)

C. **Molecular mechanisms** involved in these processes are largely unknown.

1. **Maternal gene products laid down in the cytoplasm of the ovum** *do not* **appear to be of major importance** in early mammalian embryogenesis. In invertebrates, maternal gene products are responsible for initial determinative events in the embryo.

2. **Predetermined clonal lineages** *do not* **appear to be of critical importance** in mammalian embryogenesis. In invertebrates, differentiation often occurs within specific lineages that are clonal derivatives of individual progenitor cells. Once the lineage is established, subsequent differentiation of many generations of cell progeny is largely or entirely determined.

3. In mammals, **cell fate is usually determined incrementally by a series of interactions with neighboring cells and the extracellular environment.** Although the developmental potential of an initially differentiated cell population is restricted, many alternate final fates remain possible. The ultimate differentiated state of a cell derived from this initial population depends on the **combined effect of many subsequent determinative events.**
   a. **Induction,** the process by which differentiation of one tissue is influenced by interaction with one or more other tissues, **is a central mechanism** in mammalian development.
   b. For example, a series of synergistic inductive events causes the epithelium overlying the optic vesicle to form the lens of the eye in the embryo.

4. **Once differentiation occurs, it is largely irreversible,** implying that **fixed patterns of transcription, translation, and macromolecular processing** are established.

5. **Cellular control mechanisms** important in mammalian embryogenesis include:
   a. The establishment of **morphogen gradients,** which induce qualitatively different responses of cells to different morphogen concentrations along the gradient. (A morphogen is a factor that induces the development of a particular cell type or a particular structure.)
   b. The establishment of **regulatory cascades,** in which activation or inactivation of one gene affects the function of other genes, which in turn affect the function of other genes, and so forth
   c. The remodeling of structures by means of **programmed cell death,** which is particularly important in the development of the central nervous system (CNS) and is widespread during embryogenesis

D. A few **genes and gene products** have been recognized that are **important in mammalian embryogenesis.**

1. *Hox* genes occur in clusters and are expressed along the CNS and limb buds of the embryo in temporally specific and spacially specific patterns.
   a. Certain *Hox* genes are **expressed** in the embryonic CNS **in overlapping regions extending in an anterior-to-posterior direction.**
   b. The **order of expression of the *Hox* genes along the developing neural axis is the same as the 3' to 5' order** of the genes within the cluster on the chromosome.
   c. A very similar correlation between gene order on the chromosome and spacial and temporal order of expression occurs for homologous genes in *Drosophila,* suggesting that the mechanism of anterior–posterior specification has been maintained through evolution.
   d. The order of *Hox* gene expression within the mammalian limb bud demonstrates a similar temporal and spacial order.
   e. Hox genes contain a conserved DNA sequence called a **homeobox** that codes for a **DNA-binding domain** in the corresponding proteins. Hox proteins are thought to function as transcription factors that control gene expression.

2. *Pax* genes bear some similarities to *Hox* genes. Both were originally identified through developmental mutations in *Drosophila,* both are involved in the formation of segmentation patterns in insect embryos (although in different ways), and both encode transcription factors.
   a. *Pax* genes encode proteins with a helix-turn-helix motif that acts as a **DNA binding site.**
   b. Mutations of certain human genes that encode a Pax helix-turn-helix motif produce congenital anomalies. Examples include **aniridia** (a serious eye malformation) and **Waardenburg syndrome** (a condition associated with deafness, pigmentary abnormalities, and wide-spaced eyes).

3. **Some proto-oncogenes** (see Chapter 11 III) have an important role in embryonic development. For example, the *ret* proto-oncogene is a receptor tyrosine kinase involved in transducing signals from the cell surface to the nucleus.
   a. Certain germ-line *ret* mutations cause multiple endocrine neoplasia type II and medullary carcinoma of the thyroid, which are dominantly inherited cancer syndromes (see Chapter 11 II).
   b. Other germ-line *ret* mutations cause a rare, dominantly inherited form of Hirschsprung disease, a developmental anomaly in which the large bowel does not function properly because it lacks ganglion cells.

4. The **genes for growth factors and growth factor receptors** are implicated in induction of embryonic differentiation in some vertebrate systems.

5. Genes coding for **signal transducers** such as retinoic acid **and their receptors** also appear to be involved in differentiation in some vertebrate tissues.

E. **Elucidation of additional genes and regulatory mechanisms** that are critical to mammalian embryogenesis will require a multifaceted approach. **Promising strategies** include:

1. **Identification and study of mammalian genes that are homologous to genes** with established roles in embryonic development **in other organisms**

2. **Isolation of the genes responsible for human malformations and malformation syndromes** by positional cloning and candidate gene approaches

3. **Production of developmental mutations in experimental animals by insertion of recoverable genetic elements** such as transposons into critical genes

4. Production of **transgenic animals** in which the structure or regulation of developmental genes has been altered so that expression occurs at the wrong time or in the wrong tissue or in an abnormal manner

5. Production of **"targeted knockout" animals** in which the function of a particular gene or genes has been selectively destroyed. Variations of this approach permit the knockout of a specific gene only in particular tissues or at particular times of development.

6. **Targeted ablation** experiments in which the effects of killing cells that express a specific gene are tested

7. **Characterization of genes expressed in pluripotent or differentiating cells** such as embryonic stem cell lines

8. Studies of **temporal and spacial patterns of gene expression** during embryogenesis

---

II. **SEXUAL DIFFERENTIATION.** For an infant to develop as a phenotypically and functionally normal male or female, a cascade of steps must take place. Elucidating the underlying mechanisms responsible for abnormal sexual differentiation in humans not only has aided the management of patients but also has allowed a gradual unfolding and understanding of the basic developmental pathway of sexual differentiation.

A. **Mammalian sex determination** is a model of a developmental switch; an indifferent gonad becomes a testis or ovary.

1. **Indifferent stage.** Although the chromosomal basis of sex is determined at the moment of conception, the internal structures are indifferent or bipotential until 6 weeks of development. These structures consist of the following.
   a. The **gonad** develops at 5 weeks after conception, primarily from mesonephric cells with the cortex from coelomic epithelium.
   b. **Primordial germ cells** migrate into the sexually undifferentiated gonad from the yolk sac via the mesentery by 6 weeks of development and will become either spermatogonia or ova. After settling in the gonad, the germ cells divide rapidly.
   c. **Wolffian (mesonephric) ducts** appear at 30 days of development and are paired structures.
   d. **Müllerian (paramesonephric) ducts** appear at 40–48 days of development and are also paired structures. The two pairs of ducts form the internal genitalia of the fetus. At 6 weeks of development, the structures are indifferent and are present in both male and female fetuses.

2. **The role of sex chromosomes.** The Y chromosome plays a crucial role in sex development; the embryo inheriting a Y chromosome develops as a male, whereas the embryo lacking a Y chromosome develops as a female.
   a. **Sex-determining genes** on the Y chromosome induce testicular development by an unknown mechanism. It is postulated that the Y-linked genes initiate a cascade effect of both X-linked and autosomal genes to promote the indifferent gonad to become a testis. The **SRY gene** (sex-determining region Y) is located on the short arm of the Y chromosome very near the pseudoautosomal border and codes for a highly conserved DNA binding protein. Several autosomal and one X-linked loci are also involved with testis formation.
   b. **In the absence of the SRY gene,** the gonad develops as ovaries, but two X chromosomes are necessary for maintenance of the ovary.

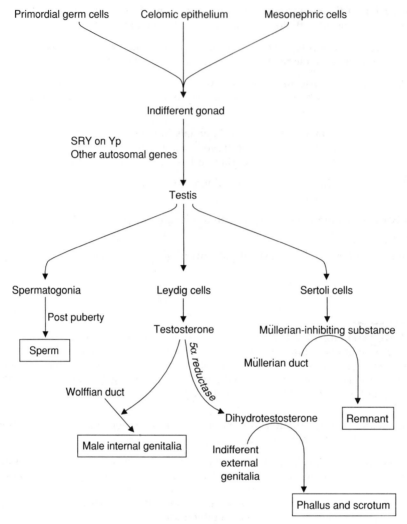

FIGURE 12-1. Differentiation of cell types involved in the development of the male genitalia. This process is influenced by the Y chromosome and begins at 6 weeks of development.

3. **Development of the early testis.** At 6 weeks of development, under the influence of the Y chromosome, the testicular cords differentiate rapidly to enclose germ cells and Leydig cells (Figure 12-1).
   a. **Sertoli cells** in the testes of the fetus produce **müllerian-inhibiting substance (MIS),** which acts locally and specifically to suppress the müllerian ducts.
   b. **Leydig cells** begin to produce testosterone by 7 weeks of development, probably under the influence of placental human chorionic gonadotropin (hCG). **Testosterone** influences the development of the wolffian duct and other sensitive structures outside the genital tract.
   c. The **germ cells** differentiate to spermatogonia, which are the stem cells of sperm production.
4. **Development of male internal and external genitalia**
   a. **Internal genitalia.** Testosterone from Leydig cells complexes with an androgen receptor and stimulates the wolffian duct to differentiate into the epididymis, the vas deferens, and seminal vesicles (male internal genitalia). This process results in the ejaculatory duct system for sperm, which is complete by 14 weeks of development.

b. External genitalia. Similar to the internal structures, the external structures are initially indifferent and consist of the urogenital tubercle, the urogenital swellings, and the urogenital folds. Testosterone is converted to dihydrotestosterone (DHT) by 5α-reductase in genital tissue. DHT acts specifically on the indifferent external structures to form the male external genitalia, which are complete by 14 weeks of development.

   (1) The **urogenital tubercle** becomes the **glans penis.**

   (2) The **urogenital swellings** fuse to become the **scrotum.**

   (3) The **urogenital folds** become the **shaft of the penis** under the influence of DHT.

5. Testosterone and DHT

   a. Testosterone initiates development of male internal structures by local diffusion and uptake by a cytosol receptor (androgen receptor). At puberty, testosterone causes changes in body hair, musculature, voice depth, and penile growth.

   b. DHT is formed from testosterone by the enzyme 5α-reductase, which is present in androgen target cells. The external genitalia and the prostate bind DHT more efficiently.

6. Development of female internal and external genitalia. In the absence of a Y chromosome or the SRY gene, testis development does not occur. The gonad becomes an ovary with epithelial cells surrounding the germ cells by 50 days of development. It is not known whether ovarian initiation is an active process.

   a. Internal genitalia. In the absence of testis-derived MIS, the müllerian duct structures continue to develop to become the fallopian tubes, the uterus, and the upper portion of the vagina. Without testosterone from Leydig cells, the wolffian duct regresses.

   b. External genitalia. In the absence of androgen, the indifferent external genitalia do not undergo fusion.

   (1) The **genital tubercle** becomes the **clitoris.**

   (2) The **urogenital swellings** become the **labia majora.** The female structures are complete by 14–16 weeks of development.

   (3) The **urogenital folds** become the **labia minora.**

B. **Abnormalities of sexual differentiation.** Development of the sexually indifferent embryo into a sexually differentiated embryo is secondary to a series of events, each of which involves a number of genes. By noting the internal and external features of syndromes with genital ambiguity or sex reversal, it is often possible to localize the nature of the problem.

1. Pure gonadal dysgenesis with sex reversal

   a. Internal features. A heterogeneous group, XY females with sex reversal may have an X-linked condition or a deletion involving the testis-determining SRY region on the short arm of the Y chromosome (Yp).

   (1) The **gonads** are streak, or rudimentary (as in Turner syndrome), because of the single X chromosome. Malignant degeneration of the gonads may occur.

   (2) Without MIS from functioning Sertoli cells, the **müllerian duct structures** develop normally into the uterus and tubes.

   (3) The **wolffian duct structures** regress without testosterone.

   b. External features. The genitalia are unambiguously female. Affected females are of normal stature but may have the shield-shaped chest and neck webbing that are typical of girls with Turner syndrome.

   c. Treatment. Gonadectomy is recommended. Replacement hormonal therapy is initiated for induction of puberty and prevention of osteoporosis.

2. Mixed gonadal dysgenesis

   a. Internal features. This condition is a variant of Turner syndrome (see Chapter 2), with mosaicism involving the Y chromosome. Most often, there are two cell lines: 46,XY and 45,X, with the proportions determining the clinical phenotype.

   b. External features. Phenotypic males may have hypospadias, dysgenetic gonads with a risk for malignancy, and the short stature and neck webbing of Turner syn-

TABLE 12-1. Types of Congenital Adrenal Hyperplasia

Form	Genitalia	Androgens	Other
21-OH deficiency	Virilized ♀	↑↑	± Salt-losing, most common
11-OH deficiency	Virilized ♀	↑↑	Hypertension
Cholesterol desmolase	Ambiguous ♂	N/A	Salt-wasting
3-β-OH steroid	Ambiguous ♂	↑↑	Lethal
17-OH deficiency	Ambiguous ♂	↓	Hypertension

Note: ↑ = increase; ↓ = decrease; ± = with or without; ♂ = male; ♀ = female.

drome. Other children may have ambiguous genitalia or a classic Turner syndrome presentation. The sex of rearing depends on the appearance of the external genitalia, particularly when there is a reasonable phallic structure.

3. **Congenital adrenal hyperplasia (adrenogenital syndrome)** includes five autosomal recessive disorders involving steroid hormone biosynthesis (Table 12-1). Several disorders can be associated with genital ambiguity, either on the basis of masculinization of a female fetus or on the basis of undermasculinization of a male fetus. The most common disorder is **21-hydroxylase deficiency,** which involves the structural gene for the adrenal cytochrome P_{450} specific for steroid 21-hydroxylation.
   a. At least three different **clinical presentations** have been associated with 21-hydroxylase deficiency:
      (1) **Salt-losing,** which can result in hypovolemia, shock, and subsequent death
      (2) **Simple-virilizing,** which leads to overgrowth and masculinization
      (3) **Late-onset,** which is rare and leads to virilization in childhood or adolescence rather than in infancy
   b. **Oversecretion of adrenal androgens,** which begins at the third month of development, masculinizes the external genitalia of female fetuses, resulting in **female pseudohermaphroditism.** The masculinization is variable, but may be severe enough to allow formation of a normal phallus. Because the gonads are normal ovaries, the internal genitalia arise normally from the müllerian duct and are female.
   c. **Diagnostic clues** include the absence of gonads in the scrotum, the presence of a uterus, elevated 17-ketosteroids (17-KS) in the urine, and a normal female karyotype.

4. **Androgen insensitivity.** The spectrum of androgen insensitivity (also called androgen-resistant syndromes) may include genital ambiguity. The androgen receptor is absent or abnormal, which results in altered binding of androgens, including both testosterone and DHT.
   a. **Clinical background**
      (1) **Complete androgen insensitivity** is associated with a normal male karyotype and unambiguous female external genitalia, whereas **incomplete androgen insensitivity** is associated with varying degrees of undermasculinization, including genital ambiguity or glandular hypospadias.
      (2) Because of the **variability of expression,** the maternal family history must be carefully evaluated, both for classic expression and for less severely affected males. About one-third of cases are sporadic, but the remainder have affected maternally related relatives.
   b. The **diagnosis** of androgen insensitivity is made by documenting a normal male karyotype and normal testicular function and by androgen-receptor studies documenting functional absence of the receptor, diminished amounts of normal receptor, or qualitatively abnormal receptor.
   c. **Genetics.** The **gene** for the androgen receptor, located at **Xq13,** has now been characterized and shows similarities with other steroid receptors (e.g., progesterone, glucocorticoid, mineralocorticoid receptors). Affected individuals may have deletions or point mutations in the gene.

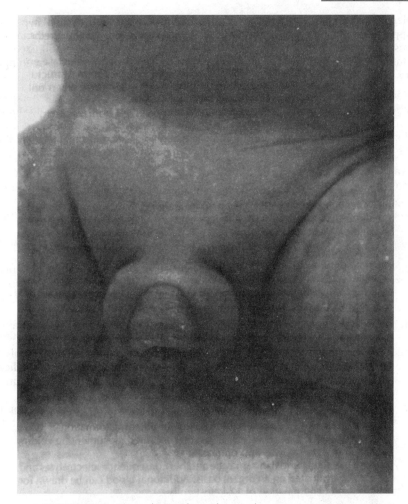

FIGURE 12-2. External genitalia with an indeterminate appearance.

    d. Treatment. The majority of those with androgen insensitivity are raised as females. Gonadectomy removes both the risk of masculinization at puberty and the risk of malignancy. Females receive replacement estrogen and progesterone therapy.

5. 5α-Reductase deficiency is also known as **pseudovaginal perineoscrotal hypospadias** because the infant usually presents with a severely hypospadic penis with the urethra opening on the perineum.

    a. Clinical background. Because of an absent or abnormal 5α-reductase enzyme, testosterone cannot be converted to DHT. The receptors of the external structures respond most efficiently to DHT and, therefore, are predominantly female when only testosterone is present. The internal genitalia will be normal male.

    b. Genetics. This syndrome is inherited as an autosomal recessive trait.

    c. Diagnosis is made by evaluating the production of DHT from testosterone in cultured genital skin fibroblasts.

    d. Treatment. If recognized early, infants can now be treated specifically with DHT, and a good response is expected.

C. **Clinical presentation.** A mental checklist is helpful when examining the external genitalia of a newborn. Genitalia with an indeterminate appearance (i.e., large clitoris, severely hypospadic penile structure, partial scrotal fusion, undescended testes) should prompt further investigation (Figure 12-2).

1. **Newborn males.** Most term male infants will have descent of testes at least into the upper scrotum at the time of birth. Bilateral cryptorchidism may be associated with hypospadias, with abnormalities of the urinary tract, or with the masculinized female infant. The phallus should measure 2.5 cm in length, with the urethral opening at the tip. The scrotum has a midline raphe and is below the penis in orientation.

2. **Newborn females.** The female infant's labia majora may not completely cover the labia minora, especially in the preterm infant. The clitoral length should not exceed 1 cm, and there should not be fusion of the labia (although some degree of posterior fusion is seen at times). The vaginal orifice should be visible and is often identified by the presence of a whitish mucus.

3. **Evaluation of the infant with ambiguous genitalia.** Affected infants may have life-threatening conditions and need assessment quickly, with a thoughtful ordering of investigations.

   a. After suspicion that an infant's genital appearance is unusual or ambiguous, the infant should be carefully examined for evidence of other malformations.

   b. The adequacy of the urinary tract must be confirmed, documenting voiding and using ultrasound or cytoscopy as appropriate.

   c. Because a metabolic imbalance may be a consequence of either congenital adrenal hyperplasia or a central cause of hypogonadism, electrolytes and blood glucose should be evaluated on an urgent basis. Blood should be drawn for chromosome studies and urine should be obtained for determination of 17-KS.

   d. The presence or absence of a uterus may help differentiate the type of abnormality.

   e. While the evaluation of the infant is underway, the pregnancy and family history can be reviewed. Important points include the use of any virilizing medications (e.g., danazol), maternal virilization during the pregnancy, previous neonatal deaths, consanguinity, or family history of similarly affected children.

   f. While assessing and coming to a diagnosis or deciding the sex of rearing in the infant with genital ambiguity, a team approach and good parental support are crucial.

STUDY QUESTIONS

DIRECTIONS: Each of the numbered items or incomplete statements in this section is followed by answers or by completions of the statement. Select the ONE lettered answer or completion that is BEST in each case.

1. Which one of the following statements best describes *Hox* genes?

(A) They lie on the chromosome in a linear order that is the same as the spacial and temporal order of expression in the embryonic central nervous system (CNS)

(B) They encode structural proteins that are essential for determining the shape of the early embryo

(C) They encode growth factor receptors that are important in embryonic development

(D) They are proto-oncogenes that are also involved in embryonic development

(E) They occur in humans but not in lower organisms, such as mice and *Drosophila*

2. Which one of the following statements most accurately describes embryonic induction?

(A) It is important in invertebrate embryogenesis but does not appear to occur in mammals

(B) It is the allocation of cells into lineages that have more restricted developmental potential

(C) It is control of early embryogenesis by maternal gene products stored in the ovum's cytoplasm

(D) It is the regulatory cascade that leads to programmed cell death

(E) It is the process by which one tissue influences the developmental fate of another tissue

DIRECTIONS: Each of the numbered items or incomplete statements in this section is negatively phrased, as indicated by a capitalized word such as NOT, LEAST, or EXCEPT. Select the ONE lettered answer or completion that is BEST in each case.

3. Genes that are important in mammalian embryogenesis include members of all of the following classes EXCEPT

(A) proto-oncogenes
(B) tumor suppressor genes
(C) growth factor genes
(D) *Hox* genes
(E) signal transduction genes

4. Each of the following mechanisms appears to be of major importance in early mammalian embryogenesis EXCEPT

(A) interactions of cells with neighboring cells and extracellular matrix

(B) morphogen gradients that induce different responses, depending on local concentration

(C) regulatory cascades in which activation or inactivation of one gene affects the function of others

(D) maternal gene products laid down in the ovum that trigger early determinative events

(E) establishment of fixed patterns of transcription

5. Androgen insensitivity could be suspected in all of the following situations EXCEPT

(A) an infant with ambiguous genitalia and no evidence of a uterus on ultrasound

(B) a phenotypic female infant

(C) the child with chromosome mosaicism (46,XY/45,X) and female genitalia

(D) a male infant with hypospadias

6. A 21-hydroxylase deficiency (congenital adrenal hyperplasia) may be associated with all of the following EXCEPT

(A) phenotypically normal male infants

(B) nondevelopment of müllerian duct structures in affected females

(C) variably masculinized female infants

(D) severe electrolyte abnormalities

(E) variable clinical expression

ANSWERS AND EXPLANATIONS

1. The answer is A [I D 1 a–e]. *Hox* genes are expressed in a fixed temporal and spacial (anteroposterior) order during embryogenesis of the central nervous system (CNS) and limb bud. This order is the same as 3′ to 5′ order of the *Hox* genes within a cluster, indicating that the control of *Hox* gene expression is probably related to chromosomal location. *Hox* genes encode a DNA binding domain and are thought to function as transcription factors. *Hox* genes are widely conserved in evolution; they were first identified in *Drosophila melanogaster*.

2. The answer is E [I B, C 1–4]. Embryonic induction, one of the most important processes in mammalian development, occurs when one tissue influences the developmental fate of another tissue. The effects of induction may vary, depending on the tissues involved and the developmental timing. In some cases, a new structure may arise; in other cases, cells with a more restricted (but not completely determined) developmental potential may result; and in still other cases, the interaction may lead to programmed cell death. Control of early embryogenesis by maternal gene products stored in the ovum's cytoplasm is important in invertebrates but appears to be less critical to mammalian development.

3. The answer is B [I D 1–5]. Tumor suppressor genes are not known to be important in mammalian embryogenesis. Several proto-oncogenes appear to be involved in embryogenesis. Growth factors and signal transducers such as retinoic acid can induce differentiation. *Hox* genes play an important role in embryonic pattern formation.

4. The answer is D [I C 1–5]. Neither maternal effect genes (which lay down products initiating differentiation in the cytoplasm of the egg) nor cell differentiation through specific

lineal antecedents appears to be crucial to mammalian embryogenesis. Cell–cell interactions, cell–environment interactions, morphogen gradients, regulatory cascades, and the establishment of fixed patterns of transcription are all critical to embryonic development in many species, including mammals.

5. The answer is C [II C 4]. Androgen insensitivity may be complete or incomplete when the androgen receptor for both testosterone or dihydrotestosterone (DHT) is completely absent, present but nonfunctional, or dysfunctional with poor activity. This leads to a variety of clinical presentations, from an undermasculinized male with hypospadias to a phenotypic female. Because the gonad has developed normally to form a testis and both testosterone and müllerian duct-inhibiting substance function normally, the müllerian duct structures never develop and a uterus is not seen. The problem is not with the chromosomal makeup of the child; one would expect 46,XY in these infants.

6. The answer is B [II C 3]. A 21-hydroxylase deficiency is associated with underproduction of cortisol, excessive androgens, and sometimes a defect in aldosterone production. This leads to variable degrees of masculinization of chromosomally female fetuses, with the most severe degree being male external genitalia with absent testes. Male infants, although phenotypically normal, may have an increase in pigmentation of the scrotum or a larger phallus, but this is generally not noticed. Diminished aldosterone production leads to salt wasting and severe electrolyte abnormalities. In female infants, the increased androgens are from the adrenal glands and occur after development of the internal genitalia from the müllerian duct. Therefore, such females will have normal development of the ovaries, uterus, and fallopian tubes and are potentially fertile females.

Chapter 13

Clinical Genetic Evaluation

J.M. Friedman
Barbara McGillivray

I. **APPROACH TO CLINICAL GENETICS.** To provide accurate information regarding the natural history and the recurrence risks of a disease to the family seeking counseling, a precise diagnosis is needed. Assessing an infant with malformations or dysmorphic features requires knowledge of the normal condition and an appreciation for the alteration of clinical presentations with maturation.

A. **Initial referrals** for evaluation and counseling are usually made by the family physician or a specialty physician. However, concerned families may self-refer, or the referral may come from a variety of other health professionals (e.g., a public health nurse) who are involved in the care of an infant with problems.

1. **Fetal abnormalities** command an urgent referral, but counseling may be hampered by limited accessibility of the fetus except through detailed ultrasound or fetal karyotyping. Components of the findings that may concern the parents include:
   a. The natural history of a particular ultrasound finding (e.g., if the problem is lethal, as is the case with renal agenesis)
   b. The extent of malformations present in the fetus
   c. Whether mental retardation may be expected

2. In a **stillborn** infant, the most serious problem in establishing a diagnosis may be the condition of the fetus and the placenta (i.e., the state of maceration, whether it is fixed in formalin, whether the placenta and membranes are available).
   a. The **autopsy findings** may determine whether the geneticist can make a diagnosis.
   b. If an autopsy is incomplete (i.e., the fetus may have been examined only externally), counseling is constrained by the available information.

3. A **dysmorphic infant or child** may be referred urgently if the anomalies are life-threatening.
   a. The **purpose of the assessment** may be to determine the course of treatment (aggressive therapy versus just providing warmth and comfort) and only later involve counseling the family. The infant may be transported away from the birth hospital, resulting in parents not being able to see the infant or meet with the physician who is caring for the infant for several days, if at all.
   b. Details of the pregnancy and family history, as well as visual comparison to the family may be lacking.

4. A **dysmorphic adult** or an **adult with a suspected genetic abnormality** may be referred for advice on reproductive options (including sterilization). Evaluation of dysmorphic features may be limited by:
   a. Lack of knowledge of the appearance of certain syndromes in the adult population
   b. Lack of information about earlier investigations
   c. Death of family members who would have been able to provide details about family history

B. **Gathering information.** A number of pieces of information are necessary to arrive at the most likely diagnosis and the recurrence risk. Families may be reluctant to divulge details of family members with problems or may not be aware of affected members in earlier generations. The stigma attached to being affected with a genetic disorder may be difficult to overcome at the time of counseling. Establishing a feeling of trust and confidentiality is crucial. All data must be recorded as completely and accurately as possible.

1. **Constructing the pedigree.** Even with the advent of sophisticated molecular analysis, the starting point of information gathering is still the pedigree, or the charting of the

family history. A pedigree is a graphic method of representing the generations of a family, with various symbols used for relationships or for particular clinical findings (Figure 13-1).

  a. Steps to taking pedigrees include the following.

   (1) Give simple instructions to the patient as to the information expected and why the information is being sought.

   (2) Use clearly defined symbols with a key for interpretation. These symbols may be used to denote different conditions found within the family (see Figure 13-1).

   (3) Identify the informant, the historian, and the date of the interview, so that the pedigree remains meaningful to others at a later date and can be amended as necessary. The pedigree is usually taken from the person who requested the counseling, but use of other family members (e.g., parents) and documentation (e.g., church records) may be appropriate as well.

   (4) Ask not only about those alive and affected in a family but also about spontaneous abortions, stillbirths, children relinquished for adoption, and deceased individuals. Such details are essential for understanding conditions that are lethal or are associated with reproductive losses.

   (5) Ask for details such as place of birth, size of towns, and the presence of consanguinity to help define recessive conditions.

  b. Analysis of the pedigree is only possible if both affected and unaffected individuals are shown. Patterns of inheritance may then be clear, and differential expression in one sex may be noted.

 2. Reviewing past records. With the modern problem of limited record storage space, crucial medical records may be destroyed after a number of years. For this reason, obtaining details of past medical information may be a challenge.

  a. After obtaining written permission from the individual (or the closest surviving relative) regarding his or her medical records, documentation may be sought from hospital medical records' departments, physicians' offices (more likely to be kept for extended periods), coroners' records, or other institutions.

  b. Often, medical information is available on biologic relatives of an adopted person from the appropriate provincial or state facility.

  c. Types of documentation that are most useful include:

   (1) Autopsy findings

   (2) Reports of surgical procedures

   (3) Discharge summaries, which should review all of the pertinent investigations from that admission

   (4) Laboratory investigations, such as chromosome studies

   (5) Family photographs, which are very helpful when trying to assess physical characteristics or judge whether another family member was affected

 3. Clinical assessment may involve multiple family members. Important findings should be documented by diagrams, clinical photographs, or videotape (if pattern of movement is a distinguishing feature).

  a. Visual assessment. Before touching the patient, observe the overall presentation (i.e., Is the individual behaving in an age-appropriate manner? Does the individual have peculiar movements, facial expressions, or limitations in movement?). All examinations should be done with the patient disrobed, although this may be done in a progressive fashion.

  b. Measurement. Standard physical measurements should be documented (e.g., head circumference, height, weight), as well as any other measurements appropriate to the situation. Measurements can then be compared to published standards for age, sex, and racial origin, if possible. Family comparisons may be valid (e.g., a child with a large head and other features may have many normal family members with macrocephaly).

  c. Extended family. If the diagnosis is unclear, examination of other affected or potentially affected family members may help. For example, if a child is suspected of having tuberous sclerosis, the family cannot be adequately counseled regarding recurrence risks unless the parents have been examined.

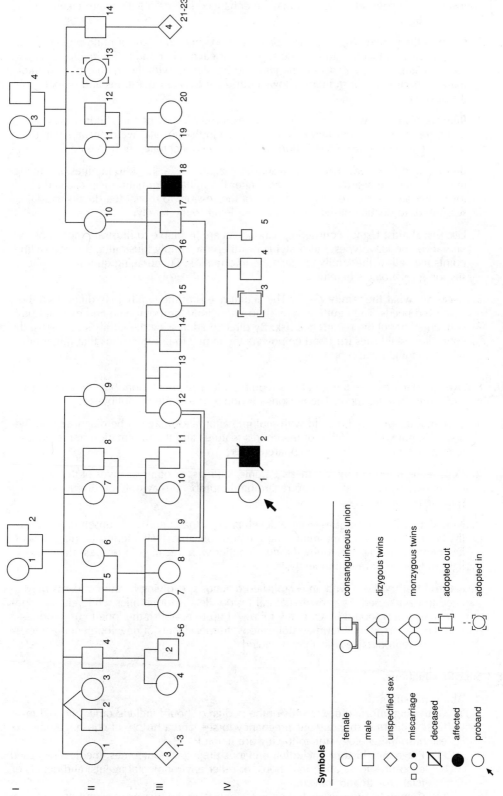

FIGURE 13-1. Sample pedigree showing a variety of symbols.

C. **Counseling.** The counseling session may be enhanced if certain actions are taken (see Chapter 15 I).

1. **Counsel the parents together.** The parents of an affected infant or child need to hear the information together to provide support for each other and to fill in gaps of knowledge. Making arrangements for the father to be present with the mother to hear information about a newborn infant allows both parents to ask questions and be part of the session.

2. **Remove distractions.** For the counseling session itself, having the children playing apart from the parents or finding a quiet space in the hospital ward ensures that the parents can be free from distractions and able to concentrate on the session.

3. **Be prepared to repeat.** Receiving a serious diagnosis is a shock to families. Realizing that little may be heard or remembered after the initial information is presented allows the counselor to review at the end of the session, to repeat the details at a later session, or to document the discussion in a letter to the family.

4. **Use visual aids.** Useful counseling handbooks are available to illustrate modes of inheritance and karyotypes, but drawing or otherwise simply illustrating the counseling points may allow the family to grasp the information. Encouraging questions as the session goes along is helpful.

5. **Ascertain what the family needs.** The actual needs of the family may differ from the perceived needs. The family may wish to know long-term outcome and may not be concerned about the recurrence risk. By directly addressing the family's concerns, the counselor establishes trust and empowers the family to ask questions that might otherwise be thought inappropriate.

D. **Follow-up.** Many counseling situations require only a single session, but some families may return for reassessment. The reasons for doing so include the following.

1. **Lack of a diagnosis.** The child with multiple anomalies may not be diagnosed on the first visit, but with evolution of the child's features and the information in the literature, a diagnosis may become apparent later.

2. **Counseling other family members.** Parents, siblings, or other relatives of the original family may be seen. Information regarding the proband may only be discussed with specific permission.

3. **New diagnostic techniques.** Future developments may improve counseling to a family. For example, when the molecular methods became available for the diagnosis of Duchenne muscular dystrophy (DMD), families were recalled to reassess their risks in light of linkage or mutation analysis.

4. **Natural history.** Even with an established diagnosis, evolving health concerns may need to be assessed. To provide natural history details for families, children with specific syndromes should be carefully followed up to establish the long-term information. Unsuspected long-term complications, further details of developmental achievements, or reproductive risks may be noted.

E. **Specific situations**

1. **Abnormal stillbirth**
   a. **Gathering information.** Details of the pedigree should include other affected infants, stillbirths, spontaneous pregnancy losses, and a history of consanguinity. To establish the etiology, the following are helpful:
      (1) **Pregnancy history,** including previous pregnancy outcomes; medications used; exposures to alcohol, infections, or other environmental agents; and details of fetal growth and movement
      (2) **Complete autopsy,** including examination of the membranes and placenta, radiologic studies of the fetus, and photographs

       (3) **Laboratory investigations** of the fetus and parents, including chromosome studies and other appropriate investigations (e.g., thalassemia evaluations when the fetus has hydrops to rule out α-thalassemia)

  b. Counseling the family. Usually, counseling after a stillbirth is an emotionally charged session because the parents are grieving, have feelings of guilt, and have feelings of anxiety regarding the outcome of future pregnancies. Returning to the hospital is stressful, and parents may view the counseling session as a necessary hurdle before planning another pregnancy.

       (1) **The literature should be reviewed** to help establish a diagnosis.

       (2) **The findings should be reviewed** with the parents, who may request a copy of the autopsy results.

       (3) **The diagnosis and recurrence risk should be explained.**

       (4) **Reproductive options** in subsequent pregnancies, including whether prenatal diagnosis would be available, should be discussed.

       (5) **The grief response should be assessed** and further supportive counseling should be offered as appropriate.

       (6) **Appropriate literature** regarding grief and pregnancy loss **should be provided.**

2. Developmental delay

  a. Gathering information. Diagnosing the child with developmental delay is often difficult because there are a number of prenatal and postnatal causes to be considered. The family may come to the session frustrated about the time taken to recognize that their child was, in fact, delayed and irritated about the limitations of service available. Alternatively, the geneticist may be the individual first confirming the clinical suspicion of delay. The initial assessment and counseling session are enhanced with:

       (1) **A careful review of the pregnancy,** with particular attention paid to drug, chemical, or infectious disease exposures. Severe bleeding may suggest loss of a twin or a placental abruption, both of which could be associated with fetal compromise. Significant prematurity implies a number of risk factors for developmental delay.

       (2) **Previous pregnancy history.** Recurrent pregnancy losses or a similarly affected child may suggest a chromosome or single gene etiology.

       (3) **Family history.** Other affected individuals, pregnancy losses, and consanguinity or incest are details that help to outline a cause for the delay.

       (4) **Results of all investigations** (e.g., developmental assessments, hearing and visual testing, laboratory testing) **or surgical procedures** should be reviewed.

       (5) **Physical examination** to observe growth (e.g., to rule out microcephaly), dysmorphic features, and abnormal movements. The physical appearance should be documented with photographs, especially if the child is likely to be seen over a period of time to establish a diagnosis.

       (6) **Further investigations.** Developmental delay in an infant may prompt evaluation of possible intrauterine infection [e.g., organism-specific immunoglobulin G (IgG) and IgM levels], metabolic abnormalities, or a chromosome abnormality. An older child, especially if male, may undergo DNA studies for fragile X syndrome. If all children of a couple are affected, either maternal phenylketonuria (PKU) or mitochondrial inheritance should be considered.

  b. Counseling. The information discussed during the counseling session varies, depending on whether a diagnosis can be made. If no diagnosis is made, the family may be seen again, but empiric recurrence risks may be valuable in the interim. If a specific diagnosis is established, the geneticist needs to consider the emotional impact on the family, as well as the future implications. With a specific diagnosis, the parents will require appropriate medical information (e.g., natural history, possible health concerns), recurrence risks for themselves and other family members, and information regarding lay support groups. Contact with another family who has a child with the same disorder may be helpful. The availability of specific prenatal diagnosis should be covered.

II. CALCULATING GENETIC RISKS

A. Inferring genotypes from phenotypes

1. **The most frequent error made in clinical genetics is providing counseling or prenatal testing on the basis of the wrong diagnosis.** A correct and precise diagnosis is essential for accurate genetic counseling or prenatal testing.

2. **The possibility of genetic heterogeneity**—the production of the same phenotype by more than one abnormal genotype—must always be considered. For example, retinitis pigmentosa may be transmitted as an autosomal recessive, autosomal dominant, or X-linked recessive trait in various families.

3. When confronted with several different phenotypic abnormalities in a patient or in a family, the possibility of **pleiotropy**—the production of multiple phenotypic abnormalities by a single gene or gene pair—must always be considered. Often, the physical abnormalities in a genetic condition are not obviously related. This is the case, for example, in:
   a. **Nail-patella syndrome** (nail dysplasia, absent patellae, nephropathy)
   b. **Myotonic dystrophy** (weakness and atrophy of distal and facial muscles, myotonia, cataracts, cardiac conduction defects, frontal balding, endocrine abnormalities)

4. When assessing a family with a genetic disease or congenital anomaly, **it is important to determine who is affected and who is not.** This is information about the **phenotype**. To calculate genetic risks, however, it is necessary to know each individual's **genotype**. In some diseases, DNA diagnosis or other kinds of testing permits direct demonstration of the genotype in family members. More often, it is necessary to infer genotype from phenotype and the family history.

5. **When inferring genotypes** within a family, **the most likely case should be assumed** unless there is good reason to do otherwise.
   a. **Individuals with autosomal dominant diseases can generally be assumed to be heterozygotes** rather than homozygotes.
      (1) Homozygotes for dominant diseases occur much less frequently than do heterozygotes (see Chapter 7 I B 5).
      (2) A homozygote for an autosomal dominant disease should be recognized by the fact that both parents are affected with the disease.
      (3) The phenotype of the homozygote for most autosomal dominant diseases is much more severely abnormal than the phenotype of the heterozygote.
   b. **Normal parents of a child with an autosomal recessive disease generally can be assumed to be heterozygous carriers of the abnormal gene.**
      (1) A parent who is homozygous for an autosomal recessive disease would be expected to exhibit the abnormal trait.
      (2) The population frequency of heterozygous carriers of autosomal recessive diseases is much greater than the frequency of new mutations for the corresponding genes (see Chapter 7 I B 6).
   c. **One of the parents of a carrier of an autosomal recessive disease generally can be assumed to be a carrier.** Although it is possible that both parents of a heterozygote are themselves carriers, this is unlikely unless there is also a homozygote among their children or there is consanguinity.
   d. In a family exhibiting an **X-linked recessive disease, a woman can be assumed to be a carrier if she has more than one affected son or if she has an affected son and other male relatives** who are related to her through their mothers.
   e. If a woman is the mother of only one boy with a serious X-linked recessive disease and there is **no history** of the condition in the family, she **may or may not be a carrier** (see Chapter 7 I B 7).

B. Linkage

1. For some **autosomal or X-linked recessive conditions** [e.g., cystic fibrosis (CF), DMD] and for **pre-symptomatic individuals with some late-onset dominant disorders** (e.g.,

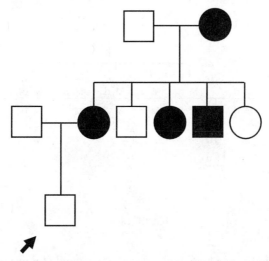

FIGURE 13-2. Pedigree of an autosomal dominant, adult-onset, degenerative neurologic disease. The proband is indicated by the *arrow*.

Huntington disease, myotonic dystrophy), direct DNA diagnosis permits unequivocal identification of carriers in most families. In some other mendelian diseases, **direct DNA diagnosis is either impossible or impractical.** In these circumstances, **linkage may be useful.**

2. **Linkage can be used to estimate the probabilities of alternative genotypes** in individual members of a family (see Chapter 5 I). For example, consider the following pedigree for an autosomal dominant, adult-onset, degenerative neurologic disease (Figure 13-2). The proband is an adult who is too young to manifest symptoms of the disease.
   a. On the basis of the information provided in the pedigree, the chance that the child has inherited the disease gene is 50%. If, however, the disease gene locus (*D*) is known to be linked to the locus for a genetic marker (*M*), such as a short tandem repeat polymorphism (STRP), the family can be typed for the marker to determine the most likely genotype of the proband at the disease locus. In this family, the typing produces the results shown in Figure 13-3.
   b. It is necessary to determine which allele of the marker locus is on the same chromosome as the abnormal allele of the disease gene. This is called assigning the

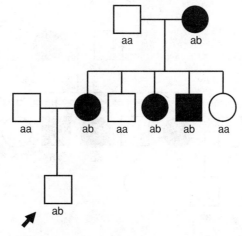

FIGURE 13-3.

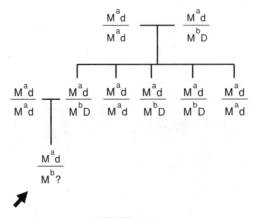

FIGURE 13-4.

phase of the linkage and can be done in this family by inspection (Figure 13-4). M^a indicates the a allele at the marker locus, M^b indicates the b allele at the marker locus, d indicates the normal allele at the disease locus, and D indicates the abnormal allele at the disease locus.

c. If it is also known that the **recombination distance** between the M locus and the D locus is 5 centimorgans (cM), then the risk of the proband having inherited the disease gene is 95%.

(1) If the chance of recombination between a particular pair of alleles at the M and D loci is 5%, then the chance that this pair of alleles will be transmitted together without recombination in meiosis is 100% − 5% = 95%.

(2) Note that when linkage is used, the **50% chance of transmission related to genetic segregation is not included in the calculation** because linkage depends on knowing which alleles went to the gamete that produced a given individual. Such information is only available *after* segregation has occurred.

(3) Also note that **the particular alleles involved at the marker locus are irrelevant** as long as the locus is informative. The allele at a marker locus found to be in coupling with a linked disease gene varies from family to family.

(a) In this example, the same information could have been obtained if the proband's unaffected maternal aunt, uncle, and grandfather had all typed M^b/M^b instead of M^a/M^a (Figure 13-5).

(b) In this case, however, the phase of the linkage would be reversed, and M^a would be on the same chromosome as the abnormal allele of the disease gene so that the affected individuals would all be M^aD/M^bd (Figure 13-6).

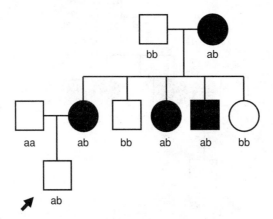

FIGURE 13-5.

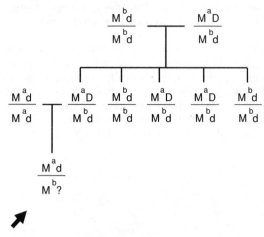

FIGURE 13-6.

(c) The proband would have a 5% chance of being affected if found to be M^a/M^b.

C. The **Bayesian method** is the use of information that alters the relative probabilities of prior events to estimate current risks.

1. The Bayesian method is used extensively throughout medicine as well as in everyday life, but its use is generally not explicit. In clinical genetics, an explicit Bayesian approach is **used to modify risk calculations.**
   a. As an **example of the everyday use of the Bayesian method,** consider a medical student who looks out of her window at 5:30 P.M. and notices that it is dark. She will interpret this observation differently depending on the time of the year.
      (1) If it is summer, she may be concerned that there is about to be a thunderstorm.
      (2) If it is winter, she will not find the darkness unusual and is unlikely to be concerned about a thunderstorm.
      (3) In both cases, the observation is the same, but the likelihood that darkness at 5:30 P.M. portends a thunderstorm is very different in the summer and winter.
   b. As an **example of intuitive but inexplicit use of the Bayesian method** in medicine, consider a laboratory report showing a very high serum potassium level.
      (1) If the patient is a healthy man who is being tested as part of a routine physical examination, it is likely that the result is erroneous, and a physician would probably just repeat the test for verification.
      (2) However, if the patient is in renal failure, the elevated potassium may be an ominous sign that hemodialysis is necessary.
      (3) Again, the observation is the same, but the interpretation is very different because of additional information.

2. **Conditions for use of the Bayesian method in calculating genetic risks**
   a. The **genotype cannot be determined with certainty** from the pedigree or by testing.
   b. **Additional information is available** that makes one interpretation of the genotype more or less likely.

3. **Explicit use of the Bayesian method in clinical genetics** is illustrated in the following sample case. Case 7 provides a more realistic example from clinical genetics.

4. **Sample case:** Use of the Bayesian method in CF
   a. **Presentation.** A 4-year-old boy has just been diagnosed as having CF, which is an autosomal recessive condition (i.e., *cc* genotype). His only sibling is a 1-year-old sister.

    b. Questions. What is the risk that the sister is a heterozygous carrier (i.e., *Cc* geno-
type) of the CF gene? What is the chance that the patient's clinically normal sister
is a carrier for CF?

    c. Discussion. The risk of the sister being a heterozygous carrier of the CF gene is
50%. After gathering more information, a Bayesian calculation is necessary, because knowing that the sister is clinically normal changes the probabilities of other
outcomes. It is not possible that the sister has the *cc* genotype, so the only possibilities remaining are that she has a genotype of *Cc* or *CC*. The final probability (*P*)
that the sister is a heterozygous carrier is the chance that she is a heterozygote divided by the sum of all of the probabilities that remain possible (*Cc* or *CC*).

$$P = \frac{\frac{1}{2}}{\frac{1}{2} + \frac{1}{4}}$$

$$P = \frac{\frac{2}{4}}{\frac{2}{4} + \frac{1}{4}}$$

$$P = \frac{\frac{2}{4}}{\frac{3}{4}}$$

$$P = \frac{2}{3}$$

STUDY QUESTIONS

DIRECTIONS: Each of the numbered items or incomplete statements in this section is followed by answers or by completions of the statement. Select the ONE lettered answer or completion that is BEST in each case.

Questions 1 and 2

Mrs. S. is 32 years old and 28 weeks pregnant. She consults a physician because her sister's son has just been found to have hemophilia B (an X-linked recessive condition). Mrs. S's pregnancy has been uncomplicated. She had an ultrasound examination last week and was told that her fetus appears normal and is a male.

On taking the family history, the physician learns that two of Mrs. S's brothers bled to death in early childhood. Further inquiry reveals that they almost certainly had hemophilia B. Mrs. S. has three normal sons and a normal daughter.

1. What is the chance that the fetus Mrs. S. is carrying has hemophilia B?

(A) 1/2
(B) 1/4
(C) 1/9
(D) 1/18
(E) 1/32

2. The family undergoes testing for linkage to DNA markers, which are informative for a short tandem repeat polymorphism (STRP) located 2 cM from the hemophilia B gene. The results of the typing for this marker are shown below.

On the basis of this additional information, what is the chance that Mrs. S's fetus has hemophilia B?

(A) 0
(B) 2%
(C) 25%
(D) 50%
(E) 98%

3. Mrs. H., a 25-year-old woman, consults a physician because she has a brother and a half-brother who are both profoundly mentally retarded. Further assessment reveals that both have severe hydrocephalus due to stenosis of the aqueduct of Sylvius. In some families, including this one, this kind of hydrocephalus is inherited as an X-linked recessive trait. DNA linkage studies are performed, and a marker 5 cM from the disease gene is found to be informative in the family. The results are shown below. (The numbers underneath the pedigree symbols indicate different alleles at the marker locus).

What is the chance that Mrs. H. is a heterozygous carrier for the X-linked hydrocephalus gene?

(A) 0
(B) 2.5%
(C) 5%
(D) 50%
(E) 95%

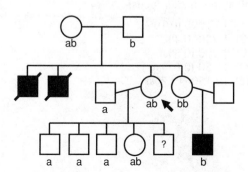

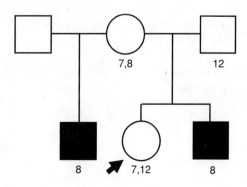

4. Measurement of the serum creatine phosphokinase (CPK) level can detect about 75% of obligate carriers of Duchenne muscular dystrophy [(DMD), an X-linked recessive disease that is lethal in males]. Ms. P., a 26-year-old woman, has a brother who died of DMD at age 18. There is no other family history of DMD. CPK testing is done on Ms. P. and is normal. If she has a son, what is the risk that he will have DMD?

(A) 1/24 (4.2%)
(B) 1/18 (5.6%)
(C) 1/10 (10%)
(D) 1/8 (12.5%)
(E) 1/4 (25%)

5. Huntington disease is an autosomal dominant condition characterized by progressive dementia and uncontrollable movements. The age of onset is variable. Approximately 10% of individuals carrying the Huntington disease gene are clinically affected by age 30, approximately 50% by age 45, approximately 80% by age 50, and almost 100% by age 70. Mr. C., the proband in the family shown below, has just had a completely normal neurologic examination. (The numbers below the pedigree symbols indicate each individual's age in years.)

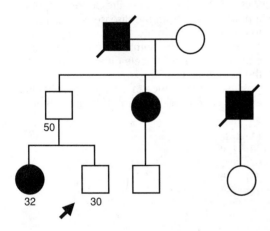

What is the chance that Mr. C. carries the gene for Huntington disease?

(A) 1/20 (5%)
(B) 9/119 (7.6%)
(C) 1/4 (25%)

(D) 9/19 (47.4%)
(E) 1/2 (50%)

Questions 6 and 7

Retinoblastoma, a malignant tumor of the eye, may be inherited as an autosomal dominant trait. Penetrance in such families is about 4/5 (80%). Ms. R's paternal grandmother, father, and brother had retinoblastoma, but Ms. R. herself is unaffected. She is 12 weeks pregnant.

6. What is the risk of retinoblastoma in Ms. R's fetus?

(A) 1/4 (25%)
(B) 1/12 (8.3%)
(C) 1/15 (6.7%)
(D) 1/20 (5%)
(E) 1/25 (4%)

7. DNA linkage studies are done on Ms. R's family. The results for a marker known to be linked to the retinoblastoma locus at a distance of 5 cM are shown below.

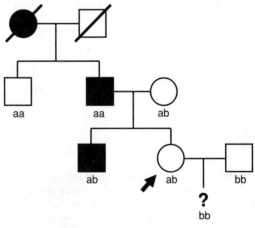

What is the risk of retinoblastoma developing in Ms. R's fetus if the fetus is shown to be *bb* at the marker locus?

(A) 19/1000 (0.19%)
(B) 1/250 (0.4%)
(C) 1/200 (0.5%)
(D) 1/150 (0.67%)
(E) 19/150 (12.7%)

ANSWERS AND EXPLANATIONS

1–2. The answers are: 1-D [II C; Case 7], **2-A** [II B 2; Case 7]. The pedigree is shown below.

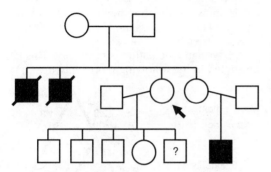

Mrs. S. has an a priori risk of 1/2 of having inherited the abnormal hemophilia B gene that is segregating in her family. However, the fact that she has had three sons, none of whom has hemophilia B, makes it less likely that she is a carrier. The only way that the fetus could have inherited the abnormal gene would have been for Mrs. S. to have inherited the abnormal gene and to have passed it on to the fetus but *not* to any of her three sons.

The other possibilities that must be considered are that Mrs. S. did not inherit the abnormal gene from her mother or that Mrs. S. did inherit the abnormal gene but did not transmit it to the fetus.

Because all three of Mrs. S's sons are unaffected, the chance that she inherited the abnormal gene and transmitted it to one, two, or all three of her sons must be excluded from the calculation.

The chance of a carrier woman transmitting an abnormal X-linked gene to her son is 1/2. If she has three sons, the chance that all three would be affected is (1/2 × 1/2 × 1/2) = 1/8.

The chance that two sons would be affected and one unaffected is 3 x (1/2 × 1/2 × 1/2) = 3/8. There are three ways this could happen: (1) The first son could be unaffected and the other two affected; (2) the second son could be unaffected and the other two affected; or (3) the third son could be unaffected and the other two affected.

The chance that two of Mrs. S's sons would be unaffected and one affected is 3 × (1/2 × 1/2 × 1/2) = 3/8. Again, there are

three ways this could happen: (1) only the first son could be affected; (2) only the second son could be affected, or (3) only the third son could be affected.

The chance that all three sons would be unaffected is (1/2 × 1/2 × 1/2) = 1/8. Only this last possibility is compatible with the information given; the others must be excluded from the calculation.

One must perform a Bayesian calculation to determine the overall risk that Mrs. S's fetus is affected with hemophilia B.

The solution can be illustrated with a probability tree.

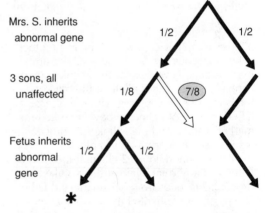

The probability that Mrs. S's male fetus has hemophilia B is

$$P = \frac{\frac{1}{2} \times \frac{1}{8} \times \frac{1}{2}}{\left(\frac{1}{2} \times \frac{1}{8} \times \frac{1}{2}\right) + \left(\frac{1}{2} \times \frac{1}{8} \times \frac{1}{2}\right) + \frac{1}{2}}$$

$$P = \frac{\frac{1}{32}}{\frac{1}{32} + \frac{1}{32} + \frac{16}{32}}$$

$$P = \frac{\frac{1}{32}}{\frac{18}{32}}$$

$$P = \frac{1}{18}$$

Mrs. S's mother is an obligate carrier for hemophilia B. Testing for the linked marker reveals that she is heterozygous *ab* at the marker locus. The *b* allele is likely to be the one that is in coupling with the hemophilia B disease allele, because Mrs. S's nephew who has hemophilia B has this marker allele.

There is almost no risk that Mrs. S's fetus will have hemophilia B. Mrs. S. must have inherited a *b* allele at the marker locus and a normal allele at the hemophilia B locus from her father. This means that she inherited the *a* allele at the marker locus from her mother. This is likely to be the allele in her mother that is in coupling with the normal allele at the hemophilia B locus. Although there was a 2% chance that Mrs. S. inherited the *a* allele at the marker locus and the hemophilia B disease allele from her mother as a result of recombination, this did not occur in this case because all three of Mrs. S's sons have the *a* allele she received from her mother, and none of them has hemophilia B. If Mrs. S. did not inherit the hemophilia B disease gene, she could not transmit it (barring a new mutation).

3. The answer is C [II B 2]. Mrs. H's mother is heterozygous for the *7* and *8* alleles at the marker locus as well as for the X-linked hydrocephalus gene. The *8* allele at the marker locus must be in coupling with the disease allele because both affected boys inherited the marker *8* allele and the X-linked hydrocephalus disease allele from their mother.

Mrs. H. inherited a *12* allele at the marker locus and a normal allele at the X-linked hydrocephalus locus from her unaffected father. She must have inherited the *7* allele at the marker locus from her mother. Since the *7* allele at the marker locus and the normal allele at the X-linked hydrocephalus locus are in coupling, and since the two loci are separated by a recombination distance of 5 cM, Mrs. H. has only a 5% chance of being a carrier of the abnormal allele for X-linked hydrocephalus. This is the chance of recombination between the marker locus and the X-linked hydrocephalus locus on the X chromosome that Mrs. H. received from her mother.

Note that the usual 50% risk of Mrs. H. transmitting the gene for X-linked hydrocephalus does *not* apply here. The use of linked markers provides information regarding how segregation actually occurred, so the 50% risk related to random segregation is no longer relevant.

4. The answer is B [II C; Ch 7 II E 2; Case 7]. Duchenne muscular dystrophy (DMD) is an

X-linked recessive disease that is genetically lethal. In this instance, the family history is negative except for Ms. P's affected brother. There is a 2/3 chance that Ms. P's mother carries the abnormal gene and a 1/3 chance that Ms. P's brother with DMD represents a new mutation. If Ms. P's mother is a carrier, there is a 1/2 chance that Ms. P. inherited the abnormal DMD gene. However, her creatine phosphokinase (CPK) test is normal, and this test is known to be abnormal in about 75% of carriers. This decreases the likelihood that Ms. P. is a carrier.

A Bayesian calculation is necessary. This is illustrated in the following probability tree.

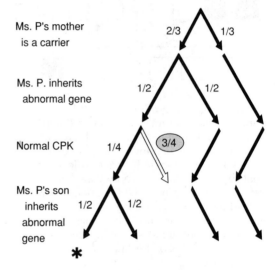

Ms. P. can only have an affected son if her mother was a carrier of the abnormal gene, Ms. P's mother transmitted the abnormal gene to Ms. P., Ms. P. is among the 25% of carriers whose CPK tests are normal, and she transmits the abnormal gene to her son.

The other possibilities that must be considered are: (1) that Ms. P's mother was not a carrier (i.e., Ms. P's affected brother represents a new mutation); (2) that Ms. P's mother was a carrier but did not transmit the abnormal gene to Ms. P.; and (3) that Ms. P's mother was a carrier and transmitted the abnormal gene to Ms. P. who has a normal CPK test, but Ms. P. does not transmit the abnormal gene to her son.

The remaining possibility, that Ms. P's mother was a carrier and transmitted the abnormal gene to Ms. P. who has an abnormal carrier test, is not applicable here and must be removed from the calculation.

The chance that Ms. P's son would have DMD is

$$P = \frac{\frac{2}{3} \times \frac{1}{2} \times \frac{1}{4} \times \frac{1}{2}}{\left(\frac{2}{3} \times \frac{1}{2} \times \frac{1}{4} \times \frac{1}{2}\right) + \left(\frac{2}{3} \times \frac{1}{2} \times \frac{1}{4} \times \frac{1}{2}\right) + \left(\frac{2}{3} \times \frac{1}{2}\right) + \frac{1}{3}}$$

$$P = \frac{\frac{2}{48}}{\frac{2}{48} + \frac{2}{48} + \frac{2}{6} + \frac{1}{3}}$$

$$P = \frac{\frac{2}{48}}{\frac{2}{48} + \frac{2}{48} + \frac{16}{48} + \frac{16}{48}}$$

$$P = \frac{\frac{2}{48}}{\frac{36}{48}}$$

$$P = \frac{2}{36} = \frac{1}{18}$$

5. The answer is D [II C 2; Case 7]. Mr. C's father must carry the abnormal gene, despite the fact that he does not yet manifest the disease, because he has an affected daughter. There is thus a 50% chance that Mr. C's father has transmitted the abnormal gene to Mr. C. The fact that Mr. C is clinically unaffected at age 30 makes it a little less likely that he carries the abnormal gene.

A Bayesian calculation is necessary to determine the risk.

This is shown in the following probability tree.

Mr. C. inherits abnormal gene from father

Clinically unaffected at age 30

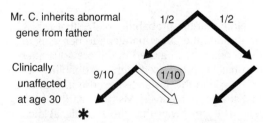

Either Mr. C. inherited the abnormal gene and does not yet express it or he did not inherit the abnormal gene. The remaining possibility, that he inherited the abnormal gene and already expresses it, did not occur and must be removed from the calculation. The chance that Mr. C carries the gene for Huntington disease but does not express it at age 30 is

$$P = \frac{\frac{1}{2} \times \frac{9}{10}}{\left(\frac{1}{2} \times \frac{9}{10}\right) + \frac{1}{2}}$$

$$P = \frac{\frac{9}{20}}{\frac{9}{20} + \frac{10}{20}}$$

$$P = \frac{\frac{9}{20}}{\frac{19}{20}}$$

$$P = \frac{9}{19}$$

6–7. The answers are: 6-C [II C; Case 7], **7-D** [II B 2, C; Case 7]. Ms. R's father carries the abnormal gene for retinoblastoma. She had a 1/2 chance of inheriting the abnormal gene from him, but she shows no evidence of it. This makes it much less likely that Ms. R carries the abnormal gene, but this possibility cannot be excluded because 20% of carriers of the retinoblastoma gene do not develop eye tumors.

The necessary Bayesian calculation is illustrated in the following probability tree.

Ms. R. inherits abnormal gene

Ms. R. is clinically unaffected

Abnormal gene transmitted to fetus

Fetus affected

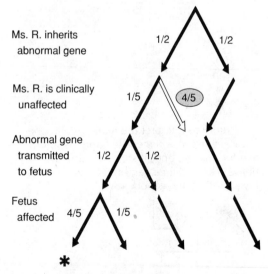

Notice that if Ms. R is a carrier of the abnormal gene, is unaffected, and transmits the abnormal gene to her fetus, there is only an 80% chance that the fetus will be affected by the disease because of incomplete penetrance. The other possibilities that must be considered are: (1) Ms. R did not inherit the abnormal gene from her father; (2) Ms. R did inherit the abnormal gene despite not showing any sign of it but did not transmit it to her fetus; and (3) Ms. R did inherit the abnormal gene despite not showing any sign of it and did transmit it to her fetus who also will not show any sign of it.

The possibility that Ms. R inherited the abnormal gene from her father and developed retinoblastoma is contrary to the information known in this family and must be excluded from the calculation.

The chance that Ms. R's fetus will develop retinoblastoma is

$$P = \frac{\frac{1}{2} \times \frac{1}{5} \times \frac{1}{2} \times \frac{4}{5}}{\left(\frac{1}{2} \times \frac{1}{5} \times \frac{1}{2} \times \frac{4}{5}\right) + \left(\frac{1}{2} \times \frac{1}{5} \times \frac{1}{2} \times \frac{1}{5}\right) + \left(\frac{1}{2} \times \frac{1}{5} \times \frac{1}{2}\right) + \frac{1}{2}}$$

$$P = \frac{\frac{4}{100}}{\frac{4}{100} + \frac{1}{100} + \frac{1}{20} + \frac{1}{2}}$$

$$P = \frac{\frac{4}{100}}{\frac{4}{100} + \frac{1}{100} + \frac{5}{100} + \frac{50}{100}}$$

$$P = \frac{\frac{4}{100}}{\frac{60}{100}}$$

$$P = \frac{4}{60} = \frac{1}{15}$$

In order to interpret the marker data, one must determine whether the family is informative for linkage, and, if so, determine the phase. The pedigree can be redrawn as follows to show the genotypes.

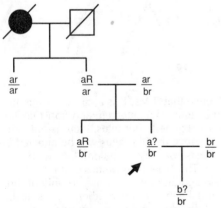

Note that the linked marker is uninformative regarding whether Ms. R inherited the abnormal gene from her father. He is homozygous for the *a* allele at the marker locus, so one cannot determine from the information provided which allele at either the marker locus or the retinoblastoma locus he transmitted to Ms. R. The fact that she does not exhibit the disease makes it more likely (but not certain) that she inherited the normal allele at the retinoblastoma locus. The linked marker is informative with respect to the fetus. Ms. R transmitted to the fetus the allele at the marker locus that she received from her mother, not the one received from Ms. R's father.

A Bayesian calculation is necessary. This is illustrated in the following probability tree.

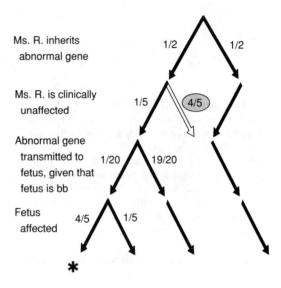

Note that the probability of 1/2 that Ms. R transmitted the abnormal gene to her fetus in the probability tree used in the previous question has been replaced with a probability of 1/20 (5%) in this instance because it is known that the fetus received Ms. R's marker *b* allele. The only way that the *b* allele at the marker locus could be associated with the abnormal allele at the retinoblastoma locus (assuming that Ms. R inherited it) would be for a recombination to have occurred. The probability of such an event is 1/20 between two loci that are 5 cM apart. The fetus would develop hereditary retinoblastoma only if Ms. R inherited her father's abnormal gene, she did not express it, she transmitted it to her fetus with the *b* allele at the marker locus by recombination, and expression occurred in the fetus.

The other possibilities that need to be considered are: (1) that Ms. R inherited the abnormal gene, she did not express it, she passed it on to her fetus with the *b* allele at the marker locus by recombination, but expression did not occur in the fetus; (2) that Ms. R inherited the abnormal gene, she did not express it, and she did not pass it on to her fetus with the *b* allele at the marker locus (i.e., no recombination occurred between the two loci); and (3) that Ms. R did not inherit the abnormal allele at the retinoblastoma locus from her father.

The remaining possibility (i.e., that Ms. R inherited the abnormal allele at the retinoblastoma locus and did express it) is contrary to the information provided in this case and must, therefore, be excluded from the calculation.

The chance that Ms. R's fetus will develop retinoblastoma, given that it has been found to be *bb* at the marker locus is

$$P = \frac{\frac{1}{2} \times \frac{1}{5} \times \frac{1}{20} \times \frac{4}{5}}{\left(\frac{1}{2} \times \frac{1}{5} \times \frac{1}{20} \times \frac{4}{5}\right) + \left(\frac{1}{2} \times \frac{1}{5} \times \frac{1}{20} \times \frac{1}{5}\right) + \left(\frac{1}{2} \times \frac{1}{5} \times \frac{19}{20}\right) + \frac{1}{2}}$$

$$P = \frac{\frac{4}{1000}}{\frac{4}{1000} + \frac{1}{1000} + \frac{95}{200} + \frac{1}{2}}$$

$$P = \frac{\frac{4}{1000}}{\frac{4}{1000} + \frac{1}{1000} + \frac{95}{1000} + \frac{500}{1000}}$$

$$P = \frac{\frac{4}{1000}}{\frac{600}{1000}}$$

$$P = \frac{4}{600} = \frac{1}{150}$$

Chapter 14

Prenatal Diagnosis

Barbara McGillivray

I. **INTRODUCTION.** Prenatal diagnosis is a rapidly developing field encompassing both screening [e.g., maternal serum α-fetoprotein (MSAFP)] and definitive testing. In Europe and North America, the development of reliable methods of contraception and the planned reduction in family size have placed a greater emphasis on an optimal outcome of each pregnancy. Also, physicians have recognized the need to assess the genetic and environmental risks facing a pregnancy and the need to be aware of available prenatal diagnostic services. Before a prenatal diagnostic technique (e.g., early amniocentesis) is offered as a service, several criteria need to be met.

A. **Safety** is related to the experience of the operator of the technique and requires the following assessments:

1. **Maternal and fetal morbidity** as compared with a similar background population

2. **Fetal loss rates,** both immediate and long-term, following the procedure, as compared with loss rates without the procedure

B. **Accuracy** requires that the operator of the technique be aware of its limitations as well as the risk of false-positive and false-negative results.

C. **Identification of at-risk populations.** Screening tests may be offered to the entire pregnant population, whereas more invasive or specific analyses are offered only to those with a defined risk factor (e.g., fetal karyotyping to pregnant women older than 35 years).

D. Ongoing **quality control** is necessary, including pregnancy outcome and development of standards for procedures and laboratories.

E. **Known diagnostic limitations.** Offering prenatal diagnosis may not always be appropriate. For example, the tissue sample may be obtained easily, but appropriate diagnostic testing on tissue may not be practical (e.g., if sequencing a very large gene in fetal DNA is the only way to make a particular diagnosis).

II. **DIAGNOSTIC TECHNIQUES**

A. **Ultrasound** was first used as a method of prenatal diagnosis in 1972 for anencephaly. Since then, many fetal structural anomalies have been diagnosed using this technique. Common uses of ultrasound in pregnancy are listed in Table 14-1.

1. Ultrasound may be used as a **screening procedure** for fetal viability, growth, and detection of fetal anomalies. The best time for screening ultrasound is between 16 and 18 weeks' gestation.

2. **Detailed ultrasound** is used when there are risks for specific anomalies.

3. The detection by ultrasound of a placental or fetal anomaly **may prompt additional studies,** including karyotyping. A number of subtle fetal features are associated with an increased risk of either chromosome abnormalities or single gene conditions (Table 14-2).

TABLE 14-1. Uses of Ultrasound in Pregnancy

Trimester	Uses
First	Dating of pregnancy
	Investigating bleeding
	Determining viability of fetus
Second	Determining presence of twins
	Determining placental position
	Screening for fetal anomalies
	Aiding procedures (e.g., chorionic villus sampling)
	Screening for suspected fetal anomalies
	Checking high-risk situations (e.g., a family history of structural abnormalities or maternal disease associated with an increased risk for fetal anomalies)
Third	Measuring interval growth
	Determining fetal size and positioning
	Screening for suspected fetal anomaly

B. **Doppler analysis** involves the generation of flow velocity waveforms with a continuous wave unit. The technique is used to evaluate blood flow in the umbilical and placental fetal circulation. Fetal cardiac pathology can be defined with Doppler analysis of fetal blood flow patterns.

1. In **normal pregnancy,** the circulation in the cord and placenta is high flow with low resistance.

2. In **growth-retarded infants,** placental blood flow may be abnormal with high resistance.

C. **Chorionic villus sampling (CVS)** is a first-trimester method of prenatal diagnosis involving either transcervical or transabdominal biopsy of the developing placenta (the chorionic villi), using a flexible catheter or needle (Figure 14-1). First developed in the 1960s, CVS was not commonly used until the availability of improved ultrasound.

1. **The chorion differentiates** into the chorion frondosum, which becomes part of the placenta and is biopsied during CVS, and the chorion laeve, which becomes part of the fetal membranes.

TABLE 14-2. Fetal Features Associated with an Increased Risk of Abnormalities

Feature	Abnormality
Large placenta	Triploidy
	Hydrops fetalis
	Thalassemia
Early growth retardation	Trisomies
	Triploidy
Abnormality of body shape	
"Lemon sign" of brain	Neural tube defect
Talipes	Neurologic problems
	Trisomies
Clefting of lip and palate	Trisomies or triploidy
Nuchal skin thickening	Turner syndrome
	Down syndrome

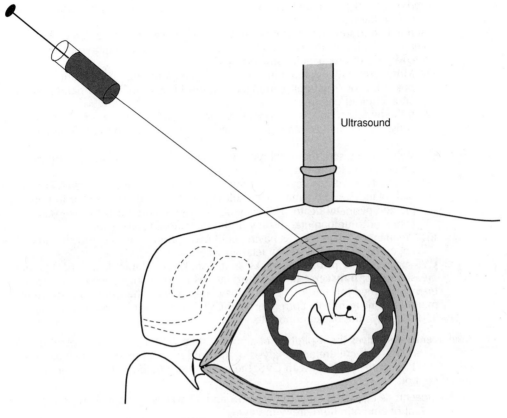

FIGURE 14-1. Chorionic villus sampling.

   a. The **frondosum** is mitotically very active. The villi are derived from three different
      cell lineages: polar trophectoderm, extraembryonic mesoderm, and primitive em-
      bryonic streak.
   b. Both the extraembryonic mesoderm and the embryo proper originate from the
      inner cell mass, but only a small number of inner cell mass cells (3–8) become
      progenitors of the embryo itself.
2. CVS is routinely done between **9 and 12 weeks'** gestation. Transabdominal placental
   biopsy is possible throughout the pregnancy and may be an alternative to amniocentesis in selected instances.
3. **Sample tissue** can be analyzed directly or cultured.
   a. **Direct analysis** or **short-term culture** involves cells from the trophectoderm
      lineage.
   b. Cells in the **long-term cultures** of chorionic villi represent the extraembryonic
      and embryonic mesoderm lineages.
4. **Results** of CVS chromosome analysis usually take 2 weeks. Biochemical or DNA
   analysis results vary and depend on whether cell culture is necessary and the complexity of the analysis. Generally, CVS tissue is preferred for molecular studies.
5. **Complications** of CVS include the following.
   a. **Bleeding.** Approximately 40% of women having CVS will experience a minor
      amount of bleeding, since the sampling is from a vascular site.
   b. **Spontaneous abortion.** A randomized Canadian trial comparing CVS with amnio-
      centesis showed no difference in loss rates. The loss rate due to spontaneous abor-
      tion is usually quoted as 1% (the background rate for spontaneous abortion at this
      stage of pregnancy is 3%–5%).
   c. **Maternal contamination.** If the villi are not carefully cleaned before being ana-

lyzed, maternal cells may be present in sufficient numbers in long-term cultures to confuse the results.

d. Confined chorionic mosaicism is defined as a dichotomy between the chromosome constitution of the placental cells and the cells of the embryo (fetus). It is reported in 2% of pregnancies studied by CVS.

   (1) Mosaicism may originate in early development through nondisjunction, anaphase lag, or structural rearrangement, resulting in both a normal diploid and an aneuploid cell line.

   (2) If the mutation occurs in trophoblast or extraembryonic mesoderm progenitor cells, the mosaicism may be confined to the placenta and not extend to the fetus.

   (3) When diagnosed, the usual recommendation is to offer amniocentesis to document normalcy of the fetal karyotype.

   (4) If the fetal chromosomes are normal, the usual pregnancy outcome is a normal infant. Some pregnancies result in growth-retarded infants or in unexplained perinatal death. This may be due to the chromosomally mosaic placenta, or to uniparental disomy in the infant (see Chapter 2).

   (5) Pregnancies diagnosed as having confined chorionic mosaicism should be followed carefully for ongoing fetal growth.

e. CVS may be done **prior to 9 weeks'** gestation, but available data indicate an increased risk of **transverse limb malformations** in pregnancies in which CVS has been performed this early. The basis may be vascular. The risk of transverse limb malformations in infants born after later CVS is thought to be no more than 1/1000 above the background rate.

D. **Amniocentesis** involves the aspiration of amniotic fluid with a fine-gauge spinal needle for amniotic fluid cell culture and analysis of the fluid for fetal markers, such as α-fetoprotein (AFP) [Figure 14-2]. As with CVS, the technique should be done under ultrasound control.

   1. Amniocentesis is usually done between **15 and 17 weeks'** gestation. Approximately 15–20 ml of amniotic fluid are withdrawn.

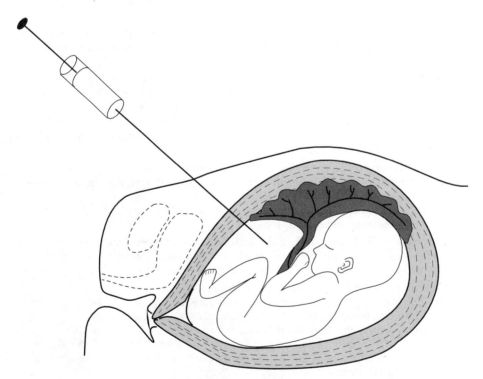

FIGURE 14-2. Amniocentesis.

2. **Results** from amniotic fluid cell culture take 2–4 weeks, depending on the culture technique used.

3. **Complications** of amniocentesis include the following.
   a. Failure to aspirate fluid may be due to a uterine contraction, which obliterates the available sampling space, or tenting of the membranes.
   b. Maternal complications include spotting or amniotic fluid leakage and are usually short-lived.
   c. The risk of fetal loss related to the procedure is 0.5% in most centers.
   d. **Fetal injury.** A potential exists to injure the fetus with the sampling needle. The risk is thought to be extremely small, especially with the use of ultrasound.

4. **Early amniocentesis** (11–14 weeks' gestation) trials are now underway. The technique is similar to routine amniocentesis but involves the removal of a smaller amount of fluid.
   a. The **major advantages** of early amniocentesis are that a procedure earlier in the pregnancy than routine amniocentesis provides earlier reassurance for most women and an opportunity for an easier and safer abortion for women who are found to have an abnormal fetus and choose pregnancy termination. Early amniocentesis allows an alternative to CVS for many women.
   b. The **risks** of the procedure appear to be no higher than those seen with routine amniocentesis, but large numbers of women have not yet been studied in controlled trials.

E. **Fetal blood sampling [percutaneous umbilical blood sampling (PUBS)]** was first developed to diagnose conditions not expressed in cells obtained by amniocentesis or CVS. As ultrasound resolution improved, the technique became more widely used as a faster method to obtain genetic information on the fetus.

1. The **technique** involves percutaneous sampling from the umbilical cord near the placental insertion under ultrasound guidance (Figure 14-3). The procedure is done from 17 weeks' gestation to near term.

2. Usually, no more than 0.5–1.0 ml of fetal blood is removed, and the sample is immediately analyzed to ensure that it is of fetal origin (maternal placental vessels are in close proximity to the sampling site).

3. **Chromosome analysis** is possible in 48 hours, so the sample is most often used for urgent fetal karyotyping. Fetal blood sampling may also be used for viral or bacterial cultures or analysis of various hematologic indices (e.g., platelet count).

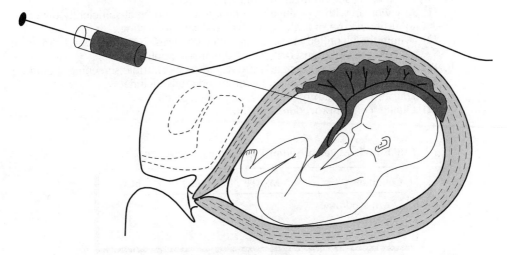

FIGURE 14-3. Fetal blood sampling [percutaneous umbilical blood sampling (PUBS)].

4. Complications of fetal blood sampling include the following.
   a. Fetal loss rates are difficult to obtain because the fetus being studied may be at increased risk for loss by virtue of the abnormalities present. However, a risk of 2% is seen with experienced centers. In pregnancies with a compromised fetus (for example, with severe growth retardation), the loss risk may be approximately 5%. Because the complications of fetal blood sampling may lead to rapid delivery of the fetus after the period of fetal viability, facilities for emergency delivery should be available.
   b. Fetal bleeding from the sampling site may continue for 1–2 minutes and is usually not a major problem.
   c. Fetal bradycardia, thought to be secondary to vascular spasm, may be documented immediately after the procedure but is usually brief.

F. **Maternal serum screening** involves the use of unique fetal markers, proteins made by the fetus during early gestation that are present in predictable levels in maternal serum throughout pregnancy.

1. AFP is the principal plasma protein in early fetal life, and is gradually replaced by albumin. Levels of AFP can be measured in fetal blood, amniotic fluid, and maternal serum.
   a. Maternal serum levels increase during pregnancy, whereas amniotic fluid levels fall. Levels, therefore, must be correlated with gestational age.
   b. Neural tube and abdominal wall defects in the fetus allow leakage of fetal serum into amniotic fluid. In the 1970s, amniotic fluid AFP measurement was introduced as a method to diagnose these conditions. Subsequently, the level of AFP was also found to be elevated in the maternal serum in most but not all cases in which there was a fetal neural tube defect.
   c. Low levels of maternal serum AFP are associated with an increased risk for Down syndrome in the fetus.

2. Unconjugated estriol (uE3) concentrations in maternal serum increase throughout pregnancy. Pregnancies with fetal Down syndrome have significantly lower uE3 levels in the second trimester.

3. Human chorionic gonadotropin (hCG) originates from the placenta, and levels decrease sharply between 10 and 20 weeks of pregnancy. Down syndrome pregnancies have higher hCG levels, and hCG levels may be the best single marker for Down syndrome.

4. Triple screening, utilizing maternal serum AFP, uE3, and hCG, is now used in many areas for risk assessment in pregnant women. Table 14-3 outlines the values seen in chromosomal abnormalities.
   a. Triple screening should meet the following **criteria.**
      (1) Any woman with a positive screening test should be at sufficiently high risk to justify the use of further invasive confirmatory testing.
      (2) Within the identified at-risk group, affected cases should be found. Arbitrarily set cutoff levels are used to define the at-risk population.
   b. Because both false-positives and false-negatives exist, triple screening should be **offered in a controlled manner.** Recommendations include:
      (1) Education of health professionals and the patient
      (2) Quality control procedures in laboratories

TABLE 14-3. Maternal Serum Triple Screening Results

Condition	MSAFP	uE3	hCG
Down syndrome	↓	↓	↑
Trisomy 18	↓	↓	↓
Turner syndrome*	↓	↓	↑

* Turner syndrome pattern of triple screen results based on limited data at present.

      (3) Adequate counseling of the patient before the screening and in the event of an abnormal result

  c. After an abnormal result, the procedure includes counseling, directed ultrasound, and amniocentesis with measurement of amniotic fluid AFP and fetal karyotyping (if the patient so chooses).

  d. Other related issues

      (1) The risks of open neural tube defects must be calculated for specific populations, because they vary racially and geographically. The incidence of neural tube defects decreases from east to west in the United States.

      (2) Other factors altering the normal levels of serum markers include maternal weight and maternal diabetes.

      (3) Screening programs generate patient-specific risk reports, which give the patient's risk before and after testing and allow both the patient and the physician a more informed decision-making process.

III. **THE COUNSELING PROCESS.** As the field of prenatal diagnosis becomes more complex, the need for a systematic approach to the care of the pregnant patient becomes increasingly necessary. Both genetic and environmental screening have now become a part of routine prenatal care. Thus, the patient who requires specific types of prenatal diagnosis can be identified and appropriately managed. Ideally, such screening should be done before the pregnancy.

A. **Parental age.** Age-related risks for chromosome anomalies should be discussed, and prenatal karyotyping by CVS or amniocentesis should be offered to women 35 years of age and older at the time of delivery (see Chapter 2 II). Paternal age older than 55 years is associated with an increased risk of dominant mutations. It may be appropriate to offer detailed ultrasound scanning to such patients.

B. **Race and ethnic background.** A particular ethnic background may indicate an increased risk for certain single gene conditions (see Chapter 3 I). Screening can be offered to the following racial groups.

  1. Ashkenazi Jewish. Test for Tay-Sachs heterozygosity with measurement of hexosaminidase A.

  2. French Canadian. Test for Tay-Sachs heterozygosity.

  3. Black. Screen for sickle-cell disease heterozygosity with hemoglobin (Hb) electrophoresis.

  4. Mediterranean. Test for β-thalassemia trait by measuring mean corpuscular volume (MCV) and by performing Hb electrophoresis.

  5. Southeast Asian, East Indian. Screen for α- and β-thalassemia by measuring MCV and complete blood count (CBC) and by performing Hb electrophoresis.

C. **Obstetric history.** Previous pregnancies may include recurrent losses, stillbirths, or livebirths with congenital abnormalities.

  1. Recurrent pregnancy losses. Consider parental translocation in cases of recurrent miscarriage.

  2. Previous congenital abnormality. After careful review of the autopsy or examination of the child, discuss the recurrence risk (if known) and the most appropriate method of prenatal diagnosis.

D. **Maternal health history.** Maternal disease may put the pregnancy at risk because of general maternal health (e.g., maternal azotemia), direct fetal effects (e.g., maternal malformation), or risk for transmission of a genetic disorder. Some **examples** of conditions to consider include:

1. **Diabetes mellitus.** Women with type I diabetes have a twofold to threefold increased risk of having a child with a major birth defect. This includes a specific risk for limb, cardiac, and neural tube defects as well as the increased risk of birth defects overall.
   a. **Poor control during very early embryogenesis** may explain some of the increased risk; therefore, optimal control of diabetes beginning before conception is important.
   b. **Prenatal diagnosis** includes ultrasound and MSAFP screening.

2. **Epilepsy.** Many commonly used anticonvulsants are associated with an increased risk of craniofacial and cardiac malformations. The mechanism is not clear, nor is the effect of the epilepsy itself. However, seizure control should be optimized with the least number of anticonvulsants, and detailed ultrasound should be offered.

3. **Maternal myotonic dystrophy.** Pregnancies in women with myotonic dystrophy, if the fetus is also affected, are complicated with polyhydramnios and difficulties with labor.
   a. In addition, affected offspring of affected mothers are more likely to have the congenital form of myotonic dystrophy.
   b. Therefore, management not only involves more frequent monitoring of the pregnancy but also may involve prenatal diagnosis.

E. **Exposure history.** The question of whether a maternal exposure increases the risk of congenital malformation must be asked in light of the already existing background risk of malformations of 3%–5%. Also, the timing of exposure and the dosage must be known. Exposures can be characterized as the following.

1. **Infections.** A number of infections put the pregnancy at increased risk for malformations [e.g., rubella, cytomegalovirus (CMV)] whereas others have a low or unknown risk. **Prenatal diagnosis** is often difficult, as documentation of the presence of the infecting organism may not give information regarding fetal effects. **Detailed ultrasound** may be appropriate as a way to assess the fetus.

2. **Medications.** After considering timing, dosage, and maternal effects, information should be sought from either written resources or teratogen information services to assess the fetal risk. **Detailed ultrasound** may be appropriate to assess particular organ systems known to be involved.

3. **Environmental hazards.** Questions regarding occupational and hobby exposures should be asked of all pregnant women. Exposures to significant radiation, organic solvents, and heavy metals may be of concern and need further assessment.

F. **Assessing the need for prenatal diagnosis.** When considering whether prenatal diagnostic techniques are appropriate for a particular patient, the physician must be aware of recognized indications for prenatal diagnosis (Table 14-4), and then decide whether the patient fits these criteria. After review of the previous and present pregnancy history, the maternal health and the family history should be considered.

1. Some of the **diagnostic modalities** are used for screening purposes, whereas others should be considered only with specific indications. Triple screening may be offered to all pregnant patients, but the results give an altered risk figure for either neural tube defects or Down syndrome, not a specific diagnosis.

2. The **decision** to have prenatal diagnosis should be made by the patient after she has heard a description of the procedures and is informed of the risks (Table 14-5) and possible complications. She should be told that prenatal diagnosis is an option and not a requirement for ongoing prenatal care.

G. **Abnormal fetus.** The most difficult situation for both the patient and the physician is the unexpected diagnosis of fetal abnormalities. The patient is referred urgently; counseling and subsequent investigations must, out of necessity, be done rapidly, and ethical concerns may arise when considering options for the remainder of the pregnancy. The sequence includes the following.

1. **Review of existing information.** This should include a history of the pregnancy to date, details of the abnormal scan or result, and any other relevant information.

TABLE 14-4. Indications for Prenatal Diagnosis

Test	Indications
Fetal karyotype	Maternal age ≥35 years at time of delivery
	Previous stillbirth or livebirth with chromosome abnormality
	Parental translocation or chromosome abnormality
	Fetal ultrasound abnormality suggestive of chromosome abnormality
	Low maternal serum α-fetoprotein (MSAFP)
Amniotic fluid or maternal serum α-fetoprotein	Previous pregnancy with neural tube defect
	Maternal diabetes mellitus
	Maternal use of sodium valproate
	Ultrasound finding suggestive of open fetal defect
Fetal blood sampling	Ultrasound abnormality suggestive of chromosome abnormality
	Hemoglobinopathies or immune deficiencies
	Diagnosis of fetal infection
Detailed ultrasound	Raised MSAFP at 16–18 weeks of gestation
	Past history of child with structural malformation
	Patient affected with, or having family history of, structural malformation
	Patient affected by medical disorder associated with increased risk for fetal structural malformation
	Environmental exposure associated with increased risk of structural malformation in fetus

TABLE 14-5. Risks of Prenatal Diagnostic Techniques

Technique	Time Performed	Risks
Ultrasound	Throughout pregnancy	None known
Chorionic villus sampling	<9 weeks	Possible transverse limb abnormalities
Chorionic villus sampling	>9 weeks	Loss risk = 1.0%
Amniocentesis	13–14 weeks	Loss risk ~ 0.5%
Amniocentesis	15–17 weeks	Loss risk = 0.5%
Fetal blood sampling	>17 weeks	Loss risk = 2.0%
Doppler	Throughout pregnancy	None known

2. **Initial counseling of the family.** The couple should be seen together, if possible. A review of the findings, possible diagnoses, and recommended further investigations should be covered. Supportive counseling and follow-up plans can be outlined.

3. **Review of pregnancy options and discussions of other services** likely to be involved in the ongoing care of the mother and infant should take place (e.g., pediatric surgery if a surgically correctable lesion has been identified).

4. **Review of pregnancy outcome.** The infant should be examined, or an autopsy should be arranged if the infant dies or the pregnancy is terminated. All findings should be reviewed with the family. Recurrence risks, if known, and information regarding prenatal diagnosis in subsequent pregnancies can be covered.

STUDY QUESTIONS

DIRECTIONS: The numbered item or incomplete statement in this section is followed by answers or by completions of the statement. Select the ONE lettered answer or completion that is BEST.

1. A couple presents for counseling during their pregnancy. The woman, who is 31, is extremely worried because her sister has just delivered a daughter with Down syndrome. The woman is now 6 weeks pregnant and wants amniocentesis. Which would be the most appropriate way to manage and counsel the family?

(A) Offer amniocentesis and schedule the procedure to be done at 15–16 weeks

(B) Offer detailed ultrasound at 8–10 weeks

(C) Ascertain chromosome results on the child affected with Down syndrome

(D) Karyotype the patient—if normal, reassure the patient; if karyotype indicates a balanced translocation, offer chorionic villus sampling (CVS) or amniocentesis

(E) Reassure the patient that no prenatal diagnosis is necessary

DIRECTIONS: Each of the numbered items or incomplete statements in this section is negatively phrased, as indicated by a capitalized word such as NOT, LEAST, or EXCEPT. Select the ONE lettered answer or completion that is BEST in each case.

2. A 32-year-old woman has blood drawn for maternal serum α-fetoprotein (MSAFP) screening. Her results indicate that she is at increased risk for a neural tube defect. All of the following actions should be taken to follow up this risk EXCEPT

(A) Check her dates

(B) Check the patient's weight; was it reported incorrectly as "kg" instead of "lbs"?

(C) Schedule a detailed ultrasound examination for assessment of fetal anatomy

(D) Arrange for fetal chromosome analysis

3. All of the following situations are indications for fetal karyotyping EXCEPT

(A) maternal age of 39 years

(B) previous child with trisomy 21

(C) a fetus shown to have a cystic hygroma on ultrasound

(D) a second cousin with spina bifida

(E) a diagnosis of a robertsonian translocation in the father

DIRECTIONS: The set of matching questions in this section consists of a list of four to twenty-six lettered options (some of which may be in figures) followed by several numbered items. For each numbered item, select the ONE lettered option that is most closely associated with it. To avoid spending too much time on matching sets with large numbers of options, it is generally advisable to begin each set by reading the list of options. Then, for each item in the set, try to generate the correct answer and locate it in the option list, rather than evaluating each option individually. Each lettered option may be selected once, more than once, or not at all.

Questions 4–8

For each case history that follows, select the most appropriate prenatal diagnostic technique.

(A) Chorionic villus sampling (CVS)
(B) Maternal serum α-fetoprotein (MSAFP) screening
(C) Amniocentesis
(D) Detailed ultrasound
(E) Fetal blood sampling

4. A 30-year-old woman with a history of a stillborn infant with normal chromosomes and multiple abnormalities, including congenital heart disease, polydactyly, and cleft palate

5. A family history of Duchenne muscular dystrophy, in which affected males have a deletion involving the dystrophin gene and the pregnant woman is a heterozygote

6. An urgent referral of a woman whose 19-week fetus was found on ultrasound to have nuchal edema and duodenal stenosis or atresia

7. A 25-year-old primigravida with an unremarkable family history but with extreme anxiety regarding her risk for Down syndrome

8. A 36-year-old healthy woman at 14 weeks' gestation

ANSWERS AND EXPLANATIONS

1. The answer is C [II F, III D 1 b]. Because the child was newly diagnosed, the chromosome results should be readily available. If the results indicate that the child has trisomy 21, there is no increased risk for the patient (or for other family members) above that associated with age. If a translocation is diagnosed, it will then be appropriate to karyotype the parents of the child. By starting with the affected child, the information is more specific for the entire family.

Detailed ultrasound at 8–10 weeks of gestation is unlikely to provide much information regarding the structural detail and would not reliably diagnose Down syndrome at any gestational age.

Because the child may have an inherited translocation as a cause for the Down syndrome, it is not appropriate to simply reassure the patient. Maternal serum α-fetoprotein (MSAFP) screening may be offered, but only after ascertaining that the woman is not at increased risk because of a translocation.

2. The answer is D [II F 1 b, 4; III D 1 b]. The normal range for maternal serum α-fetoprotein (MSAFP) varies with gestational age. If the gestational age is uncertain or incorrectly recorded in MSAFP risk calculation, the risk provided may be erroneous. If the weight given is significantly lower, (i.e., 105 lbs instead of 105 kg), the MSAFP value will be falsely elevated. If the dates are correct and therefore the results are valid, it is appropriate to schedule a level II or detailed ultrasound examination. Amniocentesis may be offered for measurement of amniotic fluid α-fetoprotein concentration, but the risk of fetal chromosome anomalies is decreased, not increased, with an elevated MSAFP.

3. The answer is D [II C 4]. Both advanced maternal age (at or older than 35 years at the due date) and a previous stillbirth or livebirth with a chromosome abnormality are indications for fetal karyotyping via either chorionic villus sampling (CVS) or amniocentesis. A cystic hygroma may be associated with a variety of chromosome abnormalities, including Turner syndrome and trisomy 21. A distant family history of spina bifida does not significantly increase the risk for neural tube defects in this pregnancy, nor does it increase the risk for chromosome abnormalities. If one parent has a translocation, there will be an increased risk for both early miscarriages and abnormal liveborn infants. A paternal robertsonian translocation is associated with a 2% risk that an ongoing pregnancy will be chromosomally abnormal.

4–8. The answers are: 4-D, 5-A, 6-E, 7-B, 8-C [II A, C, D, E, F; Table 14-4]. The woman who has a child with normal chromosomes but multiple structural abnormalities should be offered level II ultrasound, looking specifically for those malformations seen in the previous infant. Offering fetal karyotyping is not appropriate, inasmuch as the first infant did not have a chromosome abnormality.

With a family history of a genetic disorder diagnosable by molecular methods, the most efficient method of prenatal diagnosis is chorionic villus sampling (CVS). Not only is the sampling done at an earlier time, but also more tissue is available for diagnostic purposes or for faster culture.

A 19-week ultrasound abnormality requires a rapid answer to aid the parents in making a decision. In many areas, the option of pregnancy termination is available only until 20 weeks of gestation. Therefore, the most rapid method would be fetal blood sampling.

The woman with no identified risks but with anxiety could be offered maternal serum α-fetoprotein (MSAFP) screening. She should, of course, be aware of the screening nature of this test and what will happen if the result is abnormal.

The 36-year-old woman is at increased risk for chromosome aneuploidies and should be offered either CVS or amniocentesis. However, as she is already at 14 weeks' gestation, amniocentesis is more appropriate.

Chapter 15

Genetic Counseling

J. M. Friedman
Barbara McGillivray

I. **APPROACH TO GENETIC COUNSELING.** The counselor in medical genetics generally uses nondirective counseling, with the responsibility being education of the family. However, the counseling session is not merely a litany of facts (e.g., recurrence risks) but is colored with the counselor's own experiences and opinions. For the couple or the family seeking counseling, the information received may have long-term consequences and will often be used as part of the information necessary for decision-making.

A. **Indications for genetic counseling** may change with time as new methods of diagnosis become available or as specific therapies are developed. The most common indications include:

1. Advanced maternal age (prenatal diagnosis is offered to pregnant women at 35 years of age or older)

2. Known or suspected hereditary condition in the family (e.g., a malformation, mental retardation, or several relatives with a specific type of malignancy)

3. A fetus or child with birth defects, including either single or multiple malformations

4. A child with mental retardation

5. Recurrent spontaneous abortions

6. Exposure to known or suspected teratogens (in many centers, most of these referrals are handled by telephone)

7. Consanguinity

B. **Genetic counseling team.** Genetic counseling is most effectively done using a team approach to convey information to a family.

1. **The medical specialist** is often trained in a primary medical specialty (e.g., pediatrics), with additional training as a clinical geneticist. Specific medical genetics residency programs are available. The role of the medical or clinical geneticist is to establish the diagnosis and to counsel patients regarding the medical implications of the condition. In many counseling situations, the clinical geneticist plays a consultant role.

2. The **genetic counselor** may be either formally trained or experienced in the area of genetic counseling. Counselors come from a variety of backgrounds, including nursing, social work, and education. Formal training programs involve a master's degree after an undergraduate education with an emphasis on science and psychology. The role of the counselor is to be involved in the counseling process, support, and follow-up of the family.

3. **Additional members** include medical specialists consulted for specific investigations and opinions. Ongoing family support may also be given by social workers, religious support persons, and parent and lay groups. For some genetic disorders (e.g., hemophilia), counseling may be provided within disease-specific clinics by a physician or other health professional. Family physicians and primary medical specialists provide genetic counseling to patients in a number of situations.

C. **Genetic counseling facilities**

1. **Teaching or university-based tertiary care hospitals.** These centers are involved in counseling services; the education of other health professionals, fellows, and the lay public; and research into genetic conditions (clinical and basic research).

2. **Component of a specialized multidisciplinary clinic.** In such a clinic (e.g., for spina bifida), the provision of genetic counseling is part of the overall service to the family.

3. **Screening programs** (e.g., for maternal serum screening in pregnancy) provide a specific service to a large number of families. Only patients with abnormal results may be formally counseled.

4. **Outreach programs** are generally run from a tertiary care center and provide local service on an intermittent basis.

D. **The goals of genetic counseling** as defined by the American Society of Human Genetics (1975) are to help the patient or family in the following ways.

1. **Comprehending the medical facts.** After the most precise diagnosis is made, the diagnosis, prognosis, appropriate investigations needed, and ongoing management of the condition are discussed with the family. If a diagnosis is not possible, the counseling should present what is understood as well as uncertainties regarding prognosis or inheritance.

2. **Understanding the mode of inheritance and the recurrence risks.** The inheritance should be clearly explained (the use of diagrams and examples may be helpful) to the parents or to other family members. Recurrence risks may involve standard mendelian genetics, calculated risks, or risks observed in the population (empiric).
   a. The **origin of the risk** and whether it pertains to a specific diagnosis (e.g., cystic fibrosis) or to a nonspecific diagnosis (e.g., nonspecific mental retardation) should be made clear.
   b. **Couples may appreciate risks in different ways.**
      (1) **Binary.** Two states are seen: The condition will or will not happen again.
      (2) **Comparison of losses and gains.** The condition is analyzed according to whether there are positive or negative aspects to a recurrence; the balance may determine the decision to have another pregnancy.
      (3) **Numerical risk** is expressed either as a percentage (e.g., 50%) or as a fraction (e.g., $\frac{1}{2}$). The percentage may be perceived as being a larger risk than the equivalent fraction, perhaps because the numerator is a number greater than 1.

3. **Understanding the options.** When faced with a distinct recurrence risk, the reproductive options for the couple may include methods of contraception, adoption, insemination by donor sperm, use of donated ova, prenatal diagnosis with or without termination of the affected fetus, and an unmonitored pregnancy.

4. **Choosing a course of action.** The couple is encouraged to choose the best course for themselves in light of the recurrence risk, the perceived burden (i.e., psychological, social, economic), the goals of the family, and their religious and ethical standards.

5. **Adjusting to the condition.** The role of the counselor is to assess the family's reaction to the diagnosis and recurrence risk. Follow-up counseling, by either the medical genetics team or a psychologist, may be indicated to help the family deal with the condition affectively.

E. **Counseling process.** To achieve the goals of genetic counseling, the family must be able to receive the information presented and convert the facts into a part of their decision-making. The counseling team (i.e., the medical geneticist and the genetic counselor) interacts with the family most effectively by:

1. **Having information required for counseling at hand.** This may require documenting the family history, collecting records, and examining individuals.

2. **Recognizing the psychological and emotional burdens** associated with the diagnosis. Families may experience guilt and shame after the diagnosis of a genetic condition in a family member. Either situation can result in a patient who does not keep the counseling appointment, who is angry or belligerent, or who initiates a legal action.
   a. **Guilt** is a type of self-reproach to violations of inner standards. The guilty feelings may be masked by expression of "bad behaviors" (e.g., drug or alcohol abuse), by

intellectualizing the problem (e.g., the patient who converses in an abstract way about the condition), or by separating the feelings of guilt from other emotions.

(1) **Realistic guilt feelings** may exist, for example, when a woman chooses not to have prenatal diagnosis and delivers an infant with Down syndrome.

(2) **Unrealistic guilt feelings** are seen when the individual feels responsible for factors over which he or she has no control.

b. **Shame** is a response to anticipated or actual external disapproval or a response to a failure to reach certain goals and standards. Shame may be masked by denial, relabeling the losses as gains (e.g., "We were chosen to have this child because of our strength"), or by finding fault with others.

2. **Recognizing factors that affect counseling**
a. **North American society is not homogeneous;** families come from a variety of ethnic backgrounds. The importance of the extended family's involvement in the decision-making process of a young immigrant couple may demand that counseling sessions involve all appropriate family members.
b. **Socioeconomic status** influences a family's access to medical services and their understanding of the information presented.

3. **Providing nondirective counseling.** The family needs support for its decision and full disclosure of options, but not paternalistic counseling. A useful method involves using the example of other families but attaching no increased value to a particular option (e.g., "Some families choose prenatal diagnosis, whereas others feel that insemination by donor is the method for them").

4. **Helping the family relieve feelings of shame and guilt**
a. The counselor may become a figure of authority, especially early in the process of diagnosis, by stating that a particular condition "is not their fault." Later, the family member may remember this reassurance with comfort.
b. Directly addressing feelings and normalizing them by comparing the family positively to others in a similar situation may help.
c. The parents' sense of responsibility for a child's problem may be reframed as, "It's normal to feel responsible and to worry and care about the child," without placing blame for the problem itself.
d. Helping the parents to define which aspects of their child's condition they can control and which aspects are beyond their control gives them a way to feel more positive.
e. Recognizing the need for respite and encouraging such relief can enable a family to deal better with the situation.

5. **Helping the family identify its personal goals.** Asking the family its expectations of the counseling session helps to set the agenda and allows the counselor to address additional issues. Families may not understand the purpose of counseling and may feel responsible for "causing" the condition.
a. Goals are often time-related, with an early goal being to understand the medical implications and a later goal to decide on another pregnancy.
b. In this way, the family is helped to formulate the task before them, given the pertinent information and support, and then given the freedom to choose for themselves.

6. **Recognizing counselor biases.** It may be disappointing or frustrating that a family makes choices against the advice of the counselor. One way to ensure that a couple decides for themselves is to explore their opinions regarding the issues in a nonjudgmental manner. The counselor may list options regarding prenatal diagnosis in a pregnancy in no particular order and emphasize that different families choose different options.

7. **Follow-up of genetic counseling.** It is unlikely that a family will clearly understand and be able to use all of the information presented in a counseling situation. Anxiety, grief, and fear may interfere with the process of information exchange. A review counseling session, follow-up telephone call, or a review letter to the family may be helpful. Pamphlets and brochures regarding the specific diagnosis or introduction to sup-

port groups provides additional information that may be read or discussed after the session. The additional contact also reinforces the clinic's interest in the family's well-being.

F. **Problems in counseling**

1. **Genetic heterogeneity** often complicates the establishment of a precise diagnosis. Similar disorders caused by mutations at different loci or involving different alleles may have different forms of inheritance. For example, retinitis pigmentosa may be inherited as an autosomal recessive or dominant condition, as well as an X-linked condition.

2. **Phenocopies mimic genetic disorders,** are caused by environmental factors, and are, therefore, unlikely to recur. Microcephaly may have both genetic and nongenetic causes.

3. **The sporadic case is common in nuclear families.** Here, the pedigree is not helpful, and the counselor must depend on an accurate diagnosis. The advent of molecular methods of diagnosis has helped in some areas [e.g., **Duchenne muscular dystrophy** (DMD) with an identified deletion] to define a recurrence risk for the family.

4. **Nonpaternity or questioned paternity** may invalidate the risks quoted in a counseling session. Interpretation of molecular analysis is dependent upon known paternity, with the use of both direct and indirect methods (see Chapter 6). The inadvertent discovery of nonpaternity during the course of such testing creates ethical concerns regarding whether to disclose the fact.

II. GENETIC SCREENING

A. **Definition.** Genetic screening is the identification of a genetic disease, a genetic predisposition to a disease, or a genotype in an individual that increases the risk of having a child with a genetic disease.

1. **The purpose of identifying individuals with a genetic disease** is usually to **permit management** of the disease or the complications of the disease in a more effective manner than would otherwise be possible. Examples include:
   a. **Screening for phenylketonuria (PKU)** in newborn infants. Recognition of affected infants within the first few weeks of life permits institution of dietary treatment that is effective in preventing the severe mental retardation that develops in untreated PKU patients.
   b. **Serum triple marker screening** of pregnant women for Down syndrome fetuses (see Chapter 14 II F 4). In this case, no effective treatment of the fetal condition is possible. Subsequent amniocentesis that shows a woman is carrying an affected fetus gives the woman the option of terminating the pregnancy or continuing it to term and preparing for the birth of an abnormal child.

2. **The purpose of identifying individuals at increased risk of having children with a serious genetic disease** is to permit them to take advantage of reproductive options that may prevent the birth of affected children. Examples include:
   a. Detection of heterozygous carriers for **Tay-Sachs disease** among Ashkenazi Jewish populations (see Chapter 8 II B 2 c)
      (1) Identification of couples in which both partners are heterozygous carriers of Tay-Sachs disease permits them to avoid having affected children.
      (2) Such couples may choose to do so by not having children of their own, by having children via artificial insemination from an unrelated donor, or by using prenatal diagnosis with abortion of affected pregnancies.
   b. Use of DNA testing to identify women who carry the gene for DMD within the family of an affected boy provides another example (see Chapter 6 II A 3 a). Recognition of women who are carriers permits them to avoid having sons with this disease.

TABLE 15–1. Population Screening for Genetic Diseases and Carrier States

Individuals with Genetic Disease
  Newborns
    Congenital hypothyroidism*
    Galactosemia
    Phenylketonuria
    Sickle cell disease
  Fetuses
    Down syndrome
    Neural tube defects
    Trisomy 18
  Heterozygous Carriers (in High-Risk Populations)
    Sickle cell disease (African-Americans and Africans)
    Tay-Sachs disease (Ashkenazi Jews)
    α-thalassemia (Chinese, Southeast Asians)
    β-thalassemia (Greeks, Italians)

* Usually sporadic, only occasionally genetic

3. **The purpose of identifying individuals with a genetic predisposition to a disease** is to enable them either to institute measures that will prevent or delay development of the disease or to deal with the disease more effectively if it does develop. This kind of screening, which is called **predictive testing,** is discussed in Chapter 9 IV E.

B. **Criteria for screening.** There are thousands of genetic diseases, but screening is used routinely for only a few. The most frequent examples are given in Table 15–1. Genetic screening is usually undertaken only when certain conditions relating to the disease, the screening test, and the system for implementing them are met.

1. **Characteristics of the disease**
   a. The disease should be **relatively frequent** within the population screened. The more frequent the disease, the more effective will be the screening program.
      (1) Some conditions are sufficiently common in the general population to warrant screening in everyone. This is called **population screening.**
      (2) Other diseases are not common enough to justify screening the entire population but are sufficiently frequent within an **easily identifiable subgroup.** Examples include Tay-Sachs disease among Ashkenazi Jews, sickle-cell disease among African-Americans, and α-thalassemia among Southeast Asians (see Chapter 4 III).
      (3) In many uncommon diseases, genetic screening can be justified only **within families in which an affected individual has been born.** DMD is such a condition.
   b. **The disease must produce severe impairment or death.** Screening for a trivial genetic condition such as postminimal polydactyly, which produces a tiny extra digit, could not be justified because it can be safely and inexpensively treated and produces no long-term morbidity.
   c. **Some beneficial intervention must be possible** if the condition is recognized. This intervention is usually an effective treatment or prevention strategy.

2. **Characteristics of the test.** An appropriate test must exist that is capable of identifying people who have the relevant condition. Appropriate tests should be **highly sensitive and specific, have a reasonably high positive predictive value, and be relatively inexpensive** to perform.
   a. **Sensitivity** is defined as the **proportion of individuals affected by the disease** or genotype in question **who have a positive test.**
      (1) **False-negative results** are produced when individuals who have the disease or genotype have a negative test.
      (2) A good test will have a **very low frequency of false-negatives.**

   b. **Specificity** is defined as the **proportion of those who are not affected** with the disease or genotype in question **who have a negative test.**
      (1) **False-positive results** are produced when individuals who do not have the disease or genotype have a positive test.
      (2) A good test will produce **few false-positives.**
   c. **Sensitivity and specificity usually bear a reciprocal relationship to each other.** When one is increased, the other decreases, and vice versa. Thus, setting cutoff levels for a screening test usually involves finding an **appropriate balance between sensitivity and specificity.**
   d. **Positive predictive value** is the proportion of persons with a positive test who actually have the disease or genotype being tested for. The higher the positive predictive value, the lower the proportion of false-positives.
   e. **Expense**
      (1) Tests applied to large populations are usually much less expensive to perform if **automation** is possible.
      (2) Economy can often be achieved by **combining more than one screening test.** For example, newborn screening for PKU and congenital hypothyroidism (which is usually not a monogenic disorder) is often done together to decrease costs.

3. **Characteristics of the screening system.** Effective genetic screening requires the use of an appropriate test within the context of a **well-organized and comprehensive program for dealing with abnormal results.**
   a. There must be **prompt initial testing and follow-up.** A mechanism must exist to assure that abnormal results are acted upon quickly and appropriately.
   b. An ongoing **mechanism for determining the effectiveness** of the screening program must be instituted. Although a test may be theoretically valuable, its usefulness must be demonstrated in practice and must be continually reassessed in the face of changing technology and demographics.
   c. **Education** regarding the nature, usefulness, and limitations of the screening program must be provided to physicians and other health care professionals. **Public knowledge** regarding the screening should be maintained, particularly within the groups for whom the screening is intended.
   d. The **benefits** of the screening program taken as a whole **should exceed its costs.** There should, at the very least, be a favorable economic benefit-to-cost ratio; social and political costs and benefits must be considered as well.

C. Genetic screening is usually a multistep process.

   1. **To avoid false-negatives,** screening tests frequently produce a substantial number of **false-positive results.**
      a. In such circumstances, **all patients who have a positive result on initial screening require a more definitive test** to confirm that they exhibit the condition or genotype of interest.
      b. A good example is provided by **serum triple screening of pregnant women for Down syndrome fetuses** (see Chapter 14 II F 4).
         (1) **Most women with abnormal triple screening tests are *not* carrying a fetus with Down syndrome** (i.e., most positive triple screening tests are false-positives).
         (2) **Additional testing** by ultrasound and amniocentesis is required to distinguish true-positive from false-positive results.

   2. Concentrating genetic testing in certain **subpopulations known to have a higher frequency** of the condition than the general population can be thought of as initial screening that precedes the test in some cases. For example, β-thalassemia is much more common among some ethnic groups (e.g., Italians, Greeks, and Africans) than among others. **Performing genetic screening only in high-risk ethnic groups increases the efficiency** of testing.

   3. Screening is often **most effective when information obtained from various sources is combined** to determine the result. For example, the risk of Down syndrome in the

fetus of a woman with an abnormal serum triple screen depends on the absolute values obtained in the test, the woman's ethnic origin, the gestational age, her weight, whether she is carrying twins, and whether she has diabetes. All of these factors can be included in a single risk estimate.

D. **Ethical and legal concerns regarding genetic screening** (see Chapter 17)

1. Although genetic screening programs are developed to benefit patients and families, they **sometimes have a negative impact** on screened populations.
   a. For example, people found to have a certain disease or genotype have sometimes been **stigmatized** so that they are unable to obtain employment or insurance.
   b. **Education,** both professional and public, is the **most important tool in preventing stigmatization.**

2. **Genetic screening may be mandated by legislation,** which can raise issues of personal conscience, privacy, and consent.

E. **Future perspective: the genetic profile**

1. **Recent advances** in molecular genetics have increased the ability to identify individuals who have **genotypes that produce disease** (e.g., in Huntington disease), have **genetic predispositions to disease** (e.g., in hyperlipidemias), or are at **high risk for having a child with a given disease** (e.g., detection of heterozygous carriers for cystic fibrosis).

2. **Predicting most of the diseases that each individual is likely to develop or pass on to his or her children** should be possible if advances in genetic research continue.
   a. **Such knowledge would enable patients to:**
      (1) Alter their lives to **reduce nongenetic risk factors** of particular relevance and thereby forestall the diseases to which they are genetically predisposed
      (2) **Take advantage of all available reproductive options** if potential offspring carry genetic risks
   b. **Privacy.** Appropriate safeguards will be necessary to make certain that knowledge of a person's genetic endowment is maintained with strictest confidentiality and does not result in discriminatory practices against him or her.

3. When a sufficiently large number of genotypes can be identified, **every individual will be found to carry some disease-predisposing traits.** Thus, genetic screening will be used to determine the individual genetic predispositions of every person rather than to identify "normal" or "abnormal" people.

STUDY QUESTIONS

DIRECTIONS: Each of the numbered items or incomplete statements in this section is followed by answers or by completions of the statement. Select the ONE lettered answer or completion that is BEST in each case.

1. A good genetic screening test should have which one of the following characteristics?

(A) High sensitivity

(B) A high rate of false-negative results

(C) A high rate of false-positive results

(D) Low specificity

(E) Low positive predictive value

DIRECTIONS: Each of the numbered items or incomplete statements in this section is negatively phrased, as indicated by a capitalized word such as NOT, LEAST, or EXCEPT. Select the ONE lettered answer or completion that is BEST in each case.

2. A good genetic screening program has all of the following characteristics EXCEPT

(A) the overall cost of having the program is substantially less than the cost of not having the program

(B) the program includes provision for professional education regarding the screening

(C) the diseases for which patients are screened are lethal or have serious adverse consequences

(D) the diseases for which patients are screened are curable if appropriately treated

(E) the program incorporates an effective mechanism for follow-up of abnormal results

ANSWERS AND EXPLANATIONS

1. The answer is A [II B 2]. A good screening test should have high sensitivity so that all (or almost all) of those with the condition being tested for are identified. The specificity should also be high so that most of those who do not have the condition will have a negative test. The rate of false-positives should be low, and the rate of false-negatives should be very low. The positive predictive value should be reasonably high, so that among those with positive screening tests, many will actually have the condition being sought.

2. The answer is D [II B 1, 3]. Good genetic screening programs do not need to be limited to diseases that can be cured. Screening may also be valuable to help delay the onset or improve the management of genetic disease. Alternatively, screening may be justified to help couples avoid having children with a serious and untreatable genetic disease. Good genetic screening programs must have a net benefit that exceeds their cost and should deal only with diseases that cause serious morbidity or mortality. Timely and effective follow-up of abnormal results and both professional and public education are essential to a good program.

Chapter 16

Treatment of Genetic Disease

J. M. Friedman

I. INTRODUCTION

A. **Genetic disease is treatable.** Many people assume that because a disease is determined completely, or largely, by genetic factors, it cannot be treated. This is not correct.

1. **Genetic diseases generally cannot be cured,** but this is also true for most other diseases.

2. **Diagnostic precision is important** in planning and evaluating therapeutic interventions in genetic diseases.

   a. **Etiologic heterogeneity** (see Chapter 5 III) is common in genetic disease.

      (1) **Different genetic lesions,** and thus different pathogenic mechanisms, may be involved **in clinically similar conditions.**

      (2) **Effective therapy often requires knowing precisely what gene or protein is altered** in an affected patient.

      (3) For **example,** hyperphenylalaninemia, which leads to mental retardation, may be caused by deficiency of the enzyme phenylalanine hydroxylase [e.g., in classic phenylketonuria (PKU)] or by certain abnormalities of biopterin metabolism.

         (a) PKU can be treated successfully by dietary restriction of phenylalanine.

         (b) Treatment of abnormalities of biopterin metabolism by dietary restriction of phenylalanine does not prevent the development of mental retardation.

   b. Even within a single genetic entity, there may be substantial **variability in expression** (see Chapter 3 I B 2 c). For example, some patients with neurofibromatosis develop severe complications (e.g., scoliosis, brain tumors, or sarcoma) but most do not. Such variability must be considered in evaluating therapy.

B. **Treatment of genetic diseases,** particularly if based upon incomplete understanding of pathogenesis, is **often associated with unexpected problems.**

1. For example, although appropriate therapy can save patients with **hereditary retinoblastoma** from death from retinal malignancy within the first years of life, survivors frequently develop osteosarcoma as they grow older.

2. Similarly, early dietary treatment of **galactosemia** prevents the life-threatening metabolic derangements that occur in affected infants, but successfully treated individuals often manifest learning disabilities and ovarian failure later in life.

C. In genetic disease, as in medicine in general, **prevention is better than treatment.** Prevention of genetic disease may sometimes be facilitated by genetic screening (see Chapter 15 II), genetic counseling (see Chapter 15 I), or prenatal diagnosis with elective termination of affected pregnancies (see Chapter 14).

II. METHODS OF TREATING GENETIC DISEASE

A. **Amelioration of the clinical phenotype** is the method used most commonly to treat genetic diseases. This approach is **applicable to all types of genetic disease,** including chromosome abnormalities, and monogenic and multifactorial conditions.

1. **Symptomatic treatment does not require knowledge of either the pathogenesis or the specific nature of a genetic defect,** although such knowledge may permit the design of more appropriate and effective therapy.

2. **Examples are numerous** and include the following:
   a. **Surgical correction** of congenital anomalies such as cleft lip, congenital heart disease, or polydactyly
   b. **Special education** in conditions like Down syndrome or fragile X syndrome
   c. **Physical therapy** for congenital hip dislocation or congenital contractural arachnodactyly
   d. Use of **medication,** such as β-adrenergic blockers to prevent aortic dissection in Marfan syndrome (see Chapter 3 I B 3 b).
   e. **Avoidance of environmental exposures** that trigger a genetic disease. Avoidance of drugs that induce hemolysis in glucose-6-phosphate dehydrogenase (G6PD) deficiency is one example (see Chapter 9 II B 1).

B. Treatment by **amelioration of metabolic abnormalities** is often possible if the pathogenesis of a disease is understood at the biochemical level.

1. Such therapy is restricted almost exclusively to **monogenic disorders** because the necessary pathogenic understanding is not available for most chromosome abnormalities and multifactorial diseases.

2. **Several different approaches** may be used, depending on the nature of the disease.
   a. **Dietary restriction** can be used to **remove the substrate for a deficient enzyme,** if accumulation of that substrate causes disease.
      (1) One example is **PKU,** in which limitation of phenylalanine in the diet prevents development of mental retardation that results from hyperphenylalaninemia.
      (2) In **galactosemia,** removal of milk and dairy products from the diet prevents the metabolic derangements by eliminating galactose, the sugar that cannot be properly metabolized by these patients.
   b. If the pathology is produced by accumulation of a toxic metabolite, improvement may be achieved by **diverting the toxic substance to alternate metabolic pathways.** For example, administration of sodium benzoate to patients with hyperammonemia caused by **ornithine transcarbamoylase deficiency** helps eliminate nitrogen through an alternative metabolic pathway.
   c. **Removal of a substance that is being stored excessively** is effective if such storage produces disease.
      (1) In **hemochromatosis,** removal of excess iron by phlebotomy helps prevent progressive organ damage caused by iron deposition.
      (2) Similarly, removal of excess copper by administration of penicillamine is useful in preventing the neurologic and hepatic damage caused by copper accumulation in **Wilson disease.**
   d. **Activating the defective metabolic pathway** is used to treat some conditions.
      (1) **Homocystinuria** is caused by a defect in cystathionine β-synthase, which requires a pyridoxine cofactor. In some patients, activity of the defective enzyme can be increased substantially by administering very large amounts of pyridoxine (vitamin B_6).
      (2) **Familial hypercholesterolemia (FH)** is caused by abnormalities of cellular receptors for low-density lipoprotein (LDL) cholesterol. Administration of a drug such as **lovastatin** which inhibits 3-hydroxy-3-methylglutaryl coenzyme A (**HMG-CoA**) **reductase**—the enzyme that makes cholesterol—causes FH cells to increase their production of receptors to maintain adequate intracellular cholesterol pools. Blood cholesterol levels are thus reduced because circulating cholesterol is bound to the cellular receptors and internalized.

C. **Replacement therapy**

1. **Replacement of a deficient substance** is often useful if pathology is caused by absence of that substance.
   a. Several **monogenic disorders** benefit from replacement therapy.
      (1) In **classic hemophilia,** replacement of the deficient clotting protein—factor VIII—corrects the bleeding disorder.
      (2) **Hereditary isolated growth hormone deficiency,** a rare form of dwarfism, can be treated by administering growth hormone to the patients.

    b. Some **multifactorial conditions** also benefit from replacement therapy. For example, **type-I (insulin-dependent) diabetes mellitus** is treated by administration of insulin.

  2. Organ transplantation is sometimes a method of replacement therapy as well as a method of gene therapy (see II E 1).

    a. The donor organ may provide the product that is abnormal or deficient in the recipient.

    b. A donor organ can provide such product because its cells contain normal genes.

D. **Modulation of gene expression** is used to treat some monogenic disorders.

  1. The goal is to alter the pathogenic process by **activating a normal gene that has been turned off or by turning off a gene that is abnormally active.**

  2. For example, treatment of patients who have **sickle cell anemia** with **hydroxyurea** ameliorates the disease by reactivating fetal hemoglobin synthesis. The presence of fetal hemoglobin in the red blood cells helps prevent them from sickling.

  3. Antisense RNA and antisense DNA oligonucleotides can be used to block gene expression in some experimental systems. This approach may be useful in diseases that result from inappropriate or excessive gene expression. Antisense RNA or DNA oligonucleotides may also provide a means of treating mutations with dominant negative effects (see Chapter 3 II).

E. **Gene therapy** involves correction of a genetic defect by altering the genotype.

  1. Transplantation of cells, tissues, or organs is a form of gene therapy because the transferred cells continue to function on the basis of the donor genome which differs from that of the recipient.

    a. Transplantation can be used to replace a protein that is defective or absent in the recipient. This has been done, for example, in the following circumstances:

      (1) Bone marrow transplantation in patients with severe combined immunodeficiency disease (SCID) caused by **adenosine deaminase deficiency**

      (2) Liver transplantation in patients with **homozygous FH**

    b. Alternatively, **transplantation can be used to replace an organ that has been damaged** by a genetic disease. This approach is used to treat renal failure in patients with **adult polycystic kidney disease (APKD)** and cardiac failure in patients with **hereditary cardiomyopathy.**

    c. In some cases, transplantation serves **to replace both a defective protein and a damaged organ.** This occurs, for example, when liver transplantation is used to treat hepatic failure in α_1-antitrypsin deficiency.

    d. There are several **problems with transplantation** that make it a less-than-ideal method for transferring genetic material.

      (1) Availability of suitable tissue for transplantation is limited, particularly for organs such as livers and hearts.

      (2) Preparation and recovery from transplantation, as well as the procedure itself, are associated with **considerable morbidity and mortality.**

      (3) Tissue rejection or graft-versus-host (GVH) disease is an ongoing risk; immunosuppressive therapy must be continued throughout life.

      (4) Transplantation is expensive.

  2. Somatic gene therapy involves the addition, alteration, or replacement of an abnormal gene in an affected patient.

    a. Somatic gene therapy **does not affect the germ-line** because only certain somatic tissues or cells of a patient are altered. The change is not passed on to the children of a treated individual. **This is the essential difference between germ-line and somatic gene therapy.**

    b. Several approaches to somatic gene therapy have been tried or are being considered.

      (1) Addition of an appropriately functioning normal gene is applicable to diseases such as PKU or galactosemia, in which a person lacks a critical metabolic enzyme. This approach, which is called **gene augmentation,** is the only one that has been used clinically to treat genetic disease.

(2) **Replacement of an abnormal gene by a normal one** may be necessary in diseases in which the abnormal gene functions in a dominant fashion. Examples include most cases of severe osteogenesis imperfecta (see Chapter 8 II B 1) and one form of hereditary isolated growth hormone deficiency. In these conditions, the mutation exerts a dominant negative effect—the mutant gene produces an abnormal protein that disrupts the structural integrity of tissues even in the presence of a normal product from the other allele.

(3) **Correction of an abnormal gene by targeted mutagenesis** or similar manipulation is another potential method for treating diseases in which function of an abnormal gene is pathogenic. For example, such an approach might be used to inactivate an inherited mutation that causes an autosomal dominant disease by overexpression of a normal product or production of a toxic peptide.

c. Several **technical difficulties** limit the current use of somatic gene therapy, including:

(1) **Transfer of the therapeutic gene to appropriate target tissues.** An effective construct containing the gene must be prepared and inserted into the patient's cells.

(a) **Incorporation of the gene.** Insertion of the gene may be accomplished by placing it into a retrovirus, plasmid, or other appropriate vector and treating the host cells to induce uptake.

(b) **Access to target cells.** For some cell types (e.g., marrow), the patient's cells can be removed, the therapeutic gene inserted in them, and the cells returned to the patient. For other types of target cells (e.g., brain neurons), uptake of therapeutic DNA needs to be induced in situ.

(c) **Large genes.** Gene therapy is especially difficult for very large genes, such as those involved in Duchenne muscular dystrophy or neurofibromatosis type 1. The complementary DNA (cDNA) of these genes is too big to fit into conventional vectors, so a construct containing only part of the normal gene or a different method of DNA transfer must be used.

(2) **Selection of appropriate target cells**

(a) The **cell in which a gene normally functions** can sometimes be used as the target for somatic gene therapy. This is the case, for example, in thalassemia, in which therapy can be directed to marrow cells.

(b) In other instances, **a more accessible or convenient cell type** may make a better target. For example, in a disease such as α_1-antitrypsin deficiency, in which normal protein circulating in the blood is expected to have a beneficial effect, ectopic expression of a therapeutic gene in marrow cells or implants of skin fibroblasts might be useful.

(c) Neurons and other **target cells that do not normally divide** in adults present a particular problem because commonly used transfer vectors (e.g., retroviruses) are taken up only by dividing cells.

(i) Vectors that are taken up by nondividing cells must be used in these cases. Adenovirus and herpes simplex virus are examples of vectors of this type.

(ii) An alternative approach is to induce cell division in the normally quiescent target tissue. For example, partial hepatectomy can be performed to induce division of liver cells in the portion of the organ that remains.

(d) **Some cells have a limited life span.** If such cells are used as targets for gene therapy, the treatment will have to be repeated periodically.

(3) **Induction of appropriate expression** of the therapeutic gene in target tissues

(a) The **amount of expression needed** to correct the genetic defect **varies in different diseases.** In some cases, only a small amount of activity is necessary; in other cases, near-normal activity may be required.

(b) **Overexpression** of some normal genes **may be deleterious.**

(c) **Transient expression and expression at a too-low level** are frequent problems in gene therapy.

    (4) Proper regulation of the therapeutic gene. The necessity for proper regulation is also likely to vary in different diseases. Some genes need to function within normal regulatory constraints to provide therapeutic benefit; for other genes, unregulated expression seems adequate.

d. There are **many potential risks** of somatic gene therapy, but until substantial human experience is obtained, it will **not** be **known which, if any, of these risks are of practical importance.** The **theoretical risks** include the following:

    (1) Induction of neoplasia within the target tissue by action of the vector, activation of a proto-oncogene, or damage to a tumor suppressor gene (see Chapter 11 III C 2) is the greatest concern.

    (2) Damage to or inactivation of other genes in target cells seems unlikely to be a serious problem, especially with therapeutic vectors that integrate randomly in the host genome. Any abnormality produced should be restricted to a very small proportion of the target cells that have been altered.

    (3) Alteration of the germ line with risks to children of the treated patient **should not occur** if the therapeutic intervention is limited to somatic cells.

e. Clinical applications of somatic gene therapy are currently in the realm of **research,** not routine patient care. Initial applications have been undertaken in several different areas.

    (1) Autosomal or X-linked recessive diseases

      (a) Mendelian diseases that are most amenable to somatic gene therapy are those that exhibit **certain favorable characteristics.** These include:

        (i) The mutant gene has been identified and characterized.

        (ii) A cDNA clone of the normal gene is available.

        (iii) The disease produces very serious morbidity or mortality.

        (iv) No adequate alternative therapy is available.

        (v) Knowledge of disease pathogenesis is sufficient to determine that gene therapy is likely to be a successful intervention.

        (vi) An appropriate target cell and a suitable method of transfer of the gene are available.

        (vii) Studies in cultured cells and experimental animals indicate that the specific combination of gene construct, target cell, and insertion strategy being attempted is likely to be safe and effective.

      (b) Examples of diseases with such characteristics include SCID caused by adenosine deaminase deficiency, homozygous FH, and cystic fibrosis.

    (2) Malignant neoplasms

      (a) Approaches to gene therapy of malignancies include:

        (i) Introducing genes with an anticancer function into tumor cells, such as transfer of a tumor supressor gene (see Chapter 11 III).

        (ii) Transfer to tumor cells of "suicide genes," such as a diphtheria toxin gene, under the control of a tumor-specific promoter

        (iii) Altering the tumor cells so that they are more immunogenic and are therefore acted against by the body's immune system

        (iv) Altering immune cells so that they react against tumor cells more effectively

        (v) Altering normal stem cells so that they are resistant to the toxic effects of chemotherapy directed against the tumor

      (b) Clinical trials of gene therapy have been undertaken in several advanced malignancies. Examples include brain tumors, malignant melanoma, and various carcinomas.

    (3) Approaches for chronic infectious diseases, such as AIDS, for which no satisfactory treatment currently exists include:

      (a) Intracellular immunization (i.e., manipulation of cells so that they resist infection by or replication of the pathogen)

      (b) Inducing a more effective immune response, which might be done by genetic alteration of immune responsive or antigen-presenting cells

    (4) Other chronic progressive diseases. For example, Parkinson disease might be treated by injecting genetically modified dopamine-secreting fibroblasts into the brain.

    f. Some **ethical concerns** about somatic gene therapy include:

      (1) Safety. The potential risks of somatic gene therapy are not fundamentally different from the risks associated with certain other novel treatments, such as new vaccines or antineoplastic agents. Somatic gene therapies must be subjected to the same critical assessments of safety and efficacy as other new therapies, such as those required for Food and Drug Administration (FDA) approval.

      (2) Effects on future generations. Although somatic gene therapies are designed to avoid germ-line transfer of altered genes, inadvertent involvement of the germ line may still be a possibility. The risk of inducing genetic damage that could be transmitted to the offspring is not unique to gene therapy, however. Similar concerns arise with some forms of cancer radiotherapy and chemotherapy.

3. Germ-line gene therapy involves the addition, alteration, or replacement of an abnormal gene in such a manner that an individual's gamete-producing cells are modified.

    a. Examples of germ-line gene therapy include the replacement of an abnormal gene in a zygote or the transfer of a therapeutic gene to a patient in a manner that permits incorporation by the spermatogonia or oocytes.

    b. Germ-line gene therapy poses risks and raises important ethical questions beyond those inherent in somatic gene therapy because damage may be caused to future generations.

    c. Most geneticists see **no role for germ-line gene therapy in humans.**

STUDY QUESTIONS

DIRECTIONS: Each of the numbered items or incomplete statements in this section is followed by answers or by completions of the statement. Select the ONE lettered answer or completion that is BEST in each case.

1. The essential difference between somatic gene therapy and germ-line gene therapy is

(A) somatic gene therapy involves the replacement of an abnormal gene by a normal gene; germ-line gene therapy involves the addition of a normal gene
(B) somatic gene therapy does not affect the genetic makeup of the children of a treated patient; germ-line gene therapy may affect future generations
(C) somatic gene therapy is performed postnatally; germ-line gene therapy is performed prenatally
(D) somatic gene therapy requires lifelong immunosuppression; germ-line gene therapy does not
(E) somatic gene therapy is applicable only to monogenic diseases; germ-line gene therapy can be applied to chromosome abnormalities and multifactorial disorders as well

2. Which one of the following statements regarding treatment of genetic disease by organ or tissue transplantation is correct?

(A) Transplantation is an experimental therapy when applied to genetic disease
(B) Although an organ damaged by genetic disease can be replaced by transplantation, the benefit is usually transient because the disease recurs in the donor organ
(C) Liver transplantation can be used to replace a hepatic protein that is defective or absent in a recipient, even if the recipient's liver is otherwise healthy
(D) Bone marrow transplantation from a sibling unaffected by a genetic disease to a sibling affected by the disease is a form of germ-line gene therapy
(E) Tissue rejection is rarely a problem in transplantation for genetic disease because the defective genotype prevents graft-versus-host disease

DIRECTIONS: Each of the numbered items or incomplete statements in this section is negatively phrased, as indicated by a capitalized word such as NOT, LEAST, or EXCEPT. Select the ONE lettered answer or completion that is BEST in each case.

3. Clinical applications of gene therapy that are currently being evaluated include all of the following EXCEPT

(A) treatment of malignant tumors by insertion of a normal tumor suppressor gene
(B) treatment of malignant tumors by manipulations that enhance the antitumor immune response
(C) treatment of normal stem cells in patients with malignancy to make the normal cells more resistant to tumor chemotherapy
(D) treatment of acquired immune deficiency syndrome (AIDS) by targeted mutagenesis of the viral genes in infected lymphocytes
(E) treatment of AIDS by alteration of lympho-

cytes so that they are more resistant to human immunodeficiency virus (HIV) infection or replication

4. Mendelian diseases most suitable for gene therapy are those that exhibit all of the following characteristics EXCEPT

(A) the mutation produces a dominant negative effect
(B) no adequate alternative therapy is available
(C) the mutant gene has been fully characterized
(D) an appropriate target cell and method of gene transfer are available
(E) the pathogenesis of the disease is well understood

DIRECTIONS: The set of matching questions in this section consists of a list of four to twenty-six lettered options (some of which may be in figures) followed by several numbered items. For each numbered item, select the ONE lettered option that is most closely associated with it. To avoid spending too much time on matching sets with large numbers of options, it is generally advisable to begin each set by reading the list of options. Then, for each item in the set, try to generate the correct answer and locate it in the option list, rather than evaluating each option individually. Each lettered option may be selected once, more than once, or not at all.

Questions 5–9

Match the following kinds of treatment with the therapies they describe.

(A) Symptomatic treatment
(B) Removal of the substrate for a deficient enzyme
(C) Diversion of a toxic metabolite to an alternate metabolic pathway
(D) Replacement of an inactive or defective gene product
(E) Activation of a defective metabolic pathway
(F) Germ-line gene therapy
(G) Somatic gene therapy

5. Administration of growth hormone to a child with hereditary isolated growth hormone deficiency

6. Administration of phenobarbital to prevent seizures in a child with hyperammonemia resulting from ornithine transcarbamoylase deficiency

7. Placing a child with galactosemia on a diet free of galactose

8. Treating a patient with familial hypercholesterolemia (FH) with an inhibitor of 3-hydroxy-3-methylglutaryl coenzyme A (HMG-CoA) reductase

9. Treating a patient with Marfan syndrome with a β-adrenergic blocking agent to prevent aortic aneurysm

ANSWERS AND EXPLANATIONS

1. The answer is B [II E 2–3]. The essential difference between germ-line and somatic gene therapy is that in germ-line gene therapy, the manipulation affects germ cells and can be transmitted to the offspring, whereas in somatic gene therapy, the germ line is unaffected. Gene addition or replacement could, in principle, be done either in somatic tissues or in the germ line. Both germ-line and somatic gene therapy could be performed either postnatally or prenatally.

An advantage of any type of gene therapy over tissue transplantation is that recipient cells that have been treated by gene therapy should be completely compatible with the host. Thus, immunosuppression should be unnecessary unless the recipient develops an immune response to the normal product of the inserted gene. Somatic gene therapy is being used experimentally in a variety of malignancies, infectious diseases, and other chronic progressive disorders as well as in monogenic disorders. Most geneticists do not see any need for germ-line gene therapy in humans. Correction of underlying genetic defects by gene therapy is unlikely in multifactorial or chromosomal disorders in the foreseeable future because our understanding of the pathogenesis of these conditions is insufficient. However, somatic gene therapy using other approaches is being tried in some multifactorial diseases (e.g., common forms of breast and colon cancer).

2. The answer is C [II C 2, E 1]. In genetic disease, an organ without apparent damage may have to be replaced with an organ that provides a function lacking in the recipient. For example, removal of the histologically normal liver from a patient with cardiac failure because of homozygous hypercholesterolemia may be required to permit transplantation of a donor liver with normal cholesterol metabolism. Transplantation is a standard treatment in genetic conditions such as adult polycystic kidney disease (APKD) or infantile hepatic failure due to α_1-antitrypsin deficiency.

Although genetic disease may recur in a donor organ if transplantation does not correct the essential genetic defect, the disease does not recur in situations in which the essential defect is corrected. For example, if the marrow of a patient with β-thalassemia is completely replaced with normal marrow, the disease will not recur. Transplantation is not usually undertaken when it is known that the donor organ's function will be limited by recurrence of the underlying disease. Marrow transplantation between siblings is somatic therapy, not germ-line gene therapy. Tissue rejection after transplantation is no less a problem in genetic diseases than in others, unless the condition being treated is an immunodeficiency disease.

3. The answer is D [II E 2 b (3)]. Targeted mutagenesis, the correction of an abnormal gene or the inactivation of a particular gene by mutation (as in D), is not yet available clinically. Current gene therapy protocols use gene augmentation, which is the addition of a gene to target cells without alteration of cognate cellular genes. The other responses to this question are all examples of gene therapy that are currently being evaluated in patients.

4. The answer is A [II E 2 e]. Autosomal or X-linked recessive genetic diseases currently are much more amenable to gene therapy than are dominant diseases. Treatment of recessive diseases generally requires addition of a normal gene to the target cells, whereas gene therapy of dominant diseases usually requires inactivation or correction of the abnormal mutant gene. No clinically applicable method of inactivating or correcting abnormal mutant genes by gene therapy is currently available.

Gene therapy is currently most applicable for recessive diseases in which the mutant gene has been fully characterized and no adequate alternative therapy exists. Before gene therapy can be undertaken, an appropriate target tissue and gene transfer system must be developed in tissue culture and experimental animal studies. In addition, disease pathogenesis must be well enough understood to justify the proposed genetic intervention.

5–9. The answers are: 5-D, 6-A, 7-B, 8-E, 9-A [II A–C]. Administration of growth hormone to a child with hereditary isolated growth hormone deficiency is an example of amelioration of a metabolic abnormality by replacement of a missing product. Anticonvulsant therapy in a child with an inborn metabolic error and β-adrenergic blocker therapy in a patient with Marfan syndrome are examples of symptomatic treatments that do not alter the underlying genetic abnormality.

Patients with galactosemia usually lack functional galactose-1-phosphate uridyl transferase, an enzyme that is essential for the metabolism of galactose. Elimination of milk and dairy products, which contain galactose, from the diet of patients with galactosemia removes the substrate for the deficient enzyme.

Administration of a 3-hydroxy-3-methylglutaryl coenzyme A (HMG-CoA) reductase inhibitor such as lovastatin to a patient with familial hypercholesterolemia (FH) due to a deficiency of low-density lipoprotein (LDL) receptors causes cells to increase their production of LDL receptors. This is an example of activation of the defective metabolic pathway.

Chapter 17

Ethical Issues in Medical Genetics

Barbara McGillivray

I. **INTRODUCTION.** The goal of genetic counseling is to provide both information and support so that couples and families can make plans and decisions according to their own values. Generally, this is accomplished by nondirective counseling, which provides information and empathy but does not direct a course of action for the couple. At times, values may conflict, and dilemmas may arise when moral considerations for taking either of two opposing courses of action can be found.

A. **Definition of terms**

1. **Morality** is behavior according to customs or codes.

2. **Ethics** is the discipline of reflecting upon what does go, and what should go, into formulating morality, or what considerations are part of sound moral judgment. The considerations should include:
   a. **Analyzing the situation,** in terms of both consequences and alternatives
   b. **Weighing the alternatives**

B. **Models in common use.** Ethical theories are bodies of moral principles and rules that justify particular actions. The field of biomedical ethics is relatively new, and no one model fits all clinical situations. It is important to be aware that there is an increasing number of models, and that several may be combined in formulating a course of action.

1. **Utilitarianism** is a set of theories based on consequences in which the aim is to promote the welfare and protect the interests of most people (i.e., the greatest good for the greatest number of people).
   a. **Actions** may be judged in proportion to their ability to maximize happiness and minimize pain (i.e., actions are judged in retrospect). **Four criteria** are given.
      (1) The obligation is to maximize the good (utility).
      (2) Attempts should be made to reach a common good, not an individual personal good (value).
      (3) Actions are right or wrong in terms of their consequences (consequentialism).
      (4) Consequences affecting all parties should receive equal consideration (universalism).
   b. The **obligation** of utilitarianism is to benefit the community rather than the individual (i.e., individuals are sacrificed for the wider universal good). Therefore, the rights of individuals may be overridden, making utilitarianism inconsistent with the value of autonomy.

2. **Deontology (the theory of duties)** proposes that acts are right or wrong in themselves and should not be justified only by their consequences. This model emphasizes truth-telling and fidelity to promises, and it states that people have a duty to act in certain ways. The **duties** include the following.
   a. Always preserve life (duty is against suicide or euthanasia).
   b. A physician's duty is to an individual patient rather than maximizing the good to others. The doctor–patient relationship has an independent moral significance.
   c. Acts must be consistently universal. A procedure performed on one patient with a specific medical problem must be available to every patient who is in that same situation.

3. **Other theories** may be based on **virtues;** that is, the integrity of the individual and the suppression of self-interest are stressed. Theories also may be based on **rights;** that is, morality itself is designed to protect the dignity and rights of the individual. The **ethic of care** holds that moral reasoning cannot be simply finding rules to arbitrate; it can also mean finding solutions that reduce or remove conflict.

4. **In clinical genetics,** physicians may be concerned with the rights of the fetus or the rights of the malformed newborn. Physicians must recognize non-Western values in patients and their families and also recognize that there may be a difference in female morality (i.e., related more to care and compassion) and male morality (i.e., justice, duty, and rights).

II. ETHICAL PRINCIPLES

A. **Beneficence** is the duty to confer benefits and to prevent and remove harm. Biomedical research, preventive medicine, and public health interventions may be said to benefit society as a whole. In clinical genetics, somatic gene therapy could benefit by providing nonheritable cures for single gene disorders.

B. **Autonomy** is the principle of being one's own person and choosing one's own course of action, including medical treatment. The individual should not be constrained by others.

1. This principle creates difficulties with those who are incompetent (i.e., children, those with psychiatric disorders, or those who are unconscious) because it assumes that the individual has been fully informed.

2. A woman exercises autonomy when she chooses whether to have prenatal diagnosis after she has been adequately counseled. The counseling would include information regarding her indication for prenatal diagnosis, the risks of the procedure, and alternatives.

C. The principle of **justice** is defined as identical cases being treated in the same manner. **Distributive justice** refers to the fair distribution of both benefits and burdens in society and begins to occur when there are scarcities. For example, if there are limited financial resources to cover all proposed medical programs, a center may decide to offer amniocentesis only to women older than a certain age. This decision treats those with the greater risk equally but does not make the procedure available to those with the lesser risk.

D. **Nonmaleficence** is a duty derived from that of beneficence and proposes that one ought not to inflict evil or harm. This duty assumes that a physician will be competent. Withholding or withdrawing treatment to an infant or adult may be seen as harmful, except in the case in which the individual was judged to be dying.

E. **Veracity,** which is the duty to tell the truth, implies that the patient has a right to information about himself or herself.

1. **Nondisclosure** may be considered when information is thought to be harmful to the patient, but health care professionals should disclose what a reasonable patient would want to know and should fulfill the individual patient's need for information.

2. For example, when researching a new lipid-lowering drug, patients should be made aware of all the risks and benefits of such drugs before being asked to participate in a clinical trial.

F. **Fidelity** is the duty to keep contracts and promises. The physician has a duty not to neglect patients once accepting them into care. If a couple presents for prenatal diagnosis, and the fetus is found to have a chromosome abnormality, the counselor has a duty to impart the information and continue support, regardless of how difficult it may be to divulge the diagnosis.

III. MAKING DECISIONS IN THE PRESENCE OF ETHICAL DILEMMAS. As part of providing genetic counseling, the physician may be faced with having to choose between two or more incompatible courses of action and must make a moral judgment

to proceed or to provide effective counseling. It may be helpful to have a framework for such problems.

A. **Identifying the facts.** It may be helpful to order the facts into four areas.

1. **Medical indications:** What are the diagnosis, prognosis, risks, and benefits of treatment? What is the chance for success of the proposed treatment?

2. **Patient preferences:** What does the patient want? If the patient is not competent, what are the wishes of the substituted decision-maker?

3. **Quality of life:** What might the patient expect with either treatment or nontreatment?

4. **Contextual features:** What do family members want? What are the costs of treatment? Are there associated legal issues?

B. **Identify the ethical principles involved.** If one course of action is clearly dominant, then the moral problem may be solved. If not, the principles should be ordered in terms of their importance. For example, is the patient's autonomy the most important issue, or is the physician's duty of beneficence to the patient overriding? If the choice is not clear, other steps may be necessary. Using the ethic of care, one may need to consider both or all principles in conflict and negotiate a course observing the needs of all parties.

C. **Compare with similar cases.** If a similar case can be found in which one principle was found to be most important, the physician may use that example as a precedent to make a similar decision. To use such comparisons, a paradigm must exist without morally relevant differences from case to case.

D. **Use an ethics committee.** Most hospitals have an ethics committee consisting of representatives from medicine, nursing, social work, philosophy, law, religion, and the lay public. The purpose of these committees is to examine such problems around an ethical framework to help the clinician. Most committees of this type do not make decisions for the physician; instead, they offer advice and support.

E. **Realize decisions may be wrong and learn from each mistake.** Identifying and making moral decisions should be a continuous process, both as the physician learns to analyze situations and as applied ethics copes with the rapid advances in medicine.

IV. AREAS OF CONFLICT IN CLINICAL GENETICS

A. **Confidentiality and the rights of the family.** Before counseling a family, confidential material is gathered regarding medical conditions, use of medications and nonmedical drugs, relationships, and medical information on family members. Such information may not be divulged without the permission of its owner (or guardian), although knowledge of a diagnosis (e.g., Huntington disease) may be deemed important for those who are at risk to know. The autonomy of the affected individual may be in conflict with beneficence to the patient.

B. **Prenatal diagnosis**

1. If a woman chooses not to have prenatal diagnosis but is at high risk (> 25%) to have another child with a severe disorder, maternal autonomy may be in conflict with beneficence for society at large or nonmaleficence to the fetus.

2. Maternal and fetal autonomy may be in conflict when termination of the pregnancy is considered upon diagnosis of a chromosome abnormality.

3. A woman who undergoes prenatal diagnosis because she is older than 35 years may have a legal right to abort a fetus with a normal female karyotype, but this morally pits maternal autonomy against fetal autonomy.

C. **Predictive testing**

1. Either **direct or indirect molecular methods** (see Chapter 6 II, III) may allow predictive testing for single gene conditions (e.g., Huntington disease).

2. **All concerns regarding confidentiality** of results for predictive testing **must be considered.** These include:
   a. **Not conveying results to other family members** without permission
   b. **Not conveying results to outside agencies**
   c. **Autonomy of the individual** to either refuse to give blood to enable family studies or to release results
   d. **Obtaining truly informed consent** for studies
   e. **The use of minors for predictive testing.** Generally, predictive testing is not done with minors unless the condition is expected to occur in childhood or there is treatment that will prevent disease sequelae if started early.

D. **Gene therapy.** As methods develop to introduce genes into human somatic cells, the public becomes more concerned about long-term implications. Whereas the aim of such therapy is to alleviate the effects of a particular genetic condition, the lay public often wonders if such methods will be used to "further the human race." Both public education and ethical principles are essential (see Chapter 16).

STUDY QUESTIONS

DIRECTIONS: The numbered item or incomplete statement in this section is followed by answers or by completions of the statement. Select the ONE lettered answer or completion that is BEST.

1. Recently, a clinic has been made aware of a patient choosing to terminate a female fetus on the basis of sex. The genetic counseling staff is upset about this event and decides to give information pertaining only to the normalcy of the karyotype in future cases. They will no longer divulge information regarding fetal sex, because they feel this may prevent other women from choosing to terminate a female fetus. Of the following sets of ethical principles, which set contains two conflicting principles that apply to this situation?

(A) Fidelity and nonmaleficence
(B) Justice and nonmaleficence
(C) Autonomy and beneficence
(D) Autonomy and veracity
(E) Beneficence and veracity

Directions: The set of matching questions in this section consists of a list of four to twenty-six lettered options (some of which may be in figures) followed by several numbered items. For each numbered item, select the ONE lettered option that is most closely associated with it. To avoid spending too much time on matching sets with large numbers of options, it is generally advisable to begin each set by reading the list of options. Then, for each item in the set, try to generate the correct answer and locate it in the option list, rather than evaluating each option individually. Each lettered option may be selected once, more than once, or not at all.

Questions 2–6

Match the following definitions with the correct ethical principle.

(A) Autonomy
(B) Beneficence
(C) Veracity
(D) Fidelity
(E) Justice

2. The duty to keep contracts and promises

3. Disclosing what a reasonable patient would want to know

4. Respecting a patient's decision not to seek medical care

5. Not allowing harm to come to a patient

6. Treating like cases alike

ANSWERS AND EXPLANATIONS

1. The answer is C [II, IV B]. The main conflict in this case is whether the women having prenatal diagnoses can make autonomous decisions regarding the results and continuation of the pregnancy, or whether the staff should decide that the best interests of the patient (which may be the mother and is certainly the fetus) are served by withholding information. Fidelity is of lesser importance in this case, but it is involved because one could claim that the contract between the patient and the counselor is such that all information must be divulged. Nonmaleficence is involved in terms of preventing harm to the fetus but does not address the good intended to the woman or to female fetuses in general. Justice is not directly involved because none of the women will be given information regarding fetal sex. Veracity could be involved because the women will not be told the sex, but conversely, one could claim that no lies are told. Veracity does have the same weight as autonomy and beneficence in this situation.

2–6. The answers are: 2-D, 3-C, 4-A, 5-B, 6-E [II]. Fidelity refers to the often unspoken contract between the physician and the patient to be ethical and to provide information. Veracity involves truth-telling, which includes the provision of all the information that a reasonable patient is expected to ask. The principle of autonomy is one of the strongest, and it concerns the individual's right to make decisions concerning his or her own life, including health care and reproductive decisions. Beneficence involves not only the provision of benefit to the patient but also the prevention and removal of harm. Justice involves matters of fair provision of services and is concerned with both macro- and microallocation of such resources. Generally, the physician is not expected to provide all minute details, especially regarding rare or unlikely events, unless such events are potentially serious.

CASE STUDIES IN CLINICAL DECISION MAKING

Case 1: Identification of A Displaced Child

A family who has been followed by the same physician for many years brings their teenage daughter to the physician's office. The girl, who was adopted from a Latin American country at 1 year of age, is being investigated by the government of that country as a child who may have been taken from her parents illegally during a prior repressive military dictatorship. The child in question has the same birthdate as this family's adopted daughter.

The child in question's natural father was murdered, and her mother was imprisoned by the previous regime. The child herself was taken away and has disappeared. The mother, who has now been released from prison, is trying to find her child. The mother's mother and the father's parents and sister are all alive and anxious to help. The current government wishes to obtain a blood sample on this adopted child for DNA analysis.

QUESTIONS

1. *Assuming the testing is done properly, is DNA analysis a reliable means of proving whether this child is the biologic offspring of the Latin American woman and her deceased husband?*

2. *In addition to the child, who should have DNA testing to provide the most meaningful result?*

DISCUSSION

Analysis of highly polymorphic DNA markers is an extremely reliable method of establishing genetic relationships when properly performed. To establish parentage, one ordinarily would study a child and both of his or her putative parents. Since the father is not available in this case, one would test the child, the putative mother, and the putative paternal grandparents. The putative paternal grandparents should have all the DNA markers that the putative father had. If parentage is as suspected, the adopted child should have inherited one allele at each locus from the natural mother and the other allele at each locus from *either* the paternal grandmother *or* the paternal grandfather.

DNA analysis is performed on the child, the putative mother, and the putative paternal grandparents. The results are reported as follows (A, B, C, D, and E represent 5 extremely polymorphic loci; 1, 2, 3, 4, 5, and 6 are alleles at these loci):

CHILD:		PUTATIVE MOTHER:	
A	1,3	A	1,2
B	1,3	B	1,3
C	2,5	C	2,4
D	1,5	D	3,5
E	1,6	E	1,4

PUTATIVE GRANDMOTHER:	A 3,5	PUTATIVE GRANDFATHER:	A 4,6
	B 2,4		B 3,4
	C 3,6		C 3,5
	D 1,1		D 2,4
	E 3,4		E 1,6

QUESTION

1. *Is this child likely to be the biologic offspring of the putative parents (the Latin American woman and her deceased husband)?*

DISCUSSION

It is easiest to analyze these data in two stages. The first step is to ask if the child has inherited an allele at each of the marker loci from the putative mother. If not, then this cannot be the woman's child. Inspection reveals that the child has the alleles A1, C2, D5, and E1, each of which is also found in the putative mother. The child has alleles 1 and 3 at the B locus, both of which are also found in the putative mother, but only one of these alleles could actually have been inherited from the mother.

The second allele at each locus in the child must have been inherited from the father. Thus, this child's biologic father must have had A3, B1 or B3, C5, D1, and E6, all of which he must have inherited from his parents. The putative paternal grandmother carries A3 and D1. The putative paternal grandfather carries B3, C5, and E6. It is therefore likely that this child is the biologic offspring of this Latin American woman and her deceased husband. Knowledge of the precise frequencies of each allele in the local population would permit a quantitative estimate of this probability to be made.

Case 2: Presymptomatic Diagnosis of Adult Polycystic Kidney Disease

A 21-year-old woman consults her physician because she is concerned about developing adult polycystic kidney disease (APKD). She has always been healthy and has never had any problems with her kidneys or urine. However, her father has just developed renal failure, and her aunt and grandmother had renal transplants in their 40s. The woman's father, aunt, and grandmother have been diagnosed as having APKD. The patient's 28-year-old cousin also has been found to have this condition, but she is healthy. The pedigree of the family is shown below; the shaded symbols indicate individuals who have APKD; the patient is marked with an arrow.

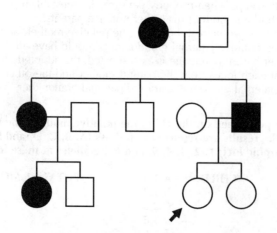

QUESTIONS

1. *What is the most likely pattern of inheritance for APKD in this family?*

2. *What is this patient's chance of developing APKD?*

DISCUSSION

APKD is an autosomal dominant condition that usually becomes symptomatic at about 40 years of age. Flank pain, renal colic, and hematuria are the most frequent presenting symptoms, and hypertension is common. The disease progresses to renal failure, usually within 10 years. Since this patient's father has APKD, her chance of having inherited the gene that causes this disease is 50%.

In most families, APKD is caused by a gene on the short arm of chromosome 16. Polymorphic DNA markers are useful for presymptomatic diagnosis in these families. Presymptomatic diagnosis is important because treatable complications, such as hypertension or impaired renal function, may be asymptomatic early in the course of the disease. Moreover, presymptomatic diagnosis is essential in family members who are being considered as potential kidney donors for an affected relative.

After appropriate counseling, the patient decided that she would like to have presymptomatic testing by linkage analysis.

QUESTION

1. *Who else in the family needs to be studied to determine by linkage whether this 21-year-old woman is likely to have inherited the APKD gene?*

DISCUSSION

To perform a study that is useful for this patient, it is necessary to find an informative linked polymorphism in her father (i.e., a marker for which he is heterozygous). It is then necessary to determine the phase of the linkage, which requires the testing of additional relatives. In this family, it would be most important to test the patient's father, paternal grandmother, paternal aunt, and paternal uncle.

DNA testing was performed, and a marker locus 1 centimorgan (cM) from that for the APKD gene was found to be informative. The results on family members who were tested are shown below. The letters *a* and *b* indicate different alleles at the marker locus.

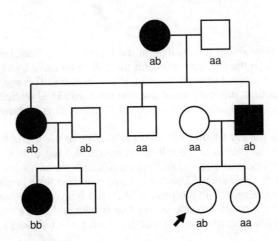

QUESTIONS

1. *Which allele at the marker locus is carried on the same chromosome as the disease allele at the APKD locus in this family?*

2. *What is the chance that the patient has inherited the gene for APKD?*

DISCUSSION

Inspection of the figure indicates that every person with APKD in the family has the *b* allele at the marker locus and that the patient's unaffected uncle has the *a* allele. It is, therefore, likely that the *b* allele at the marker locus and the disease allele at the APKD locus are being carried on the same chromosome in this family. Note, however, that the patient's aunt's husband carries the *b* allele at the marker locus but does *not* have APKD. The marker allele does not cause the disease, it simply provides a way to follow the segregation of the chromosome that carries the abnormal APKD allele in this family.

This can be seen more clearly in the next figure, in which the pedigree symbols of all tested individuals in the preceding figure have been replaced with their haplotypes at the marker and APKD loci. The alleles at these two loci on one chromosome 16 are shown above the alleles at these loci on the other chromosome 16 in each person. Letters *a* and *b* are the alleles at the linked marker locus. *D* indicates the abnormal allele at the APKD locus; *d* indicates the normal allele. The spouses of the affected individuals are all normal, so each is homozygous *dd*. The affected individuals are heterozygous *Dd*. The patient's status at the APKD locus is unknown, so that gene is replaced by a *question mark* on her father's haplotype. The same is true of her sister.

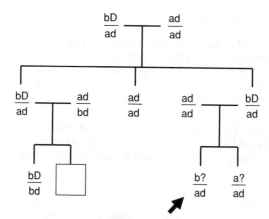

The patient has inherited the *b* allele at the marker locus from her father. Because the distance between the marker locus and the APKD locus is 1 cM, recombination can be expected to occur between them in 1% of meioses. This means that there is 1% chance that the patient did *not* inherit the abnormal APKD *D* allele from her father and a 99% chance that she did inherit the abnormal *D* allele. This is shown in the following figure.

Notice that the patient's sister inherited the *a* allele at the marker locus. For her, the situation is reversed, as shown in the following figure. She has a 99% chance of having inherited her father's normal allele *d* and only a 1% chance of having inherited his abnormal *D* allele at the APKD locus. She could have inherited the *D* mutant allele at the APKD locus *only* if a recombination event occurred between the marker locus and the APKD locus during formation of the sperm that produced her conception. The chance of this happening is 1% because the distance between these two loci is 1 cM.

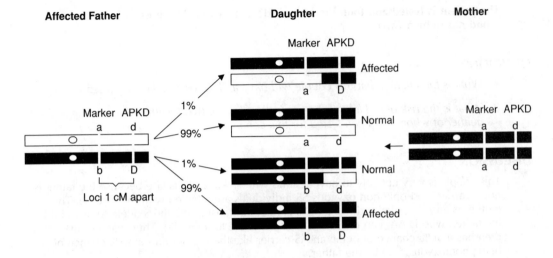

Case 3: Sickle Cell Disease

A 28-year-old woman consults her family physician because she wishes to discontinue her oral contraceptives and become pregnant. She is healthy and has never been pregnant before. Her 30-year-old husband is also in good health. Both are African-Americans, and the patient is concerned about having a child with sickle cell disease.

QUESTIONS

1. What is the frequency of sickle cell disease among African-Americans?

2. How is sickle cell disease inherited?

3. What is the chance that this woman is a carrier for sickle cell disease?

DISCUSSION

Sickle cell disease is an autosomal recessive condition that occurs with a frequency of 1/625 among African-Americans. The three genotypes are represented as AA (homozygous normal), AS (carrier), and SS (sickle cell homozygote). Only the homozygote has the disease; AS heterozygotes are called sickle cell carriers, and they are usually asymptomatic.

The Hardy-Weinberg law can be used to calculate the carrier frequency from the sickle cell disease frequency, 1/625. The disease frequency, which is also the frequency of the SS genotype, is q^2 in the Hardy-Weinberg equation. Thus,

$$q^2 = 1/625,$$

$$q = 1/25,$$

$$\text{and } p = 1 - q = 24/25 \text{ (or} \approx 1).$$

According to the Hardy-Weinberg law, the frequency of heterozygous carriers for sickle cell disease among black Americans is

$$2pq = 2(24/25)(1/25)$$

or approximately 2(1/25), which is about 8%.

The patient is tested and found to be a sickle cell carrier. Her husband is tested and found not to be a carrier.

QUESTIONS

1. *What is the chance that this couple will have a child with sickle cell disease?*

2. *What is the risk of sickle cell disease in the child of two healthy African-Americans, neither of whom has been tested for this condition?*

DISCUSSION

This couple is very unlikely to have a child with sickle cell disease because the father is not a carrier, and only homozygous SS individuals are affected with the disease. The mother is an AS carrier and has a 50% chance of transmitting the S allele to any child; the father, who is AA, can only transmit an A allele to the child. Thus, each of their children has a 50% chance of being an AS carrier like the mother and a 50% chance of being homozyous AA like the father.

The frequency of AS carriers among African-Americans is about 2/25, or 8%, as calculated above. If each member of the couple has the same chance of being a carrier, the chance that both would be carriers is

$$2/25 \times 2/25 = 4/625.$$

If both parents are AS carriers, the chance that both will transmit the S allele to a child who would then be an SS homozygote is 1/4. Thus, the overall risk for sickle cell disease in the child of healthy African-American parents is

$$2/25 \times 2/25 \times 1/4 = 1/625.$$

Case 4: Hunter Syndrome

A public health officer is asked to consider whether a new test to detect carriers of Hunter syndrome should be offered routinely to pregnant women. Hunter syndrome is an X-linked recessive mucopolysaccharide storage disease that produces progressive central nervous system (CNS) deterioration, organomegaly, joint contractures, and death, usually by 30 years of age.

QUESTIONS

1. *What information is necessary to determine the frequency of carrier females for Hunter syndrome in the population?*

2. *What other information is necessary to determine whether or not the test should be routinely implemented?*

DISCUSSION

Hunter syndrome occurs once in every 100,000 males. The gene frequency in males (q) is equal to the disease frequency and, therefore, is 1/100,000. The gene frequency in males and females is the same, so $q = 1/100,000$ in females as well. According to the Hardy-Weinberg law, the frequency of heterozygous carriers among females is 2pq, or approximately 2q, since p is almost equal to 1. Thus, the frequency of heterozygous carrier females is approximately equal to $2q = 2(1/100,000) = 1/50,000$.

The value of a routine screening test depends on a number of factors in addition to the disease frequency. These include the severity of the disease; the availability of interventions that would either prevent development of the disease or prevent mortality or morbidity if provided to presymptomatic patients; the reliability, sensitivity, specificity, and practicality of the test; the cost of the test; and the cost (both financial and social) of caring for patients with the disease.

Case 5: Anticonvulsant Use During Pregnancy

A woman consults her family physician because she thinks that she may be pregnant. Her last menstrual period was 9 weeks ago. The woman has been treated with valproic acid for the past 10 years for a seizure disorder. However, she stopped taking her medicine 1 week ago because she thought she might be pregnant. Yesterday she had a grand mal seizure, her first in 6 months.

QUESTIONS

1. *What are the risks to the fetus of a woman with epilepsy taking valproic acid during pregnancy?*

2. *What are the risks of stopping the medication in this patient?*

3. *Does stopping the valproic acid treatment in this patient decrease her chance of having a baby with a neural tube defect?*

4. *What other factors affect the risk of birth defects in this woman's baby?*

DISCUSSION

The risk of congenital anomalies among the children of epileptic women who take valproic acid in usual therapeutic doses during pregnancy is two to three times higher than in the general population. The children born to mothers taking valproic acid for epilepsy also have approximately a 2% risk of having spina bifida.

Stopping anticonvulsant therapy during pregnancy may pose a substantial hazard to both a woman and her fetus, particularly if she develops status epilepticus. In general, women with seizure disorders should plan their pregnancies. Before becoming pregnant, the woman and her physician should decide whether discontinuation of anticonvulsant therapy is safe. If it is not, the woman's medication should be adjusted to the smallest dose that will maintain effective seizure control. One anticonvulsant drug is probably safer for the fetus than are multiple drugs, so the patient should be placed on a single drug if possible. If a single-drug regimen is not possible, the woman should be given as few drugs as necessary to maintain seizure control. Studies suggest that all commonly used anticonvulsants have similar teratogenic risks, so the choice of drug should be determined largely on the basis of its effectiveness in controlling the patient's seizures.

If this patient is actually 9 weeks pregnant, discontinuing valproic acid does not affect her risk for having a baby with spina bifida. The neural tube closes completely in the human embryo by about 27 days after conception (approximately 6 weeks after the last normal menstrual period), and exposures occurring after that time do not affect neural tube closure.

Every woman in every pregnancy has a risk of at least 5% of having a baby with serious birth defects or mental retardation apparent by 1 year of age. This patient's risk is increased twofold to threefold because she is epileptic and has been taking valproic acid. This risk might be further increased if she were taking an unusually high dose of the medication, if her blood levels of the drug have been in the "toxic range," if she is also taking other anticonvulsant medications, or if there are other risk factors present. For example, her risk for having a baby with a chromosome abnormality would be increased if she were 40 years old, and her risk for having a child with fragile X syndrome would be increased if she were known to be a carrier of this condition.

Teratogen risk counseling should always be provided in the context of a patient's overall medical history, pregnancy history, and family history. Such counseling should be integrated with a patient's complete prenatal care.

The patient is 23 years of age, and this is her first pregnancy. Apart from her idiopathic epilepsy, she has been completely healthy. Her family history is noncontributory.

QUESTIONS

1. *Should prenatal diagnosis be offered to this patient?*

2. *What can be done to reduce the risk of birth defects in future pregnancies for this patient?*

DISCUSSION

Prenatal diagnosis of neural tube defects is available by means of detailed ultrasound examination and measurement of the α-fetoprotein concentration in either the maternal blood or the amniotic fluid. These tests are best performed between 16 and 18 weeks of development. Detailed ultrasound examination may also detect some other major malformations, but there is no reliable means of identifying the minor anomalies often seen among the children of women with seizure disorders treated with anticonvulsants during pregnancy.

Discontinuing anticonvulsant therapy prior to conception, if it can be safely done, is the best way to reduce teratogenic risks related to valproic acid in a future pregnancy. If the patient needs to continue taking valproic acid and she wishes to become pregnant again, administration of a folic acid supplement before conception and throughout the first 2 months of development may reduce the risk of spina bifida in the baby.

Case 6: Familial Breast Cancer

A 31-year-old woman consults her physician because she is concerned about developing breast cancer. She is currently in good health, and she has never had any breast disease. Her concern arises because her sister has just been diagnosed as having breast cancer and her mother died of breast cancer.

QUESTIONS

1. *How can one determine if the cancer in this family is likely to be a dominantly inherited predisposition?*

2. *What is this woman's chance of developing breast cancer?*

DISCUSSION

Evaluation of this patient's concern should begin with a thorough family history. Because tumors may be of many histologic types and may be either benign or malignant, it is particularly important to request medical and autopsy records to confirm tumor diagnoses in relatives reported to be affected. The following family history was obtained for this woman:

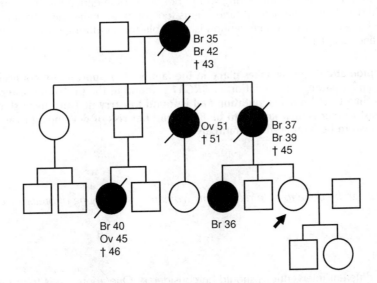

Br in this pedigree indicates carcinoma of the breast with onset at the given age; *Ov* indicates carcinoma of the ovary with onset at the given age, and "†" indicates that the individual died at the age given. All the cancers are documented by medical records.

The pattern is consistent with autosomal dominant inheritance with high penetrance. Note that the mutant gene in this family appears to be associated with both breast and ovarian cancer. The gene is transmitted through a male who is unaffected, but this is to be expected of a condition that affects the breast and ovary.

The disease exhibits characteristics of a dominantly inherited cancer predisposition—the cancers have an unusually early onset, and multiple primary neoplasms and bilateral involvement are common. The proband's mother was affected, so the proband's risk of inheriting the abnormal gene is 50%. This form of dominantly inherited breast and ovarian cancer is likely to be caused by mutation of a gene called *BRCA1*. Women who carry mutations of *BRCA1* have a risk of approximately 85% of developing breast cancer. Affected women also have a greatly increased risk of developing ovarian cancer.

The patient is counseled about her risk of developing breast and ovarian cancer. She is understandably very concerned both for herself and for her 4-year-old daughter.

QUESTION

1. How can molecular genetic testing be used to improve the counseling available to this patient?

DISCUSSION

The *BRCA1* gene has been mapped and cloned. Two approaches to presymptomatic diagnosis can be considered (see Chapter 9 IV E). Indirect molecular diagnosis using linkage can be applied if blood samples can be obtained from the proband's sister and father and tissue samples can be obtained from other affected family members for testing (see Chapter 5 I and Chapter 6 III). Alternatively, direct molecular diagnosis can be attempted if the mutation in the sister's *BRCA1* gene can be identified (see Chapter 6 II). Once the mutation in the family is known, direct testing would be available for all at-risk relatives, including the proband, her female cousin, and her maternal aunt.

It is important to provide appropriate genetic counseling to the proband and any other family members considering genetic testing *before* such testing is actually performed (see

Chapter 9 IV E). Each individual family member must volunteer to be tested, and each person considering testing should be aware of the benefits, limitations, and risks associated with it. Presymptomatic testing would not be recommended for the proband's 4-year-old daughter at the present time; she is too young to understand the implications and no beneficial medical intervention is available for her during childhood (see Chapter 9 IV E and Chapter 17).

Presymptomatic diagnosis takes place in the family after appropriate counseling is completed, and a pathogenic mutation in *BRCA1* is found in the proband's sister. The proband is then tested for this mutation and is found to carry it. Thus, her risk of developing breast cancer is now known to be 85%, and her risk of developing ovarian cancer is also known to be increased substantially.

QUESTION

1. *What can be done to help reduce this woman's risk of dying of breast or ovarian cancer?*

DISCUSSION

Several different interventions should be considered. One approach is to monitor the patient closely for development of cancer. She should be taught careful breast self-examination and encouraged to use it monthly. She should also have breast examinations performed by an experienced physician on a regular basis. Mammography can be initiated at a younger-than-usual age. Periodic abdominal ultrasound examination could be performed in an attempt to detect ovarian cancer early.

Each of these screening methods is designed to identify cancer at an early stage so that treatment will more likely be effective. Another approach is to prevent occurrence of the cancer by removing the susceptible organs. This woman should, therefore, consider prophylactic mastectomy or oophorectomy. Prevention by treatment with an agent that reduces the risk of developing cancer is another possibility. No agent has yet been demonstrated to be effective in preventing breast or ovarian cancer in high-risk women, but this is an area of active research.

Case 7: Use of the Bayesian Method in Duchenne Muscular Dystrophy

Mrs. D, a 28-year-old woman, consults her physician to find out if she is a carrier for Duchenne muscular dystrophy (DMD), which is an X-linked recessive disease. Her only son has this condition; no other family members are similarly affected.

QUESTION

1. *Based on the information provided, what is the risk that Mrs. D is a carrier of the gene that causes DMD?*

DISCUSSION

Mrs. D's a priori risk of being a carrier is 2/3; there is a 1/3 chance that her affected son represents a new mutation. This conclusion is based on recognition of the likelihood that mutation-selection equilibrium exists in this situation: it is an X-linked recessive disease that is genetically lethal in males and the family history is negative (see Chapter 7 II C 2).

Mrs. D undergoes creatine phosphokinase (CPK) testing, which detects approximately 75% of obligate female carriers of DMD. Her CPK test is normal.

QUESTION

1. Based on the information that is now available, what is the risk that Mrs. D carries a mutation of the dystrophin (DMD) gene?

DISCUSSION

Of those women who are carriers (2/3 of the total), 3/4 are expected to have an abnormal CPK test. Mrs. D does not have an abnormal CPK test, so she must either be a noncarrier or a carrier who has a normal test. The solution may be illustrated with a probability tree (Figure CS 7-1).

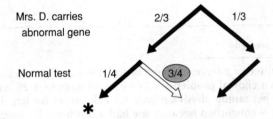

The probability of each alternative event is associated with an *arrow*. Probabilities of 1.0 (i.e., certainties) are indicated as arrows without an alternative. Possibilities contrary to the facts of the case are shown with an *unfilled arrow*. Each event is listed to the left of the probability tree. Arrows pointing toward the *left* indicate occurrence of the event. Arrows pointing to the *right* indicate nonoccurrence. The outcome of interest is indicated by an *asterisk*.

Case 8: Chromosomal Mosaicism

Mrs. Y, a 37-year-old pregnant woman, is referred for counseling because of her age and because she has a nephew with Down syndrome. This is her third pregnancy; she has two healthy children and has had no complications with this pregnancy.

QUESTION

1. What information should the genetic counselor provide to Mrs. Y at this point?

DISCUSSION

After documenting that the nephew has trisomy 21, the counselor should review the age-related risks for chromosome abnormalities and the procedure-related risks for chorionic villus sampling (CVS) and amniocentesis.

After discussion, Mrs. Y chooses CVS, and the test is performed. Mrs. Y's physician receives a call from the laboratory 2 weeks later. The CVS culture demonstrates mosaicism; half of the cells have trisomy 16 and half have a normal karyotype. After discussing the results with the family physician, the genetic counselor meets with Mrs. Y and her husband.

QUESTION

1. *What should the genetic counselor discuss with the couple?*

DISCUSSION

The chromosome findings could represent true mosaicism for the whole conceptus (i.e., including the fetus) or confined placental mosaicism, which is seen in 1%–2% of CVS cultures. The genetic counselor would offer amniocentesis to Mrs. Y to differentiate the two possibilities.

An amniocentesis is performed, and the results demonstrate only cells with a normal karyotype. Also, a detailed ultrasound shows appropriate fetal growth and no evidence of fetal anomalies. The genetic counselor reassures Mrs. Y and her husband but also recommends careful follow-up in terms of fetal growth for the remainder of the pregnancy.

Case 9: Fetal Abnormality

The ethics committee of a large teaching hospital is asked to meet urgently to provide direction on a clinical problem. A 24-year-old woman is 26 weeks pregnant. She presented to her family physician only 1 week earlier for her first prenatal visit. The woman is concerned because she had a brother with spina bifida and severe hydrocephalus who died. Because of this concern, fetal ultrasound was arranged. Unfortunately, the results indicated that the fetus has spina bifida. The woman and her partner returned 1 week later obviously distraught and demanding to terminate the pregnancy. The family physician explained that this would not be possible, at which time the woman tearfully stated that she could neither sleep nor eat and that she would end her life if she could not terminate the pregnancy.

QUESTIONS

1. *What principles are important in this moral dilemma?*

2. *What process should the committee use to evaluate this situation?*

DISCUSSION

The main principles in conflict here are autonomy (the woman's choice to discontinue the pregnancy) and beneficence (the best course for the fetus is continuation of the pregnancy until judged the most appropriate time to balance treatment of the spina bifida and the prematurity).

The committee must start with adequate information. Important issues include: (1) prognosis for the fetus, which requires the help of the local spina bifida treatment group; (2) the couple's understanding of the current treatment and prognosis for neural tube defect; (3) psychiatric assessment and possible counseling and treatment of the woman; and (4) exploration of the couple's family situation and supports.

The committee needs to explore the moral conflicts and the likely outcomes of alternate courses of action. For instance, if labor is induced, the infant will be extremely premature, and in addition to having spina bifida, it may ultimately have iatrogenic complications. If the woman is convinced to continue the pregnancy, she may decompensate further emotionally and feel that she has no choice in the situation. It may be helpful for the committee to recommend that the couple undergo counseling and meet with the spina bifida team as well as the physicians who manage premature infants. Then the committee could meet again to discuss the couple's request. Often, such requests are made while the patients are still in shock after receiving abnormal results and without having full information or support.

Case 10: Blood Samples and Family Studies

A family (a widowed mother, her two adult children, and their spouses) requests counseling and predictive testing. The father died 5 years ago of an adult-onset genetic disorder. His own father and two sisters were also affected. The sisters are still alive and are living in long-term care facilities. Linkage analysis for the condition is available, and blood samples are requested from all appropriate individuals, including the two affected sisters. The extended family has not been close, and, in fact, the husband of one affected sister refuses to allow a blood sample to be taken from his wife. The lab has determined that linkage analysis will not be informative without her blood.

QUESTIONS

1. What are the responsibilities in this situation?

2. Are there ever compelling reasons to insist that a blood sample from an affected individual be made available for family studies?

DISCUSSION

This situation is not unusual when trying to arrange family studies. The reasons may include feelings of guilt or shame on the part of affected individuals, earlier distancing of the normal individuals from the affected individuals, and a feeling that confidentiality will not be preserved. Responsibilities of the genetic counseling service are to provide information to the family members seeking counseling and, at the same time, to suggest ways to end the stalemate regarding the testing.

Outlining predictive testing, suggesting what individuals might do with the information, determining whether specific investigations or monitoring are available to the individual at high risk, or determining whether the information would make a difference in life planning are all items that are essential to the family seeking such testing. Reassuring the family that results are given individually and that there will be no discussion of another's results may alleviate the concerns regarding loss of control over personal information. It may be argued that an essential blood sample for linkage (or for specific molecular analysis) belongs to the family, but patient autonomy should always be considered first. Attempts at restoring communication within the family may help. There are no quick solutions to this dilemma and no one right course.

Case 11: The Uses of Gene Therapy

A gene for male-pattern baldness is isolated and mutations identified. A company is interested in developing gene therapy for male-pattern baldness and marketing such therapy widely. The medical community is at odds over whether this is appropriate use of this technology.

QUESTION

1. What principles are in conflict here?

DISCUSSION

Several ethical principles might be discussed with this example. Beneficence may accrue to those with baldness if treatment allows them to feel better about themselves. However, targeting baldness as an abnormal trait requiring therapy surely has the potential to stigmatize the great many who develop this normal variant of hair loss with age. As the long-term effects of gene therapy are unknown, nonmaleficence should be considered. In deciding the best use of health-care dollars, justice issues arise. Will the development of such cosmetic uses of gene therapy mean that medical uses for rare genetic conditions are jeopardized?

Comprehensive Examination

DIRECTIONS: Each of the numbered items or incomplete statements in this section is followed by answers or by completions of the statement. Select the ONE lettered answer or completion that is BEST in each case.

1. On which one of the following tissue specimens can cytogenetic analysis be performed?

(A) Products of conception that have been preserved frozen from a miscarriage
(B) Chorionic villus cultured for biochemical analysis
(C) A fixed tissue block from a malignant tumor
(D) Dried blood from a routine neonatal screening card
(E) Clotted blood from which the serum has been removed

2. Which one of the following statements about linkage and linkage disequilibrium is correct?

(A) Linkage is measured in family studies; linkage disequilibrium is measured in population studies
(B) Linkage is restricted to loci on a single chromosome; linkage disequilibrium may affect loci on different chromosomes
(C) Linked loci must be polymorphic; linkage disequilibrium may be demonstrated in both polymorphic and nonpolymorphic loci
(D) Linkage refers to alleles; linkage disequilibrium refers to loci
(E) Linkage is usually measured by restriction fragment length polymorphism (RFLP) studies; linkage disequilibrium is measured by cytogenetic studies

3. Which one of the following statements regarding the effects of medical interventions on disease gene frequencies is correct?

(A) Successful treatment of an autosomal dominant disease is likely to decrease the disease frequency substantially in future generations
(B) Successful treatment of an X-linked recessive disease is likely to decrease the disease frequency substantially in future generations
(C) Successful treatment of an autosomal recessive disease is likely to increase the disease frequency substantially in future generations

(D) Genetic counseling is likely to decrease the frequency of disease genes substantially in future generations
(E) None of the above

4. Which one of the following statements about normal phenotypic variation is true?

(A) Most normal characteristics in boys are inherited from their fathers and most normal characteristics in girls are inherited from their mothers
(B) The genes involved are the same in all populations
(C) Environmental factors play a role
(D) Most normal characteristics such as eye or hair color are transmitted as autosomal recessive traits
(E) The occurrence in a child of a more extreme phenotype than in either parent usually results from a new mutation

5. Which one of the following statements about teratogens and mutagens is correct?

(A) An agent cannot act as both a teratogen and a mutagen
(B) Exposures of either the mother or the father may produce teratogenic effects
(C) Mutagens produce their effects by alteration of the proteins of the ova or sperm
(D) Mutagens affect single cells; teratogens affect groups of cells
(E) Birth defects due to mutagens are more common than birth defects due to teratogens

6. Major events of early mammalian embryogenesis include

(A) establishment of clonal cell lineages with predetermined fates
(B) segmentation
(C) amplification of preformed maternal messenger RNA (mRNA)
(D) activation of proto-oncogenes

7. Measurement of the serum creatine phosphokinase (CPK) level can detect approximately 75% of obligate carriers of Duchenne muscular dystrophy (DMD), an X-linked recessive condition that is lethal in males. A 26-year-old woman had a brother who died of DMD at age 18. There is no other family history of DMD. CPK testing is done on the woman and the result is normal. What is the risk for DMD in her son?

(A) 1/4
(B) 1/6
(C) 1/8
(D) 1/10
(E) 1/18

8. The father of a 24-year-old male patient has a diagnosis of Huntington disease and is cared for at home. Several paternal relatives are similarly affected, and most are now in long-term care facilities. The patient and his wife request predictive testing. All appropriate blood samples are obtained, and the results obtained in duplicate indicate that there is nonpaternity; that is, the patient's biologic father is not the legal and affected father. The mother is interviewed separately and gently but does not confirm the genetic interpretation. Which one of the following approaches would best aid the patient and his wife in planning their future?

(A) Respect the autonomy of the mother and tell the patient the molecular testing was not informative
(B) Impress upon the mother the importance of divulging the results to her son
(C) Respect the autonomy of the mother, say nothing about the nonpaternity, but tell the patient the results indicate he has not inherited the Huntington allele
(D) Call the couple in and review all the results, including the nonpaternity; ask the young man not to tell his mother about the nonpaternity

9. Which one of the following statements best describes genetic polymorphisms?

(A) They usually alter protein structure and function
(B) They allow tissues from identical twins to be distinguished
(C) They reflect alterations of DNA sequence
(D) They are usually apparent on careful physical examination
(E) They are demonstrated by cytogenetic analysis

10. Which one of the following statements regarding multifactorial congenital anomalies is true?

(A) Defects typically occur with other embryologically unrelated malformations in an affected patient
(B) Defects usually have a characteristic appearance that distinguishes them from similar defects due to other causes
(C) Concordance for defects is similar in monozygotic and dizygotic twins
(D) Recurrence risks for defects are similar in the siblings and children of an affected patient
(E) Defects typically occur with equal frequency in both sexes

11. Which one of the following statements about teratogenesis is correct?

(A) The likelihood that an agent will produce a teratogenic effect can usually be predicted on the basis of its pharmacologic action in an infant
(B) The teratogenic effect of exposure to a combination of agents can usually be predicted by "adding" the effects of the individual agents in the combination
(C) The period during which the embryo is most susceptible to teratogenic effects is usually the first 2 weeks after conception
(D) Congenital anomalies are unlikely to be produced by exposure to teratogenic agents later than 10 weeks after conception
(E) The circumstances, route, and dosage of exposure are as important in determining teratogenic risk as the chemical nature of the agent

12. A woman who was affected by Rh hemolytic disease as a newborn married a man who did not have Rh hemolytic disease as a newborn but who had an elder brother and sister who died of this condition. What is the chance that their children will have Rh hemolytic disease?

(A) 0
(B) 12.5%
(C) 25%
(D) 50%
(E) 100%

13. X chromosome inactivation in females is best described by which one of the following statements?

(A) It involves all genes on the X chromosome
(B) It occurs during adolescence
(C) It is associated with demethylation of the affected chromosome
(D) It produces dosage compensation for X-linked genes
(E) It is responsible for the phenotypic abnormalities that occur in girls with Turner syndrome (45,X)

14. Which one of the following statements regarding treatment of genetic diseases is true?

(A) Genetic diseases cannot be treated if they are congenital
(B) Genetic diseases that are etiologically heterogeneous cannot be treated
(C) Genetic diseases can only be treated if they are understood at least in part at the biochemical level
(D) Diagnostic precision is often critically important in designing effective treatment for genetic diseases
(E) Treatment of genetic diseases requires proper regulation of the therapeutic gene

15. A woman was treated throughout pregnancy with Kulout, a newly introduced tranquilizer. Her infant has cleft lip and cleft palate. Which one of the following observations provides the strongest evidence that this association is causal?

(A) The frequency of cleft palate is increased among the offspring of rats treated during pregnancy with 100 times the human dose of Kulout
(B) Kulout is metabolized through the same metabolic pathway as thalidomide
(C) Six other cases of congenital anomalies among children of women who took Kulout during pregnancy have been observed: One child has congenital heart disease, one has club feet, one has hypospadias, one has Down syndrome, one has spina bifida, and one has a cavernous hemangioma
(D) The infant has several other congenital anomalies in addition to cleft lip and cleft palate, and the same pattern of anomalies has been noted in three other children whose mothers took Kulout early in pregnancy
(E) A clinical geneticist has examined the infant and says that she does not have a recognized genetic syndrome

16. Genetic disease is most often treated by which one of the following methods?

(A) Somatic gene therapy
(B) Organ transplantation
(C) Modulation of gene expression
(D) Amelioration of metabolic abnormalities
(E) Amelioration of the clinical phenotype

17. Prenatal diagnosis for neural tube defects is indicated in a pregnant woman who

(A) has long-standing, insulin-dependent diabetes mellitus
(B) had rubella during the first trimester of pregnancy
(C) has used marijuana daily throughout gestation
(D) had an abdominal x-ray early in gestation
(E) took androgenic hormones for bodybuilding before finding out that she was pregnant

18. Which of the following statements regarding the teratogenic effects of alcohol abuse is true?

(A) Maternal binge drinking a few times early in pregnancy does not pose a risk to the fetus
(B) Maternal drinking of less than 3 ounces of absolute alcohol (i.e., the equivalent of about 6 beers) per day during pregnancy is unlikely to produce an adverse effect in the fetus
(C) Behavioral abnormalities often occur in children with fetal alcohol syndrome
(D) Limb reduction defects such as phocomelia are common features of fetal alcohol syndrome
(E) Growth deficiency is common but mental retardation is uncommon in fetal alcohol syndrome

Questions 19–21

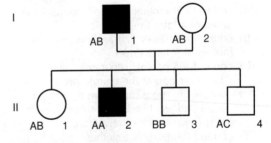

The figure above shows the DNA typing results for a family that has multiple endocrine neoplasia type II (MEN II), an autosomal dominant disease associated with a greatly increased risk for developing various tumors, including medullary thyroid carcinoma, pheochromocytoma, and parathyroid adenomas. Family member I-1 has MEN II, as does his son, II-2. Family members II-1, II-3, and II-4 want to know what their risk is of having inherited the abnormal gene. The family members have had DNA analysis with a marker approximately 2 cM from the mutation causing MEN II.

19. In comparison to her risk before testing, the risk for MEN II in II-1, knowing her DNA results is

(A) greatly increased
(B) greatly decreased
(C) mildly increased
(D) mildly decreased
(E) unchanged

20. In comparison to his risk before testing, the risk for MEN II in II-3, knowing his DNA results is

(A) greatly increased
(B) greatly decreased
(C) mildly increased
(D) mildly decreased
(E) unchanged

21. In comparison to his risk before testing, the risk for MEN II in II-3, knowing his DNA results is

(A) greatly increased
(B) greatly decreased
(C) mildly increased
(D) mildly decreased
(E) unchanged

22. In discussing the likelihood that an infant who has just been examined has Down syndrome, it is usually desirable to

(A) counsel the mother first and counsel the father at a later time
(B) counsel the father first and counsel the mother at a later time
(C) counsel the parents separately, taking whichever parent the couple prefers first
(D) counsel the more intelligent or composed parent and ask him or her to explain the information to the other parent
(E) counsel the parents together

23. Allelic heterogeneity is best described by which one of the following statements?

(A) It is most common in autosomal recessive diseases in extensively inbred populations
(B) It accounts for the occurrence of similar

phenotypes in individuals with mutations at different genetic loci
(C) It has been demonstrated in most genetic diseases for which mutations have been characterized molecularly
(D) It produces alterations of gene expression without changes in the DNA sequence
(E) It results from the effects of genes at other loci on the expression of a mutant allele

24. What proportion of early spontaneous abortions are chromosomally abnormal?

(A) 1%
(B) 5%
(C) 10%
(D) 25%
(E) 50%

25. Which one of the following combinations of active and inactive X chromosomes is found in 49,XXXXY individuals?

(A) No active and 4 inactive X chromosomes
(B) 1 active and 3 inactive X chromosomes
(C) 2 active and 2 inactive X chromosomes
(D) 3 active and 1 inactive X chromosomes
(E) 4 active and no inactive X chromosomes

Questions 26–29

Cystic fibrosis (CF), an autosomal recessive disease, occurs with a frequency of 1/2500 among people of northern European origin. What is the approximate risk of CF in a child of each of the following matings within this population?

(A) 1/25
(B) 1/50
(C) 1/100
(D) 1/400
(E) None of the above

26. A man and woman, neither of whom has a family history of CF

27. A woman with CF whose husband has no family history of CF

28. A woman whose first cousin has CF and a man who has no family history of CF

29. A man who has a child with CF by a previous marriage and a woman with no family history of CF

30. Genomic imprinting is best described by which one of the following statements?

(A) It produces differential expression of genes depending on whether they were inherited from the father or mother
(B) It affects most genes except those on the sex chromosomes
(C) It occurs only in female gametes
(D) It is reversed or removed when a cell passes through mitosis
(E) It reflects a change in the DNA sequence of affected genes

31. The Fanconi pancytopenia syndrome and Bloom syndrome are autosomal recessive conditions in which there is an increased risk of developing malignancy. Cytogenetically, both syndromes are associated with

(A) triploidy
(B) trisomy
(C) monosomy
(D) chromosome breakage
(E) fragile sites

32. The human haploid genome is composed of approximately

(A) 3 billion base pairs of DNA and 70,000 genes
(B) 3 billion base pairs of DNA and 7000 genes
(C) 3 million base pairs of DNA and 70,000 genes
(D) 3 million base pairs of DNA and 7000 genes
(E) 70,000 base pairs of DNA and 3 million genes

33. Indirect DNA diagnosis is useful only for which one of the following situations?

(A) Diseases caused by dynamic mutations
(B) Diseases that have considerable allelic heterogeneity
(C) Within populations that exhibit linkage disequilibrium
(D) Within families that have multiple affected members who are informative for closely linked markers
(E) Loci that are not polymorphic

34. Anticipation is characteristic of conditions caused by

(A) microdeletions
(B) mitochondrial inheritance
(C) genomic imprinting

(D) trinucleotide repeat expansions
(E) germ-line mosaicism

35. The differences between type I (insulin-dependent) and type II (noninsulin-dependent) diabetes mellitus include

(A) type II diabetes is associated with human leukocyte antigen (HLA)-DR3 and HLA-DR4; type I diabetes is not
(B) concordance in monozygotic twins is higher for type I diabetes than for type II diabetes
(C) islet cell autoimmunity is frequently present in patients with type I diabetes but not in patients with type II diabetes
(D) type I diabetes is usually associated with obesity; type II diabetes is not
(E) type I diabetes is usually inherited as an autosomal recessive trait; type II diabetes is usually a multifactorial condition

36. Meiosis II in the human oocyte is completed

(A) in the fetus
(B) at the time of puberty
(C) just before ovulation
(D) during ovulation
(E) just after fertilization

37. Uniparental disomy (UPD) is best described by which one of the following statements?

(A) It occurs when both chromosomes in a pair have been inherited from the same parent
(B) It means that all the chromosomes in a diploid set have been inherited from the same parent
(C) It usually is inherited from the mother in Down syndrome
(D) It is the most common cause of triploidy
(E) It may result in the expression of an autosomal recessive disease in a heterozygote

38. Linkage between two loci is considered likely if the lod score is

(A) lower than -2 at a recombination distance of less than 50 centimorgans (cM)
(B) lower than -2 at a recombination distance of more than 50 cM
(C) higher than $+3$ at a recombination distance of less than 50 cM
(D) higher than $+3$ at a recombination distance of more then 50 cM

39. Patients with tuberculosis who are treated with isoniazid and who are rapid acetylators are more likely to

(A) have allergic reactions
(B) develop neurotoxicity
(C) have recurrence of tuberculosis
(D) require just a short course of therapy

40. Most nuclear DNA in humans consists of which one of the following types of sequences?

(A) Unique sequences that function as genes
(B) Repetitive sequences such as short interspersed repeated sequences (SINES) and long interspersed repeated sequences (LINES)
(C) Introns
(D) Exons
(E) Operons

41. DNA banking is particularly useful when

(A) a specific disease mutation is known to exist within a family
(B) a child has been shown to have a genetic disease due to a new dominant mutation

(C) the gene for a particular disease in a family has not yet been identified, but its pattern of inheritance is clear
(D) a family is known to be segregating a balanced robertsonian translocation
(E) a family exhibits a genetic polymorphism that does not have any clinical manifestations

42. Ethnic differences in disease frequencies are most apparent for

(A) autosomal dominant conditions
(B) autosomal recessive conditions
(C) X-linked recessive conditions
(D) autosomal trisomies
(E) sex chromosome aneuploidies

43. Which one of the following statements best describes most malignant neoplasms?

(A) They are associated with constitutional chromosomal abnormalities
(B) They are of multifactorial etiology
(C) They are due to an inherited mutation of an oncogene
(D) They result from activation of tumor suppressor genes

DIRECTIONS: Each of the numbered items or incomplete statements in this section is negatively phrased, as indicated by a capitalized word such as NOT, LEAST, or EXCEPT. Select the ONE lettered answer or completion that is BEST in each case.

---

44. Differences between meiosis and mitosis include all of the following EXCEPT

(A) meiosis results in a reduction of chromosome number in the cell from 46 to 23, whereas mitosis does not result in a change in chromosome number
(B) mitosis is preceded by a single round of DNA synthesis; meiosis is preceded by two rounds of DNA synthesis
(C) all somatic cells undergo mitosis, but meiosis is restricted to germ cells
(D) recombination is much more common in meiosis than in mitosis
(E) chromosome pairing (synapsis) occurs in meiosis but not in mitosis

45. One member of a young couple has been found to carry a balanced reciprocal translocation. Important factors to consider in determining the risk that this couple will have a child with chromosome imbalance may include all of the following EXCEPT

(A) the number of spontaneous abortions they have had
(B) how the couple was ascertained
(C) the sex of the affected partner
(D) whether any carrier in the family has had a liveborn child with a chromosome imbalance
(E) the particular chromosome segments involved

46. All of the following statements about genetic markers are true EXCEPT they

(A) are inherited as typical multifactorial traits
(B) have alternate forms that are readily recognizable
(C) may be detected as alterations in DNA sequence or protein structure or function
(D) can be used clinically in linkage studies
(E) are used to identify individuals in forensic medicine

47. The Hardy-Weinberg law is based on all of the following assumptions EXCEPT

(A) mating within the population is completely random
(B) the genes involved are autosomal dominant
(C) there is no mutation occurring at the locus
(D) there is no selection for or against any of the genotypes at the locus
(E) there is no migration into or out of the population

48. A couple has a child with Tay-Sachs disease, an autosomal recessive condition associated with lack of the enzyme hexosaminidase A. All of the following statements are likely to apply to this family EXCEPT

(A) heterozygotes are mildly affected with Tay-Sachs disease
(B) heterozygotes can be detected because their levels of hexosaminidase A are intermediate between those of normal homozygotes and affected homozygotes
(C) prenatal diagnosis is available by measuring the level of hexosaminidase A in amniocytes
(D) siblings of the affected child are at low risk to have affected children themselves
(E) There may be a milder disease involving the same enzyme

49. All of the following infectious agents are potentially teratogenic in humans EXCEPT

(A) rubella virus
(B) gonococcus
(C) chicken pox (varicella) virus
(D) cytomegalovirus (CMV)
(E) *Toxoplasma gondii*

50. A physician is called to the nursery to examine a newborn with ambiguous genitalia. The infant has a small phallic structure with hypospadias, bilateral cryptorchidism, but no other obvious problems. All of the following studies will help to establish the diagnosis within a few days EXCEPT

(A) karyotyping
(B) urinary 17-ketosteroid levels
(C) ultrasound examination of the lower abdomen
(D) androgen-binding studies on genital skin cells
(E) serum electrolyte determinations

51. A 32-year-old woman has blood drawn for maternal serum triple screening in her first pregnancy. The result is reported with a computer-generated interpretation that indicates that her fetus has a significantly increased risk for Down syndrome. All of the following should be done to follow-up this risk EXCEPT

(A) verifying that the gestational age used in the interpretation is correct
(B) checking that the patient's correct age was included in the interpretation
(C) undertaking a detailed ultrasound examination for assessment of fetal anatomy
(D) offering the patient amniocentesis for fetal karyotyping
(E) obtaining blood from the patient for chromosome analysis

52. Genetic screening is justified in each of the following cases EXCEPT to

(A) detect female carriers of a lethal X-linked recessive disease within the family of an affected boy
(B) identify couples at high risk of having children with a life-threatening inborn metabolic error
(C) identify individuals who have a low genetic risk of heart attack so they can be provided life insurance at lower rates
(D) identify relatives likely to be affected within families of patients with a late-onset autosomal dominant neurodegenerative disease before development of symptoms
(E) detect carriers of a dominant gene that predisposes to a serious complication of anesthesia within an ethnic community with a high incidence of the disorder

53. Each of the following statements about direct and indirect DNA diagnosis of genetic disease is true EXCEPT

(A) at least part of the affected gene must be cloned before direct testing is possible
(B) direct DNA testing is more accurate than indirect testing
(C) DNA from other family members is needed for indirect approaches to DNA diagnosis
(D) genetic heterogeneity may complicate indirect approaches to DNA testing
(E) DNA polymorphisms that are closely linked to the disease gene are used in direct DNA testing

54. Each of the following statements about studies that are used to identify teratogenic effects in humans is true EXCEPT

(A) most associations observed in individual case reports are causal
(B) a causal relationship is suggested by a recurrent pattern of congenital anomalies among infants born to women with similar exposures during pregnancy
(C) most human teratogens have been recognized initially in clinical series
(D) both cohort studies and case-control studies are often subject to serious biases of ascertainment
(E) animal studies alone cannot prove that an exposure is teratogenic in humans

55. Twin studies are important tools in the analysis of multifactorial diseases, but such studies have several inherent problems. All of the following are important factors in interpreting twin studies EXCEPT

(A) accurate determination of zygosity
(B) method of ascertainment
(C) inclusion of identical numbers of monozygotic and dizygotic pairs
(D) etiologic heterogeneity

56. Examples of symptomatic treatment of genetic disease include all of the following EXCEPT

(A) restriction of phenylalanine in the diet of patients with phenylketonuria (PKU)
(B) use of hearing aids in hereditary deafness
(C) administration of antibiotics for pulmonary infections in cystic fibrosis (CF)
(D) speech therapy for a child with cleft palate
(E) plastic surgery to correct facial malformation in a dominantly inherited multiple congenital anomaly syndrome

57. All of the following statements regarding genetic mutations are true EXCEPT

(A) the mutations underlying most genetic diseases are known
(B) mutations involving only one or a few nucleotides are more common than those involving large portions of the gene

(C) deletions are common causes of mutation in Duchenne muscular dystrophy (DMD)
(D) the majority of Jewish people with Tay-Sachs disease have the same mutation
(E) the majority of persons with cystic fibrosis (CF) have the same mutation

58. All of the following statements about an association seen in an epidemiology study of birth defects are true EXCEPT the

(A) association may occur because both the child's anomaly and the mother's exposure are related to another factor
(B) association is more likely to be causal if pregnant women exposed to a much higher dose of the agent have a higher risk of having affected children than pregnant women exposed to a lower dose
(C) association is more likely to be causal if similar congenital anomalies can be induced in the offspring of rats subjected to similar exposures during pregnancy
(D) agent is likely to be an important cause of birth defects if the relative risk is less than 0.05
(E) association may be due to chance even if it is statistically significant

59. Chromosome abnormalities that develop in association with neoplasms often involve all of the following EXCEPT

(A) oncogene activation
(B) loss of tumor suppressor genes
(C) clonal evolution
(D) transmission to the offspring of an affected individual

60. Thalassemia and glucose-6-phosphate dehydrogenase (G6PD) deficiency are genetic diseases of the red blood cells that occur commonly among Africans. Each of the following statements about this association is true EXCEPT the mutant genes

(A) are thought to provide protection against malaria in some circumstances
(B) were probably selected for in some African populations
(C) are rarely seen in people whose ancestry is not African
(D) may cause disease in people living in areas in which malaria occurs
(E) may cause disease in people living in areas in which malaria does not occur

61. Certain abnormalities of the sex chromosomes have been associated with behavioral or psychiatric problems. All of the following statements regarding such associations are true EXCEPT

(A) XYY males tend to be immature and impulsive
(B) females with Turner syndrome often have psychiatric illnesses and are frequently mentally retarded
(C) Klinefelter syndrome (XXY) is associated with poor judgment and learning problems in children
(D) Klinefelter syndrome (XXY) is associated with an increased incidence of schizophrenia
(E) XXX females show an increased incidence of schizophrenia

62. A 35-year-old pregnant woman decides to have amniocentesis because of her age. The results are reported to her physician, and, although the fetus does not have Down syndrome, a chromosomal abnormality (47,XYY) was found. The physician knows that most such males are clinically normal, and he tells the patient only that her infant does not have Down syndrome. All of the following ethical principles are involved in this situation EXCEPT

(A) veracity
(B) autonomy
(C) beneficence
(D) fidelity
(E) justice

63. Each of the following statements concerning the relationship of genes and proteins is true EXCEPT

(A) every protein is encoded by one or more genes
(B) all biochemical processes are genetically controlled
(C) each step of a biochemical pathway is under the control of a different gene or genes
(D) all gene mutations result in alteration of the corresponding protein
(E) all mendelian diseases result from quantitative or qualitative abnormalities of one or more proteins

64. Microdeletion syndromes result from

small cytogenetic lesions that usually can only be demonstrated by high resolution banding studies or fluorescent in situ hybridization (FISH). All of the following conditions are often associated with chromosome microdeletions EXCEPT

(A) Angelman syndrome
(B) Cri du chat (cat cry) syndrome
(C) Miller-Dieker (lissencephaly) syndrome
(D) Prader-Willi syndrome
(E) Williams syndrome

65. Each of the following statements about mutation is correct EXCEPT

(A) somatic cell mutations play an important role in the development of cancer
(B) most mutations are recessive and are expressed only when homozygous
(C) most mutations are repaired to the normal state
(D) high-dose x-rays are mutagenic in human and experimental animal cells
(E) chemical agents that have been shown to produce transmissible gametic mutations in humans include cyclophosphamide and dioxin

66. Each of the following statements about chromosome abnormalities in malignancies is true EXCEPT

(A) acquired chromosome abnormalities occur in most leukemias, but such changes are uncommon in solid tumors
(B) the karyotype of a neoplasm tends to become more abnormal as its behavior becomes more malignant
(C) chromosome abnormalities in the affected tissue may precede clinical evidence of relapse
(D) different cells within a neoplasm often exhibit different chromosomal abnormalities
(E) individual neoplastic cells often have several different chromosome abnormalities

67. A proto-oncogene may be activated by any of the following mechanisms EXCEPT

(A) placing it under the control of another promoter
(B) chromosome rearrangement
(C) point mutation
(D) amplification
(E) deletion

68. Which of the following is NOT an indication for fetal karyotyping?

(A) maternal age of 39 years
(B) a previous child with trisomy 21
(C) a fetus shown to have a cystic hygroma on ultrasound
(D) spina bifida in the mother
(E) a robertsonian translocation in the father

69. Successful genetic counseling helps a patient or family to do all of the following EXCEPT

(A) adjust to and accept the disease in the family
(B) understand the nature, prognosis, and treatment of the condition
(C) understand the mode of inheritance and the recurrence risk
(D) understand the available reproductive options
(E) reduce the frequency of the abnormal gene in the population

---

DIRECTIONS: Each set of matching questions in this section consists of a list of four to twenty-six lettered options (some of which may be in figures) followed by several numbered items. For each numbered item, select the ONE lettered option that is most closely associated with it. To avoid spending too much time on matching sets with large numbers of options, it is generally advisable to begin each set by reading the list of options. Then, for each item in the set, try to generate the correct answer and locate it in the option list, rather than evaluating each option individually. Each lettered option may be selected once, more than once, or not at all.

Questions 70–73

For each clinical description given below, select the most closely associated kind of genetic disease.

(A) Chromosome abnormality
(B) Multifactorial inheritance
(C) X-linked recessive mutation
(D) Autosomal recessive mutation
(E) Autosomal dominant mutation

70. Disease is caused by a combination of genetic and nongenetic influences

71. Disease affects males almost exclusively

72. Disease occurs only when both genes in a pair are mutant and located on a chromosome other than X or Y

73. The mechanism responsible for most common diseases of adulthood, such as coronary artery disease and noninsulin-dependent diabetes

Questions 74–78

Match the following clinical descriptions with the most likely chromosome abnormality.

(A) Triploidy
(B) Trisomy 13
(C) Trisomy 18
(D) Trisomy 21
(E) Monosomy X

74. Flat occiput, Brushfield's spots, atrioventricular canal cardiac defect, single palmar creases

75. Small-for-age infant with small facies, congenital heart disease, peculiar hand positioning, rocker-bottom heels

76. Stillborn infant with holoprosencephaly, polydactyly, midline cleft lip and palate

77. Second trimester abortus with cystic hygroma and massive hydrops

78. Spontaneous abortus with large cystic placenta and a growth-disorganized embryo

Questions 79–83

Match the most appropriate description to the kind of genetic polymorphism it characterizes.

(A) Restriction fragment length polymorphisms (RFLPs)
(B) Minisatellites
(C) Enzyme activity variants
(D) Antigenic protein variants
(E) Chromosome heteromorphisms

79. These are often so polymorphic that two unrelated people are unlikely to share the same alleles

80. These are important in blood transfusion

81. These may produce illness if a patient is exposed to certain drugs

82. These are used in DNA fingerprinting in forensic medicine

83. These often reflect an alteration of a single nucleotide that produces gain or loss of a site recognized by certain enzymes

Questions 84–88

A deranged former employee snuck into the hospital nursery and clipped the identification bracelets from five newborn boys. In order to straighten the situation out, blood typing has been done on the infants and their parents. Match the following parents to the correct infant.

(A) Infant A: O, MN, Rh$^+$
(B) Infant B: A, MN, Rh$^-$
(C) Infant C: A, M, Rh$^+$
(D) Infant D: AB, N, Rh$^+$
(E) Infant E: B, MN, Rh$^+$

Family	Mother Blood Group			Father Blood Group		
	ABO	MN	Rh	ABO	MN	Rh
84.	B	N	Rh$^-$	A	MN	Rh$^-$
85.	B	N	Rh$^+$	AB	N	Rh$^-$
86.	AB	MN	Rh$^+$	O	MN	Rh$^+$
87.	O	M	Rh$^+$	A	M	Rh$^+$
88.	A	M	Rh$^+$	A	N	Rh$^+$

Questions 89–93

For each of the following patients, match the most appropriate form of prenatal diagnosis.

(A) Chorionic villus sampling (CVS)
(B) Maternal serum triple screening
(C) Amniocentesis
(D) Detailed ultrasound examination
(E) Fetal blood sampling

89. A pregnant woman who previously delivered a stillborn infant who had normal chromosomes but multiple abnormalities, including congenital heart disease, polydactyly, and cleft palate

90. A pregnant woman who is a heterozygous carrier of Duchenne muscular dystrophy (DMD), in a family in which affected males have a deletion involving the dystrophin gene

91. A woman identified by ultrasound to have a 20-week fetus with nuchal edema and duodenal stenosis or atresia

92. A 25-year-old primigravida with an unremarkable family history who is extremely concerned about her risk for having a baby with Down syndrome

93. A healthy 36-year-old woman who is 14 weeks pregnant

Questions 94–96

Match each description of a cytogenetic technique with the most appropriate term.

(A) Q banding
(B) G banding
(C) R banding
(D) Fluorescent in situ hybridization (FISH)

94. The most commonly used method for

chromosome analysis; the standard in most laboratories

95. A method of cytogenetic preparation in which bands that stain darkly with the standard method fluoresce brightly

96. A method that can be used to demonstrate the position of single-copy genes on chromosomes

Questions 97–101

A locus for dominantly inherited breast cancer, *BRCA1*, is located on the long arm of chromosome 17. A marker locus that is 4 centimorgans (cM) from the *BRCA1* locus has two alleles, called *1* and *2*. In a particular family with this disease, a woman with breast cancer (II-3) has an affected mother (I-1) and two affected sisters (II-1 and II-5). The genotypes in the family are shown under the symbols in the pedigree below.

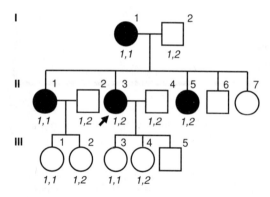

Match each of the following individuals with their risk for inheriting the *BRCA1* mutation.

(A) 2%
(B) 4%
(C) 48%
(D) 50%
(E) 96%

97. Individual II-7, who has not yet been tested for the marker

98. Individual III-3

99. Individual III-4

100. Individual III-1

101. Individual III-2

Questions 102–104

Several research methods are used to study the genetic contribution to psychiatric illness. Match each description below to the study method it best fits.

(A) Cohort study
(B) Pedigree analysis
(C) Adoption study
(D) Family interview
(E) Linkage analysis

102. Allows distinction between genetic and environmental components in psychiatric illness

103. Tends to underestimate psychiatric morbidity

104. Allows identification of mild psychiatric illness

Questions 105–109

A 5-year-old boy who presents with muscle weakness is diagnosed as having Duchenne muscular dystrophy (DMD). The physician approaches the family because she has heard about a trial of a new drug that promises to slow the rate of loss of muscle strength. The physician insists that the trial coordinator review the consent process with the child's mother before the physician herself discusses the trial with the family. Match each of the following aspects of informed consent with the ethical principle it illustrates.

(A) Veracity
(B) Autonomy
(C) Beneficence
(D) Justice
(E) Fidelity

105. The right of the family *not* to participate in the trial

106. Full discussion of the risks and benefits of the drug

107. The signatures of both the mother and the investigator on the consent form indicating acceptance

108. The initial approach to the family by their physician

109. The right to the same care should the patient refuse to enter the trial

Questions 110–115

The most common type of color blindness, green-shift, is seen in 5% of Caucasian males and is inherited as an X-linked recessive trait. The mutant allele (g) causes a shift in the absorption of a green-sensitive pigment. Females can have three different genotypes, GG, Gg, and gg, whereas males are either GY or gY. Match the most likely outcomes to the following matings.

(A) $GG \times GY$
(B) $GG \times gY$
(C) $Gg \times GY$
(D) $Gg \times gY$
(E) $gg \times gY$
(F) $gg \times GY$

110. The risk of having affected daughters is 50%

111. May have both normal and affected sons and both homozygous normal and heterozygous daughters

112. All offspring are clinically affected

113. All daughters are homozygous normal

114. All offspring are clinically normal, but daughters are all heterozygous carriers

115. All daughters are heterozygous carriers; all sons are affected

Questions 116–119

For each clinical situation described below, select the corresponding congenital anomaly.

(A) Malformation
(B) Disruption
(C) Deformation
(D) Dysplasia

116. A child has short legs because of abnormal formation of cartilage in the long bones

117. A child is born with only her right kidney because of complete loss of blood supply to the left kidney at 14 weeks of development

118. A twin has an indentation in his skull because his head and his twin's head were both tightly jammed into the mother's pelvis during the last month of pregnancy

119. A child is born with severe chorioretinitis and blindness of her right eye because of an in utero rubella infection

Questions 120–124

For each clinical presentation listed below, match the correct condition.

(A) Pure gonadal dysgenesis
(B) 21-Hydroxylase deficiency
(C) 5α-Reductase deficiency
(D) Mixed gonadal dysgenesis
(E) Androgen insensitivity

120. A phenotypic male infant is brought into the emergency room with vomiting and dehydration; he has no dysmorphic features, but the intern notices that the infant does have bilateral cryptorchidism

121. A 6-month-old female infant presents with an inguinal hernia, which at surgery is found to contain a gonad that is a normal testis

122. While an infant is being assessed for a suspected coarctation of the aorta, she is noted to have neck webbing, a shield-shaped chest, and an enlarged clitoris; her chromosomes show the presence of two cell lines

123. A 17-year-old girl presents with primary amenorrhea and is noted to have normal stature, mild neck webbing, and, on ultrasound, a normal-sized uterus but a mass in the right ovarian area; she has no breast development as yet; chromosomes are 46,XY

124. An infant is noted to have ambiguous genitalia and severe hypospadias, with the urethral opening on the perineum; gonads are present in a bifid scrotum; there is no evidence of a uterus on ultrasound; serum testosterone levels are normal

Questions 125–128

For each clinical description given below, select the corresponding pattern of anomalies.

(A) Sequence
(B) Developmental field defect
(C) Syndrome
(D) Association

125. A child has congenital heart disease, abnormal external ears, and hydrocephalus as a result of maternal treatment with isotretinoin during pregnancy

126. A child has club feet, which have resulted from decreased fetal movement because of spina bifida and consequent lack of innervation of the lower limbs

127. A stillborn female infant has lumbar vertebral defects, renal agenesis, sirenomelia (fusion of the legs into a single midline appendage), and absence of the vagina, uterus, and fallopian tubes, all of which result from abnormal development of the caudal mesoderm before the fourth week of gestation

128. A child has thrombocytopenia, bilateral absence of the radius, ulnar hypoplasia, and congenital heart disease, all of which form a pattern of anomalies known to be transmitted as an autosomal recessive trait

Questions 129–132

Match each description below with the term to which it is most closely related.

(A) Positive eugenics
(B) Negative eugenics
(C) New mutations
(D) Genetic lethals
(E) Lethal equivalents

129. Rare in the general population but common among patients with autosomal dominant diseases that reduce fertility

130. Each person carries an average of three to five of these

131. Accounts for the increased risk of some dominant diseases among the children of older fathers

132. Seeks to decrease the propagation of "less desirable" types of people

Questions 133–137

Match the descriptions with the appropriate method of DNA analysis.

(A) Allele-specific oligonucleotide (ASO) analysis
(B) DNA sequencing
(C) Electrophoresis of single-stranded DNA
(D) Fluorescent in situ hybridization (FISH)
(E) Polymerase chain reaction (PCR)
(F) Southern blot

133. Identifies mutations by hybridization using synthetic short DNA probes specific for a normal gene and for a particular known mutation of the same gene

134. The most precise way to characterize a segment of DNA completely

135. A technique that employs enzymatic amplification of a DNA fragment flanked by two specific oligonucleotide sequences

136. A technique in which fragments of patient DNA cut with restriction endonucleases are separated by gel electrophoresis and then hybridized with a specific labeled nucleotide probe

137. A technique for rapid screening of a gene for many different point mutations

Questions 138–142

Match the following diseases with the mutation-induced protein alterations with which they are usually associated.

(A) β-Thalassemia
(B) Cystic fibrosis (CF)
(C) Galactosemia
(D) Huntington disease
(E) Osteogenesis imperfecta
(F) Phenylketonuria (PKU)
(G) Tay-Sachs disease

138. Alteration of a major collagen of connective tissue

139. Alteration of a cell-membrane transport protein

140. Alteration of a protein by expansion of a segment encoded by an amplified region of tri-nucleotide repeats

141. Dysfunction of an enzyme involved in removing sugar side-chains from long-chain lipids

142. Dysfunction of an enzyme that converts one sugar to another

ANSWERS AND EXPLANATIONS

1. The answer is B [Chapter 1 IV C 1]. Cytogenetic studies require dividing cells and thus can only be performed on living tissue. Frozen, fixed, or dried material of any sort is unsatisfactory. Chromosome analysis is performed on heparinized blood specimens; clotted blood cannot be used. Cytogenetic studies can be performed on a variety of growing tissues, including specimens obtained via amniocentesis, chorionic villus sampling, or skin biopsy, or from fresh autopsy materials.

2. The answer is A [Chapter 5 I A–C]. Linkage is the occurrence of two or more genetic loci in such close proximity on a chromosome that they are likely to segregate together at meiosis. Since linkage is a result of meiosis, it can only be measured in studies in which the products of meiosis are determined (i.e., in family studies). Linkage disequilibrium is the tendency for certain alleles at linked loci to occur together more often than expected by chance. Linkage disequilibrium is demonstrated with respect to allele frequencies in a population and can only be measured in population studies.

3. The answer is E [Chapter 7 III A 1–3]. Neither treatment of genetic diseases nor genetic counseling is likely to have a substantial effect on the frequencies of disease genes in future generations. Prevention and treatment of genetic disease benefit individual patients and families. The effect on the frequencies of the disease genes in future pregnancies is generally negligible.

4. The answer is C [Chapter 9 III B]. Normal variation usually results from the combined effects of many genetic and nongenetic factors; it is multifactorial. On the average, each parent contributes half of the genetic factors involved in any particular trait to a child, regardless of sex. The genes involved in normal variation may differ in different populations. Whereas the genetic endowment of an individual determines the range of potential development of a normal trait such as intelligence, full achievement of the genetic potential depends on an optimal environment. Extreme values of a phenotype are uncommon on the basis of normal variation but may occur. Thus, a child may be taller or lighter skinned or more intelligent than her parents if she happens by chance to have inherited more of the extreme predisposing factors from both her mother and father.

5. The answer is D [Chapter 10 II A, C, D; III A, B]. Mutagens cause alteration of the genetic material (DNA or chromosomes) in a single cell. In contrast, teratogens affect the development of a tissue, organ, or structure. Many mutagens, such as irradiation with x-rays and some cancer chemotherapeutic agents, are also potentially teratogenic. Since teratogens affect the developing embryo or fetus, they typically act via exposure of the mother and not the father. Approximately 10% of congenital anomalies are thought to be due to teratogenic effects. Mutagens are rarely recognized as a cause of congenital anomalies.

6. The answer is B [Chapter 11 III A 2; Ch 12 I B, C]. The major events of early mammalian embryogenesis are cell-lineage specification (which does not occur clonally and does not predetermine precise developmental fates), segmentation, and regional specialization along the body axis. Maternal gene products in the zygote are not critically important in mammalian embryogenesis. Activation of proto-oncogenes may occur during neoplasia, not normal embryogenesis.

7. The answer is E [Chapter 13 II C 2–3]. Duchenne muscular dystrophy (DMD) is an X-linked recessive disease. Affected males usually die in the second decade of life; they do not reproduce. In this case, the family history is negative except for the affected brother. There is a 2/3 chance that the mother of the woman in the question (the proband) carries the abnormal gene and a 1/3 chance that her son (i.e., the proband's brother) had DMD as a result of a new mutation. If the proband's mother was a carrier, there is a 1/2 chance that the proband inherited the abnormal gene. However, the proband's creatine phosphokinase (CPK) test showed normal results despite the fact that the results are abnormal in 75% of carriers. This decreases the likelihood that she is a carrier.

A Bayesian calculation is necessary to determine the risk that the proband is a carrier, given that her CPK test is normal. This is illustrated in the following probability tree.

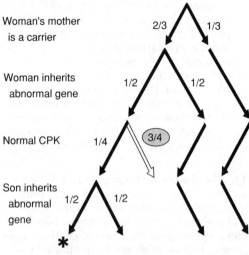

Woman's mother is a carrier 2/3 1/3

Woman inherits abnormal gene 1/2 1/2

Normal CPK 1/4 3/4

Son inherits abnormal gene 1/2 1/2

✱

The proband is unlikely to have an affected son unless: (1) her mother was a carrier of the abnormal gene; (2) her mother transmitted the abnormal gene to the proband; (3) the proband is among the 25% of carriers whose CPK test results are normal; and (4) she transmits the abnormal gene to her son. The other possibilities that must be considered are: (1) the proband's mother was not a carrier (i.e., the affected boy had a new mutation); (2) the proband's mother was a carrier but did not transmit the abnormal gene to the proband; and (3) the proband's mother was a carrier and transmitted the abnormal gene to the proband, but the proband did not transmit the abnormal gene to her son.

The chance that the proband's son has DMD is

$$P = \frac{\frac{2}{3} \times \frac{1}{2} \times \frac{1}{4} \times \frac{1}{2}}{\left(\frac{2}{3} \times \frac{1}{2} \times \frac{1}{4} \times \frac{1}{2}\right) + \left(\frac{2}{3} \times \frac{1}{2} \times \frac{1}{4} \times \frac{1}{2}\right) + \left(\frac{2}{3} \times \frac{1}{2}\right) + \frac{1}{3}}$$

$$P = \frac{\frac{2}{48}}{\frac{2}{48} + \frac{2}{48} + \frac{2}{6} + \frac{1}{3}}$$

$$P = \frac{\frac{2}{48}}{\frac{2}{48} + \frac{2}{48} + \frac{16}{48} + \frac{16}{48}}$$

$$P = \frac{\frac{2}{48}}{\frac{36}{48}}$$

$$P = \frac{2}{36} = \frac{1}{18}$$

8. The answer is C [Chapter 17 II; IV C]. There is no easy or perfect answer to this problem. The physician, through the predictive testing, has inadvertently been made privy to information that has the potential to do great damage to this family. On the other hand, the physician would like to reassure the patient that he is not at risk for Huntington disease. If the physician chooses option A, the patient still believes he is at risk when information to the contrary is available. Option B impinges on the mother's autonomy, as she has chosen not to disclose the paternity, even after a private session. Going ahead despite this could jeopardize her relationship with the family. Option D may be the most destructive as it betrays the mother's autonomy while placing a burden on the son, likely altering his relationship with his mother. Option C is not perfect but does allow the mother her privacy and gives correct information to the patient. It contravenes the principle of veracity, but there is some justification for this.

9. The answer is C [Chapter 4 I B]. All genetic polymorphisms ultimately reflect alterations of DNA sequence, but these alterations may be demonstrated in a variety of ways. Some polymorphisms affect protein structure or function, but many do not. Polymorphisms are most often demonstrated by DNA studies; very few polymorphisms are apparent either on physical examination or on cytogenetic analysis. Monozygotic twins are genetically identical and therefore cannot be distinguished by polymorphisms.

10. The answer is D [Chapter 9 III C 3–5]. Many common congenital anomalies (e.g., cleft palate, anencephaly, ventricular septal defect) may be inherited as multifactorial traits. However, these same defects also occur as features of malformation syndromes and other patterns of congenital anomalies. Multifactorial congenital anomalies usually do not differ in their appearance from similar defects seen as components of various dysmorphic syndromes, but the multifactorial anomalies are usually isolated (i.e., they occur in a child who is otherwise normal). Like other multifactorial diseases, multifactorial congenital anomalies characteristically exhibit a much higher concordance rate in monozygotic twins (who share all of their genes) than in dizygotic twins (who share only half of their genes). The recurrence risk for multifactorial congenital anomalies is similar in an affected patient's children and siblings, both of whom share about 50% of their genes with the patient.

11. The answer is E [Chapter 10 II C 1–3, 5]. The risk of teratogenic effects in a pregnancy depends not only on the chemical or pharmacologic characteristics of the agent but also upon the dose, route, and other circumstances of exposure.

Knowledge of the pharmacologic action of an agent in a child is usually insufficient to predict its teratogenic potential because different biochemical and physiologic mechanisms are often involved in the embryogenesis of a tissue and in its function once it is formed. Simultaneous exposures to several teratogenic agents may produce effects that are similar to, greater than, or less than those of exposure to the same agents individually.

The embryo is most sensitive to teratogenic effects between 2 weeks and 10 weeks after conception. Malformations are unlikely to be produced after this time, but disruptive, cytotoxic, or growth-inhibiting effects may occur.

12. The answer is A [Chapter 4 II C 3 a–b]. The woman must have been Rh$^+$ and her mother Rh$^-$ because the woman's red cells were attacked by her mother's anti-Rh antibody. The husband's mother must have been Rh$^-$ and he must be Rh$^-$ as well, because he did not get Rh hemolytic disease despite the fact that his mother was highly sensitized. Because the woman is Rh$^+$ and her husband is Rh$^-$, they are not at risk to have a child with hemolytic disease of the newborn due to the major Rh antigen.

13. The answer is D [Chapter 1 V B 3, 6, 9 c, 10, 11 c]. X-chromosome inactivation in females produces dosage compensation (i.e., reduction of the amount of X-linked gene products to approximately the amount that is present in males, who only have one X chromosome). Most, but not all, genes on the X chromosome are subject to X inactivation. X inactivation occurs early in embryogenesis, and once it takes place in a cell, all of the progeny of that cell maintain the same X chromosome in an inactive state. Inactive X chromatin is extensively methylated. The mildness of X-chromosome monosomy (Turner syndrome) in contrast to monosomy for any of the autosomes reflects the need for only one active X chromosome in most cells. X inactivation does not occur in 45,X females because they only have a single X chromosome.

14. The answer is D [Chapter 16 I A 1–2; II E 2 c (4)]. Many genetic diseases with similar phenotypic manifestations are etiologically and pathogenically heterogeneous. Effective therapy often requires knowing precisely what gene or protein is altered in an affected patient. Even if the precise diagnosis or biochemical alteration is unknown, and regardless of the age of onset, symptomatic treatment of genetic diseases is often possible. Therapeutic genes are used in somatic gene therapy, which is considered to be an experimental approach. Proper regulation of the therapeutic gene may or may not be required, depending on the specific disease being treated.

15. The answer is D [Chapter 10 II C 2, 6; IV B, C]. Most human teratogens produce a characteristic pattern of congenital anomalies rather than a single isolated defect. The observation of this pattern repeatedly within a series of infants born to women exposed to a given agent suggests that the agent is teratogenic, especially if the exposure is uncommon. Experimental animal teratology studies, particularly when performed at vastly greater doses than those used in pregnant women, are difficult to interpret in terms of human risk. Pharmacologic similarities among agents do not necessarily predict similarities in teratogenic effects, because the metabolism of embryos may differ from that of adults. Isolated case reports of infants with a variety of congenital anomalies who were delivered to women who took a medication during pregnancy are more likely to represent a chance association than a causal one, especially if use of the medication among pregnant women is common. Most congenital anomalies have multifactorial or unknown causes. Only a small proportion of birth defects results from the effects of teratogenic agents, even in infants with congenital anomalies in whom no mendelian or chromosomal cause can be recognized.

16. The answer is E [Chapter 16 II A–E]. Symptomatic treatment of genetic disease by medical, surgical, or other means is by far the most commonly used approach. Somatic gene therapy has very limited application and is considered to be experimental. Organ transplantation is used only in certain special circumstances. Modulation of gene expression is a theoretically attractive approach, but knowledge of gene regulation is currently insufficient for clinical application in most diseases. Amelioration of metabolic abnormalities is used for inborn metabolic errors, a relatively uncommon group of disorders, in which the pathogenesis is more or less well understood.

17. The answer is A [Chapter 10 II D 1 a, 2 c, 3 a, 5 b, 6 a (4)]. Neural tube defects occur in 1% to 2% of infants of women with insulin-dependent diabetes mellitus. Prenatal diagnosis for neural tube defects is, therefore, indicated in these women's pregnancies.

Although first-trimester rubella infection may be teratogenic, it does not cause neural tube defects. Maternal use of marijuana during pregnancy has not been shown to be teratogenic. Ionizing radiation may produce teratogenic effects, but the dose involved in an abdominal x-ray is unlikely to pose a significant risk to the fetus. Maternal use of androgenic hormones during pregnancy may cause virilization of a female fetus but is not associated with an increased risk for neural tube defects.

18. The answer is C [Chapter 10 II D 5 a (1)]. Common features of fetal alcohol syndrome include behavioral abnormalities, mental retardation, growth deficiency, and characteristic facial appearance. Limb reduction defects rarely occur in children with fetal alcohol syndrome.

Although women who drink only in occasional binges or who drink less than 3 ounces of absolute alcohol daily during pregnancy do not have children with classic fetal alcohol syndrome, the risk of less severe damage to their fetuses may still be substantial. The only amount of maternal drinking during pregnancy that is known to be safe is none.

19–21. The answers are: 19-E, 20-B, 21-B [Chapter 13 II B 2]. The gene causing MEN II in this family is inherited together with the A marker. However, II-1 has AB markers, and it is impossible to know whether she has inherited the A or the B marker from the affected father; therefore, her risk of having inherited the MEN II gene is not changed by the DNA testing.

II-3 has inherited marker B from his affected father and marker B from his mother. In view of the fact that the gene for MEN II is inherited together with marker A, this man's risk of being affected with MEN II is small.

II-4 has inherited an A marker from his mother, but II-4's other marker is a C. The supposed father (I-1) does not have a C marker. Therefore, it is highly unlikely that I-1 is the father of II-4. This being the case, II-4 has no risk of having inherited anything from I-1. The frequency of undisclosed nonpaternity is high (3% to 5%) and can dramatically alter risk estimates.

22. The answer is E [Chapter 13 I C 1]. It is usually best to counsel both parents together. This enables them to help each other understand the information and also facilitates mutual emotional support.

23. The answer is C [Chapter 5 III A 2]. Allelic heterogeneity, the production of similar phenotypes by different mutant alleles at a single locus, has been found for most genetic diseases studied at the molecular level. In fact, most "homozygotes" for autosomal recessive diseases are actually compound heterozygotes with two different mutant alleles for the affected locus. The exception to this is consanguineous families, in which both mutant alleles in a homozygote are usually identical by descent.

24. The answer is E [Chapter 2 I B 1]. Approximately 50% of early spontaneous abortions are chromosomally abnormal. This amounts to more than 5% of all recognized pregnancies.

25. The answer is B [Chapter 1 V B 2]. In mammalian cells, all but one X chromosome is inactivated. In a person with a 49,XXXXY karyotype, there are 4 X chromosomes, three of which are inactivated.

26–29. The answers are: 26-E, 27-B, 28-D, 29-C [Chapter 7 I B 6]. Because cystic fibrosis

(CF) is an autosomal recessive disease, it occurs in homozygotes for the mutant gene. The frequency of such homozygotes in this population is 1/2500. In terms of the Hardy-Weinberg law,

$$q^2 = \frac{1}{2500}$$

$$q = \sqrt{\frac{1}{2500}} = \frac{1}{50}.$$

The frequency of heterozygous carriers in the general population is 2pq, or approximately 2/50 = 1/25.

A man and a woman, neither of whom has a family history of CF, each have a 1/25 chance of being carriers for this condition. For the couple to have an affected child, both would have to be carriers and both would have to transmit the abnormal gene to their child. The chance of this is:

$$\frac{1}{25} \times \frac{1}{25} \times \frac{1}{4} = \frac{1}{2500}$$

A woman with CF is homozygous for the abnormal gene. All of her children must inherit this gene from her. If her husband has no family history of CF, his chance of being a carrier is 1/25, and his chance of transmitting the gene, if he is a carrier, is 1/2. Thus, the chance that this couple would have an affected child is:

$$1 \times \frac{1}{25} \times \frac{1}{2} = \frac{1}{50}$$

A woman whose first cousin is affected with CF has a 1/4 chance of carrying the CF gene herself. Her aunt or uncle (her affected cousin's parent) must carry the abnormal gene, so the woman's own parent has a 1/2 chance of being a carrier. The woman's husband has a 1/25 chance of being a carrier for CF. If both the woman and her husband are carriers, their child has a 1/4 chance of being homozygous for the CF gene. Thus, the risk that the child will have CF is:

$$\frac{1}{4} \times \frac{1}{25} \times \frac{1}{4} = \frac{1}{400}$$

A man who has a child with CF by a previous marriage must be a carrier of the abnormal gene. His new partner has a 1/25 chance of being a CF carrier. For them to have an affected child, both must transmit the abnormal gene. The chance that their child would have CF is:

$$1 \times \frac{1}{25} \times \frac{1}{4} = \frac{1}{100}$$

30. The answer is A [Chapter 1 V C]. Genomic imprinting is differential expression of a gene depending on whether it was inherited from the mother or the father. Imprinting affects only a minority of genes and occurs during early embryogenesis. Once a gene in an embryonic cell has become imprinted, it is usually transmitted in that state to all descendant cells throughout the body. Imprinting is, therefore, maintained despite many rounds of mitosis. Imprinting is a functional change of the gene; it is not associated with any alteration of the DNA sequence.

31. The answer is D [Chapter 2 IV C 1–2]. Fanconi's pancytopenia syndrome is characterized by radial limb abnormalities, patchy skin pigmentation, congenital heart disease, renal anomalies, and pancytopenia. Cultured lymphocytes show high frequencies of chromosome breakage when treated with diepoxybutane.

Patients with Bloom syndrome are small and exhibit cutaneous telangiectases. Chromosome analysis typically shows increased frequencies of chromosome breaks and rearrangements.

32. The answer is A [Chapter 5 IV A]. The Human Genome Project has as its goal the mapping of all 50,000–100,000 genes and sequencing all of approximately 3 billion base pairs of DNA in the human genome.

33. The answer is D [Chapter 6 III A]. Indirect DNA diagnosis uses polymorphic markers that are closely linked to a mutant gene to track the segregation of the mutation within a family. Linkage studies can only be performed within families and require multiple affected members who are informative for linked markers. Indirect DNA diagnosis is not usually affected by the kind of mutation, allelic heterogeneity, or the occurrence of linkage disequilibrium within a population.

34. The answer is D [Chapter 3 II F 4]. Anticipation, the occurrence of earlier onset or greater severity of a genetic disease in more recent generations of a family, is characteristic of dynamic mutations caused by trinucleotide repeat expansions. For example, Huntington disease and myotonic dystrophy, two disorders caused by dynamic mutations, frequently exhibit anticipation. Anticipation represents the enlargement of the trinucleotide repeat as it passes through meiosis. As the repeated region in the mutant gene expands more, the disease tends to become more severe and have an earlier onset.

35. The answer is C [Chapter 9 IV A 1, 2]. Both type I (insulin-dependent) and type II (noninsulin-dependent) diabetes mellitus are usually multifactorial conditions. Type I diabetes is frequently associated with islet cell autoimmunity and the presence of human leukocyte antigen (HLA)-DR3, HLA-DR4, or both. Type II diabetes is usually associated with obesity. Concordance in monozygotic twins is nearly 100% for type II diabetes but only approximately 50% for type I diabetes.

36. The answer is E [Chapter 1 III C 2 f]. All primary oocytes are produced by about the third month after conception in a female fetus. Meiosis I is initiated in utero, but the primary oocytes become arrested in the dictyotene stage of prophase. At the time of puberty, oocytes begin to be released from meiotic arrest and some mature. Meiosis I is completed and the second meiotic metaphase begun around the time of ovulation. Meiosis II is not completed until fertilization occurs.

37. The answer is A [Chapter 2 II D]. Uniparental disomy (UPD) is the inheritance of both chromosomes of a pair from the same parent, instead of one member of the pair from each parent, as normally occurs. UPD for some chromosomes, notably chromosome 7, is associated with fetal growth retardation. UPD can also account for the occurrence of autosomal recessive disease in individuals who are homozygous for a mutation carried by just one parent.

38. The answer is C [Chapter 5 I B 1–2]. The lod score is the $\log_{10}$ of the odds in favor of finding the observed combination of alleles at the loci being studied in a family if the loci are linked rather than unlinked. A lod score greater than 3 indicates that the odds favoring linkage are greater than 1000 to 1 and is considered to be strong evidence for linkage. For linkage to exist, the distance between the loci must be less than 50 centimorgans (cM); that is, the loci must be transmitted together through meiosis more than 50% of the time. Unlinked loci segregate independently and are transmitted together 50% of the time by chance. A lod score lower than −2 at recombination distances less then 50 cM is taken as evidence against linkage because this lod score indicates that the odds favoring linkage are less than 1 to 100.

39. The answer is C [Chapter 9 II A 1]. People who are rapid acetylators metabolize isoniazid more quickly and usually have lower blood levels with a given dose. They are, therefore, more likely to be treated inadequately and to have recurrent disease. Slow acetylators have higher blood levels and are more likely to develop toxic side effects of treatment.

40. The answer is B [Chapter 1 II A 2 c, B 6 a]. Most human nuclear DNA consists of repetitive sequences. Although the function of such repetitive sequences is unknown, they generally are not expressed.

Most genes are encoded by unique or single-copy DNA sequences. Exons are the functional portions of genes. Introns are noncoding DNA sequences that are interspersed between exons in genomic DNA.

41. The answer is C [Chapter 6 IV]. DNA banks are particularly useful for families segregating mendelian diseases in which the responsible mutation has not yet been identified. Storing DNA from crucial relatives in such banks can help assure that DNA testing will be available to other family members in the future.

42. The answer is B [Chapter 4 III B 2 a–b]. Differences in disease frequencies among populations are usually most apparent for autosomal recessive conditions, particularly if the population has been genetically isolated for many generations.

43. The answer is B [Chapter 11 II A, B, C 1–2; III A, B]. Most malignancies are of multifactorial etiology. A small proportion of tumors occur in patients who have strong genetic predispositions inherited as simple mendelian traits. Acquired chromosome abnormalities are found in most malignancies, but the constitutional karyotypes of these patients are usually normal. Somatic mutation often leads to activation of proto-oncogenes and inactivation or loss of tumor suppressor genes within neoplastic cell lines, but these are usually acquired and not inherited changes.

44. The answer is B [Chapter 1 III A, B]. Every mitotic cell division is preceded by a round of DNA synthesis, but a single round of DNA synthesis precedes only the first division of meiosis.

Meiosis, which only occurs in germ cells, produces haploid products (i.e., the chromosome number is reduced from 46 to 23). All somatic cells undergo mitosis, in which no change in chromosome number occurs.

Recombination is much more frequent in meiosis than in mitosis. Chromosome pairing (i.e., synapsis) occurs in meiosis but not in mitosis.

45. The answer is A [Chapter 2 III F; Table 2-3]. The cytogenetic studies may have been prompted by recurrent spontaneous abortions, but the precise number of miscarriages is not important to risk counseling once a translocation has been discovered. If any carrier in the family has had a stillborn or liveborn infant with abnormalities because of chromosome imbalance, future pregnancies for this couple might be similarly affected. This is an important consideration in counseling.

For some reciprocal translocations, the sex of the parent influences the risk of having a child with chromosome imbalance. For example, a reciprocal translocation that tends to have 3:1 segregation may have a higher risk in a female carrier.

The degree of potential imbalance associated with a translocation as well as the intrinsic nature of the rearrangement and its behavior at meiosis affect the pregnancy outcome. Risk figures should be sought from the literature or from the family itself, if enough members carry the rearrangement.

46. The answer is A [Chapter 4 I A 2, B 1]. Genetic markers are polymorphisms that are easily detected. Genetic markers are inherited in a simple mendelian fashion, not as multifactorial traits. Alternative alleles must be easy to distinguish for genetic markers to be useful. Genetic markers are most often detected by DNA-based methods [e.g., as restriction fragment length polymorphisms (RFLPs) or short tandem repeat polymorphisms (STRPs)], as protein structural variants [e.g.,human leukocyte antigens (HLAs)], or as functional alterations of proteins (e.g., the ability to taste phenylthiocarbamide). Genetic markers are useful in linkage studies and in forensic medicine.

47. The answer is B [Chapter 7 I B 2]. The Hardy-Weinberg law can be applied whether the genes involved are dominant, recessive, autosomal, or (with minor modifications) X-linked. The Hardy-Weinberg law is based on the following assumptions: (1) mating within the population is completely random; (2) there is no mutation occurring at the locus; (3) there is no selection for any of the genotypes at the locus; and (4) there is no migration into or out of the population. These assumptions are never entirely correct for any locus, but if they are nearly correct, the Hardy-Weinberg law is applicable.

48. The answer is A [Chapter 3 I C 2 a; Chapter 8 II B 2 c]. Most inborn metabolic errors are inherited as autosomal recessive traits. Heterozygotes are clinically normal, although most have intermediate levels of the enzyme.

Normal siblings of a child with Tay-Sachs disease have a 2/3 chance of being heterozygotes, but their partners are unlikely to be carriers of the same abnormal gene unless there is consanguinity or a history of the same disease in the partner's family. The risk that children of normal siblings will be affected with Tay-Sachs disease is, therefore, low.

Allelic mutations at the hexosaminidase A locus may cause disease of lesser severity. Some mutations may lead to nonproduction of the enzyme, whereas others may lead to a less efficient but functional enzyme.

49. The answer is B [Chapter 10 II D 2]. Transplacental infections with rubella virus, varicella-zoster virus, cytomegalovirus (CMV), or *Toxoplasma gondii* may cause permanent damage to the developing human embryo. Maternal gonorrheal infection during pregnancy is not known to be teratogenic, although perinatal exposure can cause neonatal ophthalmia.

50. The answer is D [Chapter 12 II C]. Androgen-binding studies on cultured genital skin cells are appropriate if the suspected diagnosis is androgen insensitivity. However, such studies often take several months, and the diagnosis may be inferred in other ways before then.

Results of karyotyping can be returned in 48 hours. If the newborn is found to be 46,XX, the infant is probably a masculinized female; an XX male with genital ambiguity is possible but extremely rare. If the infant is 46,XY, he is likely to have incomplete androgen insensitivity.

Levels of urinary 17-ketosteroids are elevated in many forms of congenital adrenal hyperplasia and can be determined quickly, but the clinician should be aware that the levels may not be greatly elevated until several days after birth.

An ultrasound examination of the lower abdomen allows determination of whether a uterus is present. If a uterus is found and the karyotype is 46,XX, the most likely diagnosis is congenital adrenal hyperplasia. Abdominal ultrasound examination also allows assessment of the urinary tract, which may be abnormal in any infant with ambiguous genitalia.

If the differential diagnosis includes congenital adrenal hyperplasia, the infant may have life-threatening electrolyte abnormalities with low serum sodium and elevated serum potassium levels. Electrolytes are also a concern in an infant who has urinary tract malformation and possible renal failure.

51. The answer is E [Chapter 14 II F]. Cytogenetic studies on the patient's blood are not useful. Her fetus is at substantially increased risk for chromosome abnormality; the patient herself is not.

Correct interpretation of the triple screen depends on knowing the correct gestational age as well as the correct age of the patient. It is, therefore, essential to make certain that this information is recorded accurately on the triple screen report. If the patient's gestational age is uncertain, it can be checked by ultrasound examination.

If the gestational age and other information used to interpret the triple screen are accurately recorded on the report, it is appropriate to perform a detailed (level II) ultrasound examination on the patient. Amniocentesis with fetal karyotyping needs to be offered because maternal serum triple screening is not a definitive test. Most positive screens are false-positives (i.e., most women with an abnormal triple screen are carrying a fetus that does not have Down syndrome). Fetal karyotyping is necessary to distinguish fetuses with Down syndrome from false positive results. Counseling is essential to make certain that the pa-

tient understands this fact as well as the benefits, risks, and limitations of amniocentesis, ultrasound examination, and the triple screen itself.

52. The answer is C [Chapter 15 II A 1–3]. Genetic screening is justified to improve the management of a genetic condition or its complications in affected patients, to prevent or ameliorate the effects of a disease in genetically predisposed individuals (as is the case in D and E), or to provide reproductive options to people at high risk of having children with a serious genetic disease (as in A and B). Screening to obtain a better rating on life insurance does not fall into any of these categories and implies that those found not to be in the genetically low-risk group will have to pay more for their insurance. This is discriminatory and, therefore, inappropriate.

53. The answer is E [Chapter 6 II A 2; III A 1, 3]. Direct testing requires that part of the affected gene has been cloned. Direct approaches to DNA diagnosis utilize a probe that is part of, or complementary to, the gene in question. The results are more accurate than with indirect testing because the involved gene itself is analyzed.

Indirect testing depends on linkage analysis, which utilizes DNA polymorphisms close to the gene of interest. DNA from numerous family members is needed for such testing. Genetic heterogeneity can complicate both direct and indirect approaches to DNA diagnosis.

54. The answer is A [Chapter 10 IV B 1–5]. Case reports are useful in raising suspicion about the teratogenic potential of an agent, but associations observed in individual case reports are usually spurious. Most human teratogens have been recognized in clinical series in which a recurrent and unusual pattern of congenital anomalies was observed among infants born to women who had similar exposures during pregnancy.

Epidemiologic studies of both the cohort and case-control type may be subject to serious biases. This must be considered when interpreting such studies.

Experimental animals differ from humans in many important ways. Consequently, a teratogenic effect observed in experimental animals is not necessarily predictive of a similar effect in women, even if similar conditions of exposure occur.

55. The answer is C [Chapter 9 III D 6]. Twin studies are a valuable method for studying complex genetic disorders. It is essential to distinguish monozygotic from dizygotic pairs in such studies so that proper comparisons can be made between the two groups. Biased ascertainment (e.g., selection in a manner that makes it more likely that twins who are concordant for a disorder will come to attention) can invalidate the results of twin studies. Small sample size is frequently a problem, but there is no need to include the same number of monozygotic and dizygotic pairs.

Diagnostic accuracy—determining who is affected and who is not—is a key feature of any genetic disease study. It is important to know if etiologic heterogeneity exists so that cases with monogenic or environmental causes can be excluded (or at least considered separately) from those with presumed multifactorial inheritance.

56. The answer is A [Chapter 16 II A, B 2 a]. Dietary restriction in patients with phenylketonuria (PKU) is designed to improve the metabolic abnormality that occurs, not just to ameliorate the symptoms. The other therapies are examples of symptomatic treatments involving an electronic device, a medication, speech therapy, and surgical intervention, respectively.

57. The answer is A [Chapter 3 II A, B; Chapter 6 II A 1, B 2 b (1), 3 b (1)]. The mutations underlying most genetic diseases are still unknown. Of approximately 4000 genetic diseases, fewer than 10% have been defined at the DNA level. Major rearrangements are uncommon causes of mutation in most genes; changes involving one or a few nucleotides are more frequent. Duchenne muscular dystrophy (DMD) and Becker muscular dystrophy (BMD) are exceptions to this rule; large deletions are common causes of mutation in these diseases.

Most people with Tay-Sachs disease are of Ashkenazi Jewish descent and have the same point mutation. Most people with cystic fibrosis (CF) have a common mutation.

58. The answer is D [Chapter 10 IV C 1–2]. Relative risk (RR) is the ratio of the occurrence rate of a condition among individuals who were exposed to an agent to the occurrence rate among individuals who were not exposed. An RR of 0.05 indicates that infants born to women exposed to an agent during pregnancy have a rate of birth defects that is one-twentieth that of infants of unexposed women (i.e., the exposure exerts a protective effect).

An association may be seen in an epidemiology study of birth defects if congenital anomalies and maternal exposures are not directly related to each other but both are associated with a common third factor. Observing a dosage effect supports the interpretation that an association between a maternal exposure and congenital anomalies in infants is causal.

Statistical significance (P) indicates how likely an observed association is to be due to chance. In studies in which many comparisons are made, some statistically significant associations are expected to occur by chance alone. For example, if $P < 0.05$ is chosen as the significance level, approximately 1/20 (5 out of 100) comparisons are expected to be statistically significant purely on the basis of chance.

59. The answer is D [Chapter 11 II C 2, D; III A 4 b, e, B 6 c]. Chromosome rearrangement is a common means of activating oncogenes in neoplastic cells. Deletions and chromosome loss frequently are associated with loss of tumor suppressor genes. Several different cytogenetic lines may be apparent within a neoplastic population, but all of the lines can usually be shown to have arisen from a common progenitor (i.e., they are clonally related).

The chromosome abnormalities that are acquired during the neoplastic process arise somatically and do not involve the germ cells. Such chromosome abnormalities cannot, therefore, be transmitted to the children of an affected person.

60. The answer is C [Chapter 4 III B 3 b]. Thalassemia and glucose-6-phosphate dehydrogenase (G6PD) deficiency are frequently seen in populations that have historically been exposed to malaria. This includes not only African populations but also non-African groups such as Greeks, Italians, Chinese, and Southeast Asians.

Selection for the genes responsible for these diseases is thought to have occurred because these genes provide protection against malaria. Protection is seen in both heterozygous carriers and affected individuals, but thalassemia major occurs only in homozygotes. G6PD deficiency, an X-linked recessive trait, usually produces disease only in affected males. Thalassemia and G6PD deficiency can produce disease whether malaria happens to occur where the affected person lives.

61. The answer is B [Chapter 9 V D 3]. Although females with Turner syndrome often are immature, they are not often mentally handicapped and do not exhibit an increased incidence of psychiatric disease. Schizophrenia is increased in males who are affected by Klinefelter syndrome and females who are affected with trisomy X. As children, XXY males demonstrate poor judgment and learning problems. XYY males tend to be immature and impulsive.

62. The answer is E [Chapter 17 II]. By acting in a paternalistic manner, even though his intentions are good, the physician has removed this woman's autonomy to make a choice regarding the results of her amniocentesis. Beneficence (the physician's decision to withhold the diagnosis from the woman to avoid worrying her) is in conflict with autonomy. The physician has not been truthful with his patient (veracity) and has not fulfilled his contract with her to inform her of results of the testing so that she can choose whether to continue her pregnancy (fidelity). Justice is not an issue, since the woman was offered a prenatal diagnosis, as any other 35-year-old pregnant woman would be.

63. The answer is D [Chapter 8 II A 1–4]. Some gene mutations have no effect on the structure or function of the corresponding protein. For example, many mutations that occur within introns or 3' or 5' untranslated regions of a gene are without effect on the protein. Similarly, synonymous mutations that change a nucleotide within a triplet without altering the amino acid for which the triplet codes have no effect on the corresponding protein.

64. The answer is B [Chapter 2 III A 2 a, 3 a, b; Table 2-1]. Angelman syndrome and

Prader-Willi syndrome are often associated with similar microdeletions of chromosome 15q11. They differ because the deleted chromosome 15 in Angelman syndrome is the one inherited from the mother, whereas the deleted chromosome 15 in Prader-Willi syndrome is the one inherited from the father. This is an example of genomic imprinting.

Miller-Dieker syndrome is associated with a microdeletion of chromosome 17p13 and Williams syndrome is associated with a microdeletion of chromosome 7q11. Cri du chat syndrome is caused by a deletion of the short arm of chromosome 5. This is not a microdeletion, however, because most cases are easily demonstrable with conventional cytogenetic techniques.

65. The answer is E [Chapter 10 III B 1–3]. No chemical agent has been proven to produce transmissible gametic mutations in humans. It is likely that such agents exist, but available studies have not demonstrated this effect. From a practical point of view, this means that remote preconceptional exposure of either parent to an apparent mutagen is unlikely to measurably increase the risk of congenital anomalies among subsequently conceived children.

66. The answer is A [Chapter 11 II C 2 a–g]. Acquired chromosome abnormalities are very common in both leukemias and solid tumors. The karyotype of a tumor tends to become more abnormal as a tumor progresses. Reappearance of a cytogenetically abnormal clone is sometimes the first sign of relapse of a malignancy. Several different chromosome abnormalities are often present within a neoplasm, and the karyotypes of individual cells frequently differ, although their cytogenetic abnormalities usually show a clonal relationship.

67. The answer is E [Chapter 11 III A 4 a–e]. Proto-oncogenes can be activated by a variety of means that result in altered gene function or in overexpression. Point mutation can cause alteration of function, and overexpression may occur, for example, when a proto-oncogene is amplified or placed under the influence of a more active promoter. Deletion of a proto-oncogene prevents its expression and so cannot activate it.

68. The answer is D [Chapter 14 III F]. Spina bifida in an otherwise normal woman does not substantially increase the risk for chromosome abnormalities in her fetus, although the fetus does have an increased risk for a neural tube defect. Both advanced maternal age (i.e., the mother is at or over 35 years of age at the due date) and a previous stillbirth or liveborn with a chromosome abnormality are indications for fetal karyotyping via either chorionic villus sampling (CVS) or amniocentesis. A cystic hygroma may be associated with a variety of chromosome abnormalities, including Turner syndrome and trisomy 21. If one parent has a translocation, there is an increased risk for both early miscarriages and abnormal liveborn infants. A paternal robertsonian translocation is associated with a 1%–2% risk that the fetus in an ongoing pregnancy will be chromosomally abnormal.

69. The answer is E [Chapter 7 III A; Chapter 15 I D 1–5]. The goal of genetic counseling is to help a family understand and deal with a specific genetic condition or congenital anomaly more effectively. Genetic counseling is concerned with the welfare of individual patients or families, not with the effects of treatment or reproductive decisions on the population's gene pool. This is not only a more compassionate approach, it is also more practical inasmuch as genetic counseling has very little effect on the frequencies of disease genes.

70–73. The answers are: 70-B, 71-C, 72-D, 73-B [Chapter 1 I B; Chapter 3 I B 1, C 1, D 1; Chapter 9 III A 1, C 3 b]. Multifactorial conditions are caused by a combination of many factors, some of which are genetic and some of which are not. In contrast, mendelian diseases are caused by single abnormal genes or gene pairs (i.e., they are unifactorial). Mendelian diseases caused by genes located on chromosomes other than the X or Y are said to be autosomal. Conditions that are expressed when just a single gene of a pair is abnormal are called dominant. Diseases that require both genes of a pair to be abnormal for expression to occur are said to be recessive.

Single gene disorders are termed X-linked if the responsible gene is on the X chromosome. X-linked recessive diseases occur almost exclusively in males.

Most common diseases of middle life are caused by a combination of many interacting genetic and nongenetic predisposing factors. Mendelian disorders and chromosome abnormalities occur in adults but are relatively uncommon.

74–78. The answers are: 74-D [Chapter 2 II A 2 a], **75-C** [Chapter 2 II A 2 c], **76-B** [Chapter 2 II A 2 b], **77-E** [Chapter 2 II B 2 b], **78-A** [Chapter 2 II E 2 a (1)]. Down syndrome (trisomy 21) may be suspected in an infant on the basis of hypotonia and typical facial features. The head is brachycephalic with a small occiput, the ears are small and squared, and there are often epicanthic folds as well as Brushfield's spots involving the irides. Approximately 40% of Down syndrome children have congenital heart disease, with the most characteristic lesion being an atrioventricular cushion defect. The hands are short and broad, and half of patients have single palmar creases.

The trisomy 18 infant is usually significantly growth retarded, with tiny facial features and prominent occiput. Because of abnormal tendon placements, there may be overlapping of the second and fifth fingers. Almost all affected infants have congenital heart disease, and many have other major malformations as well (e.g., diaphragmatic hernia).

The trisomy 13 infant, unlike the trisomy 18 infant, may be well grown. In trisomy 13, there are often midline abnormalities, including clefting of the lip and palate and midline scalp lesions, as well as congenital heart disease and omphalocele. Many affected infants also have postaxial polydactyly. The brain is frequently malformed, with the most serious lesion being holoprosencephaly.

The Turner syndrome (45,X) conceptus may abort spontaneously early in pregnancy. In the second trimester, a fetus with Turner syndrome may have a cystic hygroma (secondary to delayed development of lymph channels from the posterior neck) or overt hydrops fetalis. Internally, the fetus may have coarctation of the aorta and horseshoe kidneys.

The triploid embryo is usually the result of fertilization of a haploid oocyte by two sperm. The placenta is large and shows cystic changes like those seen with molar pregnancies. The embryo itself may be growth disorganized and tiny.

79–83. The answers are: 79-B, 80-D, 81-C, 82-B, 83-A [Chapter 4 I B 1–4]. Restriction fragment length polymorphisms (RFLPs) are inherited DNA sequence variations that can result in the gain or loss of a restriction endonuclease recognition site, often by alteration of a single nucleotide.

Minisatellites are variants that contain tandem repeat sequences of DNA 1000–30,000 base pairs in length. Minisatellites are extremely polymorphic; multilocus minisatellites exhibit so much diversity that two unrelated people are very unlikely to share the same set of alleles. This extreme polymorphism makes minisatellites useful as "DNA fingerprints" in forensic medicine.

Polymorphic enzyme activity variants may be involved in pharmacogenetic interactions. For example, some variants of the enzyme glucose-6-phosphate dehydrogenase (G6PD) predispose people to developing anemia when they take certain medications.

Polymorphic antigenic variants expressed on the surface of blood cells are responsible for transfusion reactions. Common examples of such polymorphisms include the ABO and Rh blood groups.

Chromosome heteromorphisms are heritable differences in chromosome appearance that are useful in determining the origin of chromosome rearrangements.

84–88. The answers are: 84-B, 85-D, 86-E, 87-C, 88-A [Chapter 4 II C 1–3]. The couple in family 85 can only be the parents of infant B. Infant A, C, D, or E cannot be their child because those children are Rh$^+$ and both the mother and father are Rh$^-$.

The couple in family 86 can only be the parents of infant D. The child of family 86 must have just the N antigen in the MN group. Infant D is the only infant who has just the N antigen.

The couple in family 87 could be the parents of infant B, C, or E. However, infant B must belong to family 85, and infant C must belong to family 88, since infants A, B, D, and E all have the N blood group antigen, which neither the mother nor the father in family 88 has. Therefore, infant E must belong to family 87.

The couple in family 87 cannot be the parents of infant A, who has blood type O, because the child must inherit the gene for either the A or the B antigen from his mother. The couple in family 87 cannot be the parents of infant D, because he must have inherited the gene for either the A or the B blood group antigen from his father, and the father in family 87 has the O antigen.

The couple in family 89 could be the parents of infant A or B, but infant B must belong to family 85, so infant A must be family 89's child. The couple in family 89 cannot be the parents of infant C because he did not inherit the gene for the N blood group antigen, which the father must have transmitted to his son. The couple in family 89 cannot be the parents of infant D or E because both have a

gene for the B blood group, which neither the mother nor father in family 89 has.

89–93. The answers are: 89-D [Chapter 14 II A], **90-A** [Chapter 14 II C], **91-E** [Chapter 14 II E], **92-B** [Chapter 14 II F 4], **93-C** [Chapter 14 II D]. The woman who previously delivered a stillborn infant with normal chromosomes but multiple malformations should be offered detailed II ultrasound examination, looking specifically for the malformations that were seen in the previous infant. Offering fetal karyotyping is not appropriate, because the first infant did not have a chromosome abnormality.

With a family history of a genetic disorder diagnosable by molecular methods [e.g., Duchenne muscular dystrophy (DMD)], the most efficient method of prenatal diagnosis is chorionic villus sampling (CVS). Not only is the sampling done at an earlier time, but more tissue is available for diagnostic purposes or for faster culture.

The 20-week fetus shown by ultrasound to have an abnormality requires a rapid cytogenetic test to aid the parents in decision-making. In many areas, the option of pregnancy termination is not available after approximately 20 weeks of development. The most rapid method of prenatal cytogenetic diagnosis is fetal blood sampling.

The 25-year-old primigravida could be offered maternal serum triple screening because it is not an invasive procedure but does detect most (but not all) cases of Down syndrome. She should, of course, be made aware of the screening nature of this test and that further testing will be necessary if the results are abnormal.

The fetus of a healthy 36-year-old woman is at increased risk for chromosome aneuploidy because of the mother's age. The woman should be offered either CVS or amniocentesis. However, since she is already 14 weeks pregnant, amniocentesis is more appropriate.

94–96. The answers are: 94-B, 95-A, 96-D, [Chapter 1 IV C 1 b (1)–(7)]. G banding is the standard method of cytogenetic analysis used in most laboratories. The pattern of staining produced by Q banding is similar to that in G banding, with brightly fluorescent Q bands equivalent to darkly staining G bands. Fluorescent in situ hybridization (FISH) is a method by which labeled DNA probes are made to hybridize with complementary sequences on the chromosomes. FISH can be used to identify individual single-copy genes.

97–101. The answers are: 97-D, 98-E, 99-B, 100-D, 101-D [Chapter 5 II A; Chapter 13 II B 2]. To interpret the linkage data, the phase of the linkage must be determined. Each person who carries the mutant *BRCA1* gene also carries the *1* allele at the marker locus. The genotypes in the family can be substituted for the symbols, and the pedigree redrawn as shown below. The genotypes at the *BRCA1* and marker locus on one chromosome are shown above the line for each individual; those on the other chromosome are shown below the line. *B* is used to indicate the abnormal allele at the *BRCA1* locus; *b* is used to indicate the normal allele.

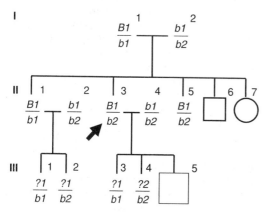

Individual II-7 has not been tested at the marker locus, but her mother carries the *BRCA1* mutation. II-7's chance of inheriting this abnormal gene is 50%.

III-3 has inherited a *1* allele at the marker locus and a normal allele at the *BRCA1* locus from her father. From her mother, she has inherited a *1* allele at the marker locus as well. Since II-3 carries the disease allele at the *BRCA1* locus on the same chromosome as the *1* allele at the marker locus, and since the two loci are separated by recombination only 4% of the time [i.e., they are 4 centimorgans (cM) apart], there is a 96% chance that III-3 inherited the disease allele at the *BRCA1* locus with the *1* allele at the marker locus. The usual 50% risk of transmitting an abnormal gene does not figure into this calculation because transmission has already occurred. It is known which allele at the marker locus was transmitted; therefore, the likelihood that the disease allele at the *BRCA1* locus was also transmitted can be calculated from the recombination fraction.

III-4 has inherited a *2* allele at the marker locus and a normal allele at the *BRCA1* locus

from her father. From her mother, she has inherited a *2* allele at the marker locus. Since III-3 carries the disease allele at the *BRCA1* locus on the same chromosome as the *1* allele at the marker locus, the only way that she could have transmitted the disease allele to III-4 is if recombination had occurred. The chance of this is only 4%.

II-1 is homozygous for the *1* allele at the marker locus. Thus, it cannot be determined from the marker locus which chromosome is transmitted to her children. Both her normal allele and her disease allele at the *BRCA1* locus are coupled with a *1* allele at the marker locus. One must revert to the chance probability of transmission of the disease allele at the *BRCA1* locus. This 50% risk is not influenced by the marker allele transmitted by II-1's husband (II-2) because both of his chromosomes 17 have normal alleles at the *BRCA1* locus.

102–104. The answers are: 102-C, 103-B, 104-D [Chapter 9 V A 1, 3]. Adoption research in psychiatric disease can be done in different ways, but basically it compares the risk for disease among individuals raised with biologic relatives (who typically are affected) to the risk among individuals raised with adoptive relatives (who usually are not affected). These studies then attempt to separate genetic from environmental contributions to the disease.

A pedigree analysis (family history) is easy to obtain but has important limitations. If diagnoses are made on the basis of second-hand information obtained from a proband, it is often imprecise or inaccurate. Mildly affected relatives may be missed in the history, giving falsely low family morbidity figures.

Family interviews often include unaffected relatives as well as affected relatives and, thus, are more likely to identify mildly affected family members. Testing of family members may be conducted in association with the interviews.

105–109. The answers are: 105-B [Chapter 17 II B], **106-A** [Chapter 17 II E], **107-E** [Chapter 17 II F], **108-C** [Chapter 17 II A], **109-D** [Chapter 17 II C]. The patient's mother, acting on his behalf, should be free to make the decision of whether to enter the trial or discontinue participation at any point (autonomy).

All important information regarding the drug, including side effects and complications, should be discussed, and the patient's and mother's questions should be answered.

If the patient is to be entered in a double-blind trial with placebo, the mother must be made aware that the child may receive a placebo. Such information is all part of veracity.

Not only the signed consent form but also the verbal consent are part of the contract with the patient and mother (fidelity). The consent form must be kept by the investigator.

Beneficence involves decisions on the part of the physician to involve her patient in research. She may believe that there is a good chance for response to the drug. She may believe that the clinical research ultimately benefits all children with muscular dystrophy, and she may believe that undertaking such a trial will not be detrimental to her patient. All of these beliefs concern the patient's best interests.

Should the child leave the study, justice ensures that he still has the right to standard care that is equally available to other boys with Duchenne muscular dystrophy (DMD).

110–115. The answers are: 110-D, 111-C, 112-E, 113-A, 114-B, 115-F [Chapter 3 I D 1]. Matings of $Gg \times gY$ and $gg \times gY$ are both rare situations that can result in affected daughters. Since both parents are affected in a $gg \times gY$ mating, all offspring will also be affected. In a mating of $Gg \times GY$, sons and daughters may inherit the mutant allele in equal proportions, but the daughters will have normal vision. For a mating of $GG \times GY$, all offspring are normal; in particular, all daughters are homozygous normal since there is no opportunity to inherit a mutant allele from either parent. In a mating of $GG \times gY$, all daughters will inherit the mutant allele from the father, whereas the sons will inherit the Y chromosome; therefore, all of the children will have normal vision and all of the daughters will be carriers. In a mating of $gg \times GY$, all daughters will be heterozygous (Gg) carriers, and all sons will be affected hemizygotes (gY).

116–119. The answers are: 116-D, 117-B, 118-C, 119-B [Chapter 9 VI B 1–4]. The child with short legs has a dysplasia because his structural defect is related to abnormal organization of cells within the cartilage.

The child with only one kidney and the child with chorioretinitis and blindness have disruptions. In both cases, there was destruction of a structure that had already formed, presumably in a normal fashion.

The child with an indentation in his skull has a deformation because his skull has been misshaped by mechanical pressure.

None of these children has a malformation, which is a morphologic defect resulting from an intrinsically abnormal developmental process.

120–124. The answers are: 120-B, 121-E, 122-D, 123-A, 124-C [Chapter 12 II C 1–5; Figure 12-1]. The form of congenital adrenal hyperplasia characterized by 21-hydroxylase deficiency may be associated with salt loss, which leads to electrolyte abnormalities and severe dehydration. Affected males have normal genitalia, and affected females have normal internal structures. Externally, affected females are masculinized by the excessive androgens and may appear to have a phallic structure with undescended testes. Because of cortisol deficiency, affected children may not survive acute episodes such as that described in question *121* without replacement therapy.

Complete androgen insensitivity implies that androgen receptors are absent or nonfunctional. Affected males have normal formation of testes with functioning Leydig and Sertoli cells. The testosterone cannot be utilized by the wolffian duct, which regresses. The müllerian duct actively regresses through action of müllerian duct inhibiting substance (MDIS). Therefore, the phenotypic female discussed in question *122* has no uterus. The external genitalia cannot respond to dihydrotestosterone (DHT) and will be female. An affected infant may present with a hernia that contains the normal testis.

The infant in question *123* has features typical of Turner syndrome: a cardiac lesion, neck webbing, and possible lymphedema. However, the clitoral enlargement suggests the presence of a Y chromosome in at least some of the cells. Mixed gonadal dysgenesis is a highly variable condition, and if the proportion of the 46,XY cell line is small, the overall phenotype will be female. It is important not to miss the diagnosis, since the gonads should be removed because of the risk for malignancy.

Females with XY karyotypes (those with sex reversal) are a heterogeneous group. In the situation in question *124*, a nonmosaic 46,XY karyotype is present in a girl with a uterus, which implies a lack of MDIS from the Sertoli cells. Pure gonadal dysgenesis is associated with a normal male karyotype, and, in some cases, deletion of the sex-determining region on the short arm of the Y chromosome (Yp). The gonads may initially start out as ovaries, but the lack of the second X chromosome inhibits continued development. The pelvic mass is worrisome, since it may represent a gonadal tumor (most likely a gonad-oblastoma).

The infant with 5α-reductase deficiency and a 46,XY karyotype has normal male internal genitalia (i.e., the gonad has developed as a normal testis and produces both testosterone and MDIS). There is suppression of the müllerian ducts, and, therefore, there is no uterus. Because testosterone cannot be converted to DHT, the external structures respond only minimally to hormone stimulation. In this situation, there are normal androgen receptors but an abnormal testosterone/DHT ratio. This condition is now treatable if recognized early. DHT is available and allows penile growth. The potential for fertility may be reasonably good as well.

125–128. The answers are: 125-C, 126-A, 127-B, 128-C [Chapter 9 VI C 1–4]. Both the child with congenital heart disease and abnormal ears and the child with thrombocytopenia have syndromes. In the child with congenital heart disease and abnormal ears, all of the anomalies have resulted from the teratogenic action of isotretinoin. In the child with thrombocytopenia, all of the anomalies are the consequence of a pair of mutant genes.

The child with spina bifida and club feet exhibits a sequence. The primary error of morphogenesis is the spina bifida. The club feet are a secondary anomaly that developed as a result of the primary defect.

The stillborn infant had a developmental field defect because all of her anomalies resulted from disturbed morphogenesis in a developmental field—the caudal mesoderm of the 3- to 4-week embryo.

None of these children exhibits an association, which is a pattern that is diagnosed only after a syndrome, sequence, and developmental field defect have been excluded. Recognition of an association requires knowledge that the anomalies seen in an individual occur together more often than expected by chance.

129–132. The answers are: 129-C, 130-E, 131-C, 132-B [Chapter 7 II B 1–3, C–D; III B 1–2]. Eugenics is the improvement of humankind by selective breeding. Eugenic proposals are said to be positive if they seek to increase the propagation of "more desirable" types of people and negative if they seek to decrease the propagation of "less desirable" types.

New mutations occur when a mutant allele that was not present in either parent is present in a child. New mutations are typically found with a frequency of only 10^{-6} to 10^{-4} per locus per generation. Clinically, they are commonly encountered among people who have autosomal dominant diseases that reduce fertility, because people with such diseases represent a very small subset of the total and all of the new mutations are contained within this subset. The paternal age is substantially older than expected among children with diseases due to some new dominant mutations.

A gene or gene pair that causes an individual to die or otherwise be incapable of reproducing is said to be a genetic lethal. A lethal equivalent is defined as a gene that is lethal to all homozygotes, or two genes, each of which is lethal to half of homozygotes, or three genes, each of which is lethal to $1/3$ of homozygotes, and so forth. Each normal person carries three to five lethal equivalents.

133–137. The answers are: 133-A, 134-B, 135-E, 136-F, 137-C [Chapter 6 I A–E]. Allele-specific oligonucleotide (ASO) analysis uses two synthetic oligonucleotides—one for the normal gene and one for a particular mutation. Patient DNA is hybridized to these two probes to determine whether the patient has two copies of the normal sequence, two copies of the particular mutant sequence, or one copy each of the normal and mutant sequence. ASO analysis is an efficient means of diagnosing a genetic disease that is always or almost always caused by a single specific mutation, as occurs, for example, in sickle cell anemia.

DNA sequencing is the most precise method of characterizing a segment of DNA completely. Sequencing is a relatively time-consuming method that is used primarily for research.

Polymerase chain reaction (PCR) is used for enzymatic amplification of a DNA segment that lies between two specific sequences. Oligonucleotides complementary to these sequences on opposite strands of the DNA molecule are used as primers in sequential rounds of polymerization and strand separation.

Southern blotting is performed by cutting patient DNA with a restriction endonuclease and separating the fragments by gel electrophoresis. The DNA is then denatured and blotted onto a membrane to which a labeled specific DNA probe is added to identify the fragment(s) with a complementary sequence.

Electrophoresis of denatured (single-stranded) DNA is used as a rapid screening method for point mutations or small deletions, insertions, or rearrangements in a specific gene. This technique is usually applied to gene fragments that have been amplified by PCR.

138–142. The answers are: 138-E [Chapter 8 II B 1 a], **139-B** [Chapter 8 II B 1 e], **140-D** [Chapter 3 III F], **141-G** [Chapter 8 II B 2 c], **142-C** [Chapter 8 II B 2 b]. β-Thalassemia results from mutations that cause decreased synthesis of β-globin chains of hemoglobin. As a result, red blood cells are deficient in hemoglobin, and oxygen transport to the tissues is compromised.

Osteogenesis imperfecta involves a defect in production of type I or type III collagen in bone and other connective tissues. Affected individuals have weak bones that are unusually susceptible to fractures.

Huntington disease is one of several degenerative neurologic diseases caused by expansion of a CAG repeat in the coding region of the gene. Huntington disease is inherited as an autosomal dominant trait.

Tay-Sachs disease is caused by deficiency of the enzyme hexosaminidase A. This enzyme normally is involved in removing sugar side-chains from ceramide, a branched lipid molecule. In patients with deficient hexosaminidase A, there is massive accumulation of ceramide in brain cells, which causes the dysfunction of brain cells.

Galactosemia usually results from galactose-1-phosphate uridyl transferase deficiency. Affected infants are unable to convert galactose, which is a component of lactose, the sugar in milk, to glucose. Untreated infants with galactosemia develop hepatomegaly, jaundice, and hypotonia.

Index

Note: Page numbers in italics denote illustrations, those followed by (t) denote tables, those followed by Q denote questions, and those followed by E denote explanations.

A

ABO blood group, 72–73, 73(t), 78Q, 79E
Abortion, spontaneous, from chromosomal anomalies, 29–30, 50Q, 51E, 258Q, 273E
Absolute risk, vs. relative risk, 155, 262Q, 278E
ACE (angiotensin-converting enzyme) inhibitors, and teratogenesis, 152, 157Q, 160E
Acetylation, genetic effects on, 123, 260Q, 275E
Achondroplasia, mutations in, 107
Acquired myelocytic leukemia (AML), acquired chromosomal abnormalities and, 162
Acute myelocytic leukemia (AML), acquired chromosomal abnormalities and, 162
Adenomatous polyposis, of colon, autosomal dominant traits in, 161
Adoption studies, of behavioral disorders, 133(t), 134, 266Q, 282E
Adrenal hyperplasia, congenital, 178, 178(t)
ethnic distribution of, 75(t)
Adrenogenital syndrome. *see* Adrenal hyperplasia, congenital
Affective disorders, 135–136, 141Q, 144E
AFP (α-fetoprotein), 206, 209(t), 210Q, 211Q, 212E
Agammaglobulinemia, X-linked, immunodeficiency syndromes and, 162
Age, and genetic counseling, 207
maternal, and trisomy, *33*, 33–34, 34(t), 221Q, 222E
paternal, effect of, 108, 221Q, 222E
Agyria, 39–40, *40*
Albinism, frequency of, 110Q, 113E
Alcohol, and teratogenesis, *150*, 150–151, 156Q, 159E, 257Q, 273E
Alleles, definition of, 53
Allele-specific oligonucleotide (ASO) probe analysis, in cystic fibrosis, 98
in deoxyribonucleic acid (DNA) diagnosis, 95, *95*, 102Q–103Q, 104E, 268Q, 284E
Allelic heterogeneity, 85, 87Q, 89E, 258Q, 273E
Allelic mutations, in biochemically based disease, 118, 119Q, 121E
α-fetoprotein (AFP), 206, 209(t), 210Q, 211Q, 212E

Alu deoxyribonucleic acid (DNA) sequence family, 4
Alzheimer's disease, deoxyribonucleic acid (DNA) diagnosis of, 99
Amniocentesis, *204*, 204–205, 211Q, 212E, 263Q, 265Q, 279E, 281E
Amniotic band disruption(s), in limbs, *138*
Anaphase, 10, *11*, 13
Androgen insensitivity, 120Q, 121E, 178–179, 181Q, 182E, 267Q, 283E–284E
Anemia, Fanconi, 49
Anencephaly, ethnic distribution of, 75(t)
Aneuploidy, mosaic, 35–36, *36*
Angelman syndrome, 19(t), 263Q, 279E
Angiotensin-converting enzyme (ACE) inhibitors, and teratogenesis, 152, 157Q, 160E
Animal experiments, in epidemiology of congenital anomalies, 154
Anticipation, 64, 259Q, 274E–275E
Anticonvulsants, and teratogenesis, 151
Antigenic variants, in polymorphism, 71, 265Q, 280E–281E
Antisense DNA/RNA oligonucleotides, for blockade of gene expression, 225
Anxiety disorders, 136
Aqueductal stenosis, recurrence risk in, 111Q, *112*, 114E
ASO (allele-specific oligonucleotide) probe analysis. *see* Allele-specific oligonucleotide (ASO) probe analysis
Associations, 139–140, 154, 268Q, 284E
Ataxia-telangiectasia, 49
autosomal recessive traits in, 162
Atherosclerosis, premature, multifactorial inheritance of, 132, 142Q, 145E
Attributable risk, 155
Autonomy, as ethical issue, 234, 237Q, 238E, 266Q–267Q, 282E–283E
Autosomal dominant inheritance, *54*, 54–56, 67Q, 68E, 220Q, 222E, 264E, 280E
Autosomal dominant traits, 1
mutation-selection equilibrium in, 108
in populations, 105–106
in predisposition to cancer, 161
Autosomal recessive inheritance, 56–57, 67Q, 68E, 119Q, 121E, 220Q, 221Q, 222E, 261Q, 264Q, 276E, 280E

Autosomal recessive traits, 1
in ataxia-telangiectasia, 162
gene therapy in, 227, 229Q, 231E
in populations, 106, 110Q, 113E

B

Banding, for chromosomal analysis, 18–19, *20–21*, 26Q, 28E, 265Q–266Q, 281E
Barr bodies, in X chromosome inactivation, 23
Bayesian method, for calculation of genetic risks, 191–192
for Duchenne muscular dystrophy, case study of, 248–249
Becker muscular dystrophy, direct deoxyribonucleic acid diagnosis of, 96–97
Behavioral disorders, 133–137
adoption studies of, 133(t), 134, 266Q, 282E
family studies of, 133(t), 133–134
Beneficence, as ethical issue, 234, 237Q, 238E, 266Q–267Q, 282E–283E
Biochemically based disease, 115–121
diagnosis of, 117–118
Bipolar affective disorder, 135–136, 141Q, 144E
Blood, typing of, 72(t), 73(t), 74(t), 72–74, 78Q, 79E, 265Q, 272E, 281E
Bloom syndrome, 49, 259Q, 274E
Breast cancer, case study of, 246–248
locus heterogeneity in, 266Q, 282E
multifactorial inheritance of, 131
phase of linkage in, 266Q, 282E
Burkitt's lymphoma, chromosomal abnormalities and, 162
proto-oncogenes in, 164

C

Cancer. *see also specific sites*
abnormalities of deoxyribonucleic acid (DNA) in, 162
chromosomal abnormalities and, 162–163, 168Q, 170E, 262Q–263Q, 278E–279E
chromosome repair abnormalities in, 162
clonal origin of, 163
of colon, progression to malignancy in, 167, *167*, 168Q, 170E
gene therapy in, 227
genetic basis of, 161–171
as genotype, 163–167